MW01156495

"This book belongs in every home, church, synagogue, and religious temple around the world. I could not put this book down. It is filled with some of the most enlightening, spellbinding, and scientifically proven information truly written by the hand of God."

James A. L. Dussault, N.D., D.D., Ph.D.
President, World Natural Health Organization


"The most brilliant game of connect-the-dots ever put into print. All of the evidence is there. *Healing Codes* has left nothing out. . . . You are left completely shocked by revelations that go far beyond exposing the genocidal intentions of a few evil men. If you want to know why so many people are sick today, what the true causes of our disease epidemics are, and how to prepare yourself physically and spiritually to defend yourself against the coming plagues, read this book. "

Don Harkins, Editor
Book Review, *The Idaho Observer*


"Delightful . . . A true masterpiece of the Lord! . . . This book confirms the awareness that we are being persecuted by organized criminals. . . . Congratulations on a work that scientifically and divinely protects the lives that honest and dedicated health professionals are devoted to saving."

Jonathan W. Bailey, N.D., D.N.B. (Prov.)
President, International Colon Hydrotherapy Foundation


"At critical junctures in history, certain key literary works come along to act as a catalyst to awaken people and provoke new learning and understanding. *Healing Codes for the Biological Apocalypse* is definitely such literary work. . . . This potent and timely work ultimately serves God in this critical, transitional, historical sequence of planetary evolution. In the final analysis, love is the driving force . . . bring[ing] about an end to the darkness that has seemingly prevailed during these last few decades. The days of darkness are numbered, and the days of true glory are before us, aided by the inspiration and higher input from Drs. Horowitz and Puleo. For all humanity, thank you! "

Rick Martin
Book Review in
*THE SPECTRUM*

"A roller coaster read awakening us to the biological perils of the New Millenium and the New World Order. Healing Codes for the Biological Apocalypse is an unprecedented mix of biblical prophesy, mysticism, and medical conspiracies, with startling revelations of an out-of-control biotechnology wedded to secret government genocidal agendas."

Alan Cantwell, Jr., M.D.
Author of *AIDS and the Doctors of Death*

"A pleasure to read and study. . . . A phenomenal work by two truly remarkable humanitarians. Five stars ★★★★★."

Mr. Wells W. Whitney
Chairman, Publication Review Committee
*WNHO Endorsement Magazine*

"A very important book that traces and documents the history of those who operate behind the scenes—some vastly wealthy and powerful people who direct a sizable part of earth's resources to now control the world's population. Protect yourself from the coming plagues by reading this book!"

Richard E. Lloyd, Ph.D.
Nutritional Scientist and Lecturer

"One of the most fascinating books I have ever read. . . ."

George Nori
KTRS Radio Talk Show Host
St. Louis, MO

"In the vast cornucopia of conspiracy books now available, I have not found information as sincerely intriguing and useful as that within the pages of *Healing Codes for the Biological Apocalypse*. . . . The most alluring facet of the book lay in the definitions of Noah Webster's famous dictionary. . . . Amazing as they are, such important revelations as the crystalline structure of 'prions' as disease transmitters effected by electromagnetic frequencies generated by Project HAARP to create and manipulate disease are astonishing, yet quite within the range of actuality."

Jaye C. Beldo
Freelance Book Reviewer
from Amazon.com

"Drs. Horowitz and Barber are two men on a mission to save the world from what is tantamount to biological warfare on the people. . . ."

Book Review<br>
NEXUS Magazine

"Critical, lifesaving, meticulously documented information that is precisely timed for the spiritual and natural healing renaissance. Vital reading for people who wish to take personal responsibility for their healthcare. "

Douglas J. Price, D.C.<br>
Chiropractic Physician and Clinic Director

"This publication is a must read, a phenomenal eye opener!"

Dr. Nicole S. Sacks<br>
Officer, International Association for Oxygen Therapies<br>
American Society of Medical Missionaries

"This fascinating book really gives you two books in one. The 'healing codes' in the first half of the book provides solutions to the extraordinary problems posed by the second half. This is an inspiring and easy to read book containing meticulously documented information that you will want to refer to frequently. "

Book Review<br>
Consumer Health Newsletter<br>
Consumer Health Organization of Canada

"A billiant compilation/synthesis of the hidden agendas and perspectives referencing bibical, scientific and health breakthroughs, past to present. Applause to you for your contributions (and great sacrifices as researchers and educators. "

Sandar Sitzmann, M.S., C.M.T<br>
and Lawrence Kennedy, Ph.D.

"I connot compliment you enough on your book, Healing Codes for the Biological Apocalypse. So many of the correlations within this fit into our research. . . [and] this was right under our nose all the time. Once again, thank you . . . I will certainly distribute this information to our students here at the academy."

Dr. Sir Peter Guy Manners<br>
The Bretforton Academy<br>
Worcestershire, England

# Healing Codes
### For The
# Biological Apocalypse

Leonard G. Horowitz, D.M.D., M.A., M.P.H.
and Joseph Puleo, N.D.

**Tetrahedron Publishing Group**
Sandpoint, Idaho

BY LEONARD G. HOROWITZ

Deadly Innocence

Taking Care of Yourself

Dentistry in the Age of AIDS

AIDS, Fear and Infection Control

Healing Codes for the Biological Apocalypse

Emerging Viruses: AIDS & Ebola—Nature, Accident or Intentional?

# History of Medicine

2000 B.C. – Here, eat this root.
1000 A.D. – That root is heathen. Here, say this prayer.
1850 A.D. – That prayer is superstition. Here, drink this potion.
1940 A.D. – That potion is snake oil. Here, swallow this pill.
1985 A.D. – That pill is ineffective. Here, take this antibiotic.
2000 A.D. – That antibiotic doesn't work anymore. Here, eat this root.
2010 A.D. – That root is contaminated. Here, practice energy medicine.

**—Adapted from *Qigong Newsletter***

DEDICATED TO GOD
AND THE 144,000 WHO WILL SOON SING
THESE MAGICAL TONES IN UNISON;
thus returning the Earth and His people
to everlasting harmony.
May this work herald the coming
thousand years of world peace.

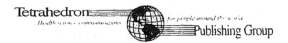

Tetrahedron
Health science communications
...to people around the world
Publishing Group

Cover designed by Sam Concialdi
Manufactured in the United States of America


10   9

Horowitz, Leonard G.
  *Healing Codes for the Biological Apocalypse*
  p.    cm.
  Includes bibliographical references and index.
  1. Popular Works;                      2. Religious History—
  —Christianity—Bible Codes;             3. Freemasonry;
  4. Epidemiology—Prion Diseases—World Health Organization—
  —Fungal Diseases;                      5. Biological Weapons—CIA
  —British Secret Service, MI6;          6. Political Science
  7. Project HAARP                       8. Mind Control
  9. Population Control                   10. Aerospace technology
  I. Title.


Library of Congress Control Number 2001 130588
ISBN: 978-0-923550-39-4


Additional copies of this book are available for bulk purchases.
For more information, please contact:
Tetrahedron, LLC • Suite 147, 206 North 4th Avenue • Sandpoint, Idaho 83864,
1-800-336-9266, Fax: 208-265-2775, E-mail: tetra@tetrahedron.org,
URL web site: http://www.tetrahedron.org


Twelfth Printing, 2013

# IMPORTANT NOTICE:

The information contained in this book is intended for educational purposes only. It is not provided in order to diagnose or treat any disease, illness, or injury of the body, mind, or spirit.

Rather, it is intended to slay Earth's deadliest dragon— a beast that breathes God's power and expires pestilence and pain on His people.

The authors, publisher, and distributors of this work accept no responsibility for people using or misusing the potentially empowering information and revelations in this book.

Individuals suffering from any disease, illness, or injury should, as Hippocrates prescribed, "learn to derive benefit from the illness," and consult with appropriate health care professionals as soon as possible.

# Contents

# Illustrations

## Figures

# Preface

In the beginning, God spoke the world into existence in six days. Then he created man in his image. He did not create man to fall victim to a cataclysmic demise. The eternal purpose of God was to create a people who would be happily married to Him; who would be a companion for Him, or His "bride." For this "joy," as told in Hebrews 12:2, Jesus "endured the cross." This joy *was* the redemption of His people—to return the "bride" to her Husband, the Creator. Godly people, who fell away through ignorance of the law and violations of it, that is, "sin," would turn from their destructive ways, return to the law, and thus be "saved."

The importance of *Healing Codes for the Biological Apocalypse* is clear. The saving or survival of millions, if not billions of people worldwide may depend on learning, telling, and acting on the information presented herein—information that is undoubtedly "stranger than fiction." For this reason, to reach the widest audience, the testimony of the main character and co-contributor—Dr. Joseph "Joey" Puleo (a pseudonym, Dr. Barber, had been used in the limited edition printing) was labored over. The scientific and technical aspects of this book, of great interest to health professionals, scientists, and lay persons alike, were written using nontechnical language, whenever possible, for all to better understand.

This book celebrates and foreshadows humanity's salvation. It is a book about the fall and redemption of "mankind"—the return of "mankind" to "Godkind" as Joey describes it. It is a celebration of the accelerating spiritual recovery that is happening today within the "bride" to which this book bears witness. As a growing number of people experience an increasing number and depth of spiritual experiences, these events, as well as others, foreshadow the reunion of God and man. It is prophesied destiny being fulfilled.

Among its distinct contributions, this work exposes previously published books such as *The Bible Code,* as being disinformative. Some authors have presented "codes" contained in the Bible as "God's codes." They have argued that the mathematical codes and encrypted messages in the Bible were divine inspirations. Evidence presented here challenges some of these authors, and their notions, by unveiling mathematical codes in the Bible that were not included in the original Torah, but were added along with chapter verses during the original translation of the Jewish Scriptures into the Greek *Septuagint*. The evidence, along with common sense, suggests these newly discovered codes were placed there and utilized by powerful men in secret societies. Implicated in this text is King James of Scotland and England and Sir Francis Bacon, authors of the *Authorized King James Bible*, and leaders of a powerful secret society known as the Prieuré de Sion, better known by its modern relatives, the Freemasons. These were people who, like today's most resourceful "inside traders," hid economic and spiritual wealth, including God's most precious and powerful mathematical truths from the masses, for financial gain, self preservation, and even spiritual warfare.

Disclosed here are some of the most important Bible codes for "miracles," including healing, creation, and destruction. Since this knowledge is most powerful, these codes were hidden in the Bible to be recognized only by the cryptocracy—the occult oriented leaders of the secret societies. For centuries their descendants have used this knowledge to increase their wealth and power and to deceive the masses so that they may maintain their control over the Earth. That the truths revealed in this book have remained hidden in the Holy Bible since at least the third century B.C. is sobering. To think that even orthodox Jews and Christians would remain unaware of God's most powerful and practical truths for so long is stunning.

At the same time, this recovered knowledge is exhilarating. The good news is that people around the world can now use these important truths for the betterment of humanity. On the verge of social, economic, political, and religious chaos, these revelations foreshadow the greatest reunion of "Godkind" since the dawn of man. For these and other reasons, this work is both historic and prophetic.

For the record, despite these challenges to the *King James Bible* raised, both authors believe the original scriptures, including the vilified Protestant Apocrypha, were divinely inspired. Thus, translations closest to these earliest works remain imperative reading. In fact, with these new codes and decrypting methods, future Bible study may be even more meaningful.

Both authors wish to acknowledge their high level of spiritual sensitivity and their religious affiliations. This is stated in advance for critics to consider the potential bias of this work. Both doctors feel justified in calling themselves "Christians" in the Nasorean sense. Dr. Len Horowitz is a Hebrew who believes what few Jews believe, that Jesus Christ was a legitimate Messiah—the chosen "son of God." Dr. Joseph Puleo, reared a Catholic, given the impressionable experiences recorded here, has been brought vastly closer to Jesus and his teachings.

This work, from beginning to end, was divinely inspired. Dr. Horowitz's privileged experience in becoming the primary author of this work bears testimony to this statement. It took him three years to investigate and report on the Florida dentist, Dr. David Acer, who transmitted the AIDS virus to his patients. The result, his ninth book, *Deadly Innocence*, was a mere 335 pages. It took the same time to research and write his first best-seller, *Emerging Viruses: AIDS & Ebola—Nature, Accident or Intentional?* with almost twice the page count. Given the urgency of the matters discussed herein, God's divine guidance facilitated this research and writing. As a result, this entire work was completed in less than six months.

Dr. Puleo, an inspired healer and visionary, takes no credit for writing or organizing this book. For help he asked "Jeshua" to meet Dr. Horowitz. Weeks later, through a synchronistic series of events, Dr. Horowitz arrived at his home. As a result, what you are about to read is Dr. Horowitz's report of research principally conducted by Joey.

Joey does not wish to enjoy fame or fortune as a result of this effort. That's why, contrary to Dr. Horowitz's urging, he initially chose to use an alias. He simply wanted to remain anonymous to avoid undesired interruptions to his busy clinic schedule and precious family life.

However, following this book's limited edition first printing, Joey decided to "go public" with his real name. Days after the book's release he was shot in the chest by a laser gun that he believes, based on reputable intelligence sources, was fired by a National Security Agency (NSA) assassin. The beam, by miracle, was largely attenuated by the time it reached Joey's chest. At the moment it was fired, Joey, at home preparing a pasta dinner, lifted a thick glass bottle of cold pressed olive oil for use in his spaghetti sauce. The beam struck the bottle dead center. (This evidence and more is available to investigators, and the media, on request.) The laser melted and bubbled both sides of the container before burning Joey's chest. Soon thereafter, Dr. Horowitz and colleagues again advised Dr. Puleo to drop his alias and remain in the public eye for his own protection. He complied.

Joey currently feels compelled to continue his risky work for the benefit of humanity. As a naturopathic physician, sincerely distressed by the number of patients who are coming to him for treatment with the conditions discussed in Chapters 7 through 9 of this work, his current research involves refining the theses detailed herein, and decoding the *Book of Gen-*

*esis* as it relates to the electromagnetic frequencies of sound that you will shortly discover from the *Book of Numbers*.

There are two old sayings in medicine and psychiatry. The former is that diagnosis is required before treatment and healing. The latter is that healing follows knowledge of the initial trauma and resulting pain, and "without pain, there is no gain." Both Drs. Horowitz and Puleo have made certain "painful" sacrifices to advance this work for the purpose of healing individuals and what ails this planet. The facts presented here, easily verified by examining the two books most people have on their book shelves— the Bible and *Webster's Dictionary*—may help diagnose the greatest and most painful example of man's inhumanity towards man the world has ever witnessed. This knowledge, therefore, is presented by the authors to articulate the greatest opportunity for mass healing and world peace in almost 2,000 years.

## Fall from the Garden

To further explain why this work is so meaningful, consider Bible history and prophecy for a moment. When Adam was in the garden, the kingdom of God was in full operation. Adam had no sin, the presence, the power and the glory of God was resonant in Adam. He had a glorified body—there was no death in him. He walked holy and blameless before the Lord in love. He was immortal and uncorrupted. He had an imperishable body. All this was his until he disobeyed God, complied with the persuasive snake's prescription, and ate from the tree. (See figure 3.5.)

When Adam sinned, death entered him. God said to him, "In dying you shall surely die." In other words, when Adam chose to cut himself off from the Holy Spirit of God, the law, and the truth, he began the process of dying. He lost the presence, the power, and the glory of God. He became mortal instead of immortal, corrupted instead of uncorrupted, and suddenly he lived in a perishable body.

When Adam fell, all of creation fell as well. Up to that point in time, the lion laid down with the lamb. There were no "weeds in the garden," so to speak. With Adam's fall from grace, fallen nature erupted in its own sin.

## The Blood and the "Covenants of Promise"

God presented a plan to restore humanity to what Drs. Horowitz and Puleo in this book call "Godkind." The plan was called the *Covenants of Promise*. Ephesians 2:12 refers to this hope in the shed *blood* of Christ. The word covenant is from the Hebrew word *bereat*, which means "to cut." This implies the shedding of *blood*. The reason blood is so important is because God knew of the life and spiritually sustaining power in blood. Then, by his command and infinite grace, *blood* was shed and made the vehicle for all atonement. Thus, Christ's shed blood atoned for the sins of man.

"For the life of the flesh is in the blood," records Leviticus 17:11, "and I have given it to you on the alter, to make atonement for your souls. For it is the blood by reason of the life that makes atonement." Atonement means "at-one-ment," or becoming one with God. The authors explain the physics of this phenomenon.

Thus, not only do the life sustaining properties of blood heal and restore life, blood functions to bring about unity with God as well. The symbolic shedding of it by Christ, restored what Adam lost for Godkind. His sin imparted death, death implied mortality, mortality evidenced separation from God, but God's covenant and eternal grace now enables reunification with Him. This is the most powerful and wonderful message, and knowhow, delivered in this book.

It all revolves around the *blood*. As the authors of this important work document, the fact that humanity's blood is currently delivering horrific contaminants—infectious agents including "mad cow disease" prions, toxic fungi, and new immune-suppressive epidemics—is central to this book's thesis and our survival. Many of today's most lethal germs have been made and spread to alter human genetics and blood lines forever. Indeed, this is apropos to Bible prophecy.

Throughout history, secret societies have compulsively fixated on blood as central to their nefarious achievements. Power mongers revered blood. Pagan and demonic rituals evolved around blood sacrifices for empowerment. Records memorialize the ceremonial drinking of blood from sacrificed animals, and even children, in the quest for power. The search for the holy grail was conducted because it was believed to be filled with the blood of Christ. This blood fixation dominated the lives of the Templars, kings, and contemporary world leaders.

Today, blood holds the promise of temporal, extended, and perhaps even eternal life. Nazi scientists typed blood stolen from their captives. Blood typing was then used as a means of granting extended life or sentencing the persecuted to death. On a similarly inconceivable and hideous note, the Royal Family and contemporary world leaders have been implicated in abusive sexual and sacrificial practices using the blood of children. Blood worship, in a sense, is practiced in contemporary medicine, science, and even law. Practitioners in these fields look to reveal the secrets for extending life or, in the case of criminals identified through DNA blood analyses, to determine imprisonment or death. Blood bankers collect, freeze, and store blood in the event it is needed during life-threatening surgeries. Diets, science explains, should be predicated on *blood types*.

Indeed, it is no accident that "blood work" is central to all medical and healing applications. The blood contains oxygen-rich red blood cells and white blood cell body guards. Both are vital to health and longevity.

Not coincidentally, the Hebrew name for God is "Yah-vah," which means "to breathe is to exist." It is the breath that delivers the oxygen to the red cells, and these in turn deliver this spiritual component to every cell and tissue in the body needed for life.

Not by accident the white cells, central to the immune system, function like a metaphor for self esteem and spiritual identity. The "God consciousness" within the "temple of God" precisely reflects the functioning immune system. White blood cells, after all, are those that assess the difference between self and nonself, cancer cells versus normal cells, normal host proteins versus invading or infectious agents—bacteria, viruses, fungi and more. So if people are estranged from God—lacking spiritual identity—that is, they do not know who they are on the highest spiritual level, then their immune system cannot function optimally either. Immune cells cannot recognize the difference between self and nonself if *their hosts don't know who they are themselves*. This helps to explain the central importance of spirituality on personal health and longevity, and it is all mediated through the *blood*.

## Limitations of this book

This book is not for everyone, but it is clearly for the prophesied 144,000 Israelites who will lead the earth's intelligent, Godly minority into the messianic new age of peace and enlightenment. If you read the above sentence and balked at any of the Christian, Jewish and/or New Age themes, this work may not be for you. There are events, facts, and concepts expressed in this book that challenge Christian, Jewish, Muslim and "New Age" fundamentals.

We make no apologies for this and challenge anyone who believes they can deliver a more certain explanation for the Bible revelations discussed. Those who believe that their religion holds an exclusive monopoly on God, we further presume, are less inclined to be "saved" themselves.

Divisive beliefs and attitudes are commonly expressed by members of various religious persuasions. For example, people who call themselves "Christians" commonly assert that eternal salvation rests exclusively in a belief in Christ as Lord and savior. All others, many Christians say, are doomed to suffer until they repent and turn their allegiance to Christ.

Likewise, Jewish people, known to have been "chosen," scorn Christians and Muslims alike for their beliefs in Christ or Allah. Muslims, too, are generally threatened by Christian doctrines and, following centuries of "Holy Wars," suspect if not condemn Christians and Jews. Many gentiles blame Jews for the world's economic and political woes.

Meanwhile, "New Agers" believe that salvation rests entirely on thinking positively and focusing on inner light and love. Tending more toward isolationism, New Agers shy away from fundamentalists of every kind. Yet, New Agers are among the first to accept and adopt other dogmas, medical ones included, risky childhood vaccinations for instance. New Age thinkers commonly include the parents of vaccine injured, crippled, or killed children who thought very positively about vaccines and held modern medicine in high esteem and a "light of love."

Aspects of this book will challenge these kinds of thinkers—people who only see their concepts of truth as the key to salvation. Given the documentation provided, fundamentalists of every kind, who are brave enough to read further, may find that their most defensive and unshakable attitudes have been irreversibly changed.

This work will also challenge the medical and scientific communities to realize that many of their established practices have been largely misguided and have not only failed the world's people, but have undermined their health and safety. This work is not intended to win the approval of the scientific majority. We can, however, hope that critical scientific reviewers of this work might actually consider the ramifications of these findings and help to develop solutions to the obvious and horrific problems discussed. Predictably, a small minority of earnest researchers *will* help in resolving these issues based on increasing knowledge in the fields of physics, mathematics, biomedicine, and electromagnetism.

Other "scientific" reviewers may be offended by the anecdotal history of Dr. Puleo's Pythagorean discoveries as reported in the Prologue and in Chapter 1. We make no apologies for taking this editorial license. It happens to be the truth and if the scientific community finds fault in the truth then wherein, exactly, does the problem lie?

Others may find these sections of the book disconcerting as they relay the ease with which monumental discoveries and data were revealed to Dr. Puleo by spiritual beings, including, perhaps, Jesus himself. Scientists are familiar with intuitive breakthroughs. Christians are able to relate to divine revelations. Yet, the editor of this book recommended striking these sections to bolster the scientific nature of the work and to make it more politically palatable. In other words, the editor advised us to appeal to fundamentalists and scientists so that they may be led directly to the meat of this book without first having to digest an esoteric, truthful, yet potentially distasteful, appetizer.

The truth is the truth and people will make of it what they will. The inclusion of the Prologue and Chapter 1 of this work will offer a personal introduction to Dr. Puleo's unique and gifted character. It is vital to the totality of this work that the reader fully appreciate the divinely-inspired direction that contributed to the timely publication of this material.

We offer *Healing Codes for the Biological Apocalypse* for critical review in the hope that it may contribute to meaningful social, cultural, religious, scientific, political, and military reforms appropriate for the coming millennium of divine peace.

Leonard G. Horowitz, D.M.D., M.A., M.P.H.
and Joseph Puleo, N.D.

## Limitations of this book

This book is not for everyone, but it is clearly for the prophesied 144,000 Israelites who will lead the earth's intelligent, Godly minority into the Messianic New Age of peace and enlightenment. If you read the above sentence and balked at any of the Christian, Jewish and/or New Age themes, this work may not be for you. There are events, facts, and concepts expressed in this book that challenge Christian, Jewish, Muslim and "New Age" fundamentals.

We make no apologies for this and challenge anyone who believes they can deliver a more certain explanation for the Bible revelations discussed. Those who believe that their religion holds an exclusive monopoly on God, we further presume, are less inclined to be "saved" themselves.

Divisive beliefs and attitudes are commonly expressed by members of various religious persuasions. For example, people who call themselves "Christians" commonly assert that eternal salvation rests exclusively in a belief in Christ as Lord and savior. All others, many Christians say, are doomed to suffer until they repent and turn their allegiance to Christ.

Likewise, Jewish people, known to have been "chosen," scorn Christians and Muslims alike for their beliefs in Christ or Allah. Muslims, too, are generally threatened by Christian doctrines and, following centuries of "Holy Wars," suspect if not condemn Christians and Jews. Many gentiles blame Jews for the world's economic and political woes.

Meanwhile, "New Agers" believe that salvation rests entirely on thinking positively and focusing on inner light and love. Tending more toward isolationism, New Agers shy away from fundamentalists of every kind. Yet, New Agers are among the first to accept and adopt other dogmas, medical ones included, risky childhood vaccinations for instance. New Age thinkers commonly include the parents of vaccine injured, crippled, or killed children who thought very positively about vaccines and held modern medicine in high esteem and a "light of love."

Aspects of this book will challenge these kinds of thinkers—people who only see their concepts of truth as the key to salvation. Given the documentation provided, fundamentalists of every kind, who are brave enough to read further, may find that their most defensive and unshakable attitudes have been irreversibly changed.

This work will also challenge the medical and scientific communities to realize that many of their established practices have been largely misguided and have not only failed the world's people, but have undermined their health and safety. This work is not intended to win the approval of the scientific majority. We can, however, hope that critical scientific reviewers of this work might actually consider the ramifications of these findings and help to develop solutions to the obvious and horrific problems discussed. Predictably, a small minority of earnest researchers *will* help in resolving these issues based on increasing knowledge in the fields of physics, mathematics, biomedicine, and electromagnetism.

Other "scientific" reviewers may be offended by the anecdotal history of Dr. Puleo's Pythagorean discoveries as reported in the Prologue and in Chapter 1. We make no apologies for taking this editorial license. It happens to be the truth and if the scientific community finds fault in the truth then wherein, exactly, does the problem lie?

Others may find these sections of the book disconcerting as they relay the ease with which monumental discoveries and data were revealed to Dr. Puleo by spiritual beings, including, perhaps, Jesus himself. Scientists are familiar with intuitive breakthroughs. Christians are able to relate to Divine revelations. Yet, the editor of this book recommended striking these sections to bolster the scientific nature of the work and to make it more politically palatable. In other words, the editor advised us to appeal to fundamentalists and scientists so that they may be led directly to the meat of this book without first having to digest an esoteric, truthful, yet potentially distasteful, appetizer.

The truth is the truth and people will make of it what they will. The inclusion of the Prologue and Chapter 1 of this work will offer a personal introduction to Dr. Puleo's unique and gifted character. It is vital to the totality of this work that the reader fully appreciate the Divinely-inspired direction that contributed to the timely publication of this material.

We offer *Healing Codes for the Biological Apocalypse* for critical review in the hope that it may contribute to meaningful social, cultural, religious, scientific, political, and military reforms appropriate for the coming millennium of Divine peace.

Leonard G. Horowitz, D.M.D., M.A., M.P.H.
and Joseph Puleo, N.D.

# Prologue

---

In 1974, I quit my job as a hospital administrator to take my Aunt Betty, who I loved dearly, to Dr. Ernesto Contreras's clinic in Tijuana, Mexico. She was dying of lung cancer.

While there, Dr. Contreras asked me about my background. I had directed a hospital and had expertise in marketing.

When we entered his office, behind his desk hung a big picture of Jesus.

During my aunt's medical interview, he asked us whether or not we believed in God?

My aunt and I both said, "Yes."

"Do you believe in Jesus?"

I said, "Yes."

"Do you have faith?"

"Yeah."

"Well, I think I can help you," he reassured.

Aunt Betty had not been doing well. I had been giving her shots of Demerol every three to four hours. Her pain was excruciating. She could not walk. On the trip down from the East Coast I had to carry her into the hotels, bathe her, and feed her. Her weight dropped to eighty pounds. She could hardly breathe.

Within three weeks, after going through Dr. Contreras's laetrile treatment, she no longer needed any pain medication. Moreover, she was walking again unaided.

For the next six months, I watched patients fly in by helicopter with their guts hanging out in many cases. I met their families. I saw people getting well and walking away. I thought, "Wow! What a miracle this place is."

At the clinic, one morning, I met a man who walked up to me and said, "I know all about you. You're going to be doing some great work for God. And you'll be at a 'gathering of eagles.' Would you kneel with me and pray?"

Although we were in a waiting room packed with people I said, "Sure."

So I knelt down, he placed his hand on my head, and we prayed together. After several minutes of listening to his prayers he stopped. But I could still feel his hand on my head.

Finally, I opened my eyes and there was nobody there. It was the strangest thing. Though I could still feel his hand, he had disappeared. I asked the people all around, "Hey, did you see that guy who was kneeling and praying with me?" They all looked at me as though I was very odd and said, "No."

During the next year, my Aunt Betty's condition improved dramatically.

One day I needed to go out of town for awhile, and had to leave Betty with my cousin, Nancy, who was a nurse. She was well qualified to care for Betty. But when I returned, Nancy told me that Betty needed chemotherapy. She had taken her for treatment. Thirty days later Betty died.

Soon after I moved to San Diego, California, where I met, and moved in with, a Spanish woman. Kathy and I became intimate friends, but we were never meant to marry.

One day she said, "I want you to go to Tijuana with me. There's a seer there. He's also an herbalist. People in my Spanish club say he shares gifts from God."

"I'm not going anywhere," I replied despite the fact I was studying herbology. "I don't believe in that psychic crap. I don't want to go."

But she cried and told me she was afraid to drive to Mexico alone. So the next day, we drove over the border. We went into the mountains outside of Tijuana to a little village. There was no electricity there. The shacks had dirt floors. Big ruts grooved main street.

Soon we found the seer's herb shop and walked in. The place had no phone. Antique urns full of herbs lined the walls and interesting jars filled the shelves.

A minute later an old frail gentleman came out to greet us. He only spoke Spanish. After a few words of introduction he took Kathy into his back room for her "reading."

While they were in the back I browsed the shop examining the old glass herb jars. Then I moved to the glass counter. There was a little Aztec calender medallion inside. I looked at it and thought, "What a nice medallion. I'd like to buy it. I'll wait till they come out and ask the old guy how much he wants."

About fifteen minutes later Kathy came out with her fiery red hair blazing. The old man had told her that we wouldn't be together too much longer. "He's waiting for you to come in," she bellowed. "He wants to speak to you."

I protested, "I don't know this guy. He doesn't even have a phone. I didn't call for an appointment."

Angrily she responded, "God told him you were coming! The angels spoke to him. Now get in there!"

"Okay," I said, then we walked into the back room where he held out his hand to me. We sat down, said a prayer, and he went into a trance.

He told Kathy that she would need to translate for him. That because she was angry, and what he might tell her she may not like; she might, therefore, be inclined to mistranslate the information. He told her if she failed to translate exactly, a great curse would befall her. Then he began.

He immediately told me that I would not be living with Kathy much longer, as he had told her. I would not marry her. I suddenly understood her anger.

The old man said I would be going to the Pacific Northwest, into the mountains, to do God's work at a "gathering of eagles." He cried when he told me this. "In days to come, your blessing may become a curse."

He hugged me and said he could tell me no more even though he could see the future.

I walked out of the back room thinking, "This is all too crazy. This guy doesn't even have a phone. He's telling me he speaks to God? But this is the second time I've heard this 'gathering of eagles' business. I don't understand this."

We were about to walk out of the store when he called to Kathy in Spanish, "Hola!" He told her to tell me that he's not crazy. Nor am I. But since I didn't get it, and seemed confused, the angels spoke to him saying he has proof for me.

He walked over to the glass counter, opened it, and took out the medallion I had wanted. "You had thought upon this, cherished it, and wished for it, my friend. It is yours Señor. Let it be proof that the angels have spoken to me."

I offered to pay him for the piece. "Go with God," he responded. "I cannot take any money. Not for doing God's work. Not when someone is sent to me by Jesus." Tears filled his eyes when he told me this and he cried as I left his store.

I pondered this meeting for weeks. I figured there was no way the old guy could have known about my attraction to the medallion. Nor could he have known about the other man who predicted my attendance at a "gathering of eagles." He obviously wasn't doing this for the money.

Months later I still wondered about the encounter. Particularly when I moved to the Pacific Northwest. I was invited to take a job as marketing director for a large resort. The place was beautifully situated in the mountains east of Seattle.

Reflecting on my search for God, I had frequently read all kinds of books—from the Bible to many New Age titles.

One day, a title tabooed for Christians called *Helping Yourself With White Witchcraft*, by doctors Frost and Frost—a husband and wife team from Berkeley—arrived by mail from my book-of-the-month club. It explained how to easily "transmute energy." It really had nothing to do with "witchcraft" per se.

But as I read it one afternoon on the front porch at the resort, I suddenly heard this noise. I looked up, and over the top of the book, I saw a man quickly running toward me. He came up to the porch, grabbed my book—a hardcover—tore it in half, and threw it off the balcony. All before I could even gather my thoughts.

"Don't ever read that kind of stuff!" he shouted. "Don't you know who you are?"

I said, "Yeah, I know who I am. I'm the guy who's gonna kick your butt for tearing my book in half. Meet me by the picnic tables down by the pond after work and I'll show you who I am."

After work I went down to the pond fully intending to break the guy's nose.

Suddenly, there he was. "Hello, I'm Larry Morris," he said. He held out his right hand for a shake. In his left hand he held a six-pack of beer. "On my way I thought I'd stop at the store to get us some brew."

I thought, "How can I pop a guy who's bringing me a six-pack?"

Then he totally mesmerized me when he said, "You had two previous messages. This is your third."

I said, "What are you talking about?"

"Think about the 'gathering of eagles.'"

"My God! Mexico in '74 at Dr. Contreras's, and the old man outside of Tijuana in '82."

"God has plans for you," he replied. "Not far from here you'll be at a 'gathering of eagles.'"

"Oh really now," I said as I thought, "This guy is really cuckoo. Either I'm losing my mind, or he's losing his."

It was just dusk. The sun was setting. There was no wind whatsoever. He reached out his hands and began to speak in a foreign tongue. I knew it was a prayer because he mentioned God here and there. Much to my amazement, as he moved his hands the bushes moved. When he moved his hands to the left, the bushes bent to the left and stayed that way. Then he moved his hands to the right and the bushes bent to the right. When he stopped, they stopped and stayed. Then his hands went to the middle and came down. The bushes went back to normal. Suddenly a strong wind blew down from the mountains.

He extended his arms again, this time with his palms up. He told me to reach out and place my palms down upon his. Then he grasped my hands. All at once it felt like I got hit with a million volts of lightning. I just stood there shaking and vibrating for what seemed to be several minutes.

"I'm glad I didn't take a swing at this guy," I thought. "Because if this is any indication of what he's capable of doing, I'd be in deep trouble now."

Then he said, "You just don't get it do you? You don't really know who you are."

"Okay. So I don't know who I am. So what? Who are you?"

"A messenger," he replied. He told me that he would speak with me again and then he quickly walked away.

I got into my car, drove down the mountain, and passed my house five times. I was in some kind of shock. I could see everything but couldn't think of anything. It was like I was in my body but not really. Finally, when I pulled my car into the driveway Kathy was standing there waiting. I told her what happened, and as I did, I started crying. Tears ran down my face. They were tears of joy.

Time passed. I got another job at another resort higher up the mountain. A few months later, as I was on my way to work, I hit a traffic jam.

"There's no sense sitting in line," I thought. So I took the next exit. There was a Denny's restaurant right in front of me. I hadn't had breakfast yet so I pulled in and parked.

I walked into the place and there was a reception sign that read: "Please wait to be seated." So I waited. A few moments later a hostess walked up to me and asked, "Would you please follow me? Your friend is waiting for you."

I said, "Excuse me?"

"Your friend's waiting for you."

"She must be talking to someone else," I thought, so I looked behind me to see if anyone was there. I was alone.

"You're talking to me?"

"Of course I'm talking to you," she replied. "Your friend saw you pull up. He's been waiting for you."

So I followed her, zigzagged around a few tables, and there was Larry Morris sitting in the corner.

"Don't worry," he said as I sat down. "Nobody got hurt on the highway. God works in mysterious ways. That's why the traffic stopped and you're here.

After a brief pause he said, "You just don't get the picture do you? Look, you don't know who you are. You've got to start knowing who you are. God has great plans for you."

"Really," I said sarcastically, then turned to look out at the bumper to bumper traffic that blocked the freeway.

As though he could read my mind he said, "Don't worry. I said nobody's been hurt. Believe me."

"You did this?" I asked.

"Well. You might say that."

I said, "Liar. Who the hell are you? If I don't know who I am, at least tell me who you are."

"I'm kinda what you might call an angel incarnate," he replied. "And I have to leave here soon to go to East Berlin to make sure the wall falls."

"I don't know what the hell you're talking about," I rebutted. "But they ought to call you Voltaire because you sure shocked the crap out of me."

He said, "Look, I want to tell you this. This is my last visit with you. I have to leave now. Something important will happen in Berlin. Think upon me when you learn of it."

"This is really cuckoo," I thought.

He must have heard my thought. "What'd you say? You still don't believe me? I'll show you."

Then he began to light up before my eyes. He started glowing a bright violet purple like ultraviolet light.

I sat there stunned. But I still had the presence of mind to think, "I wonder whether he's wearing some kind of electronic device?"

He said, "You're really thick! Do you need another electric shock to convince you, Joey?"

"No Larry. That's okay. I really believe you."

"Well, you're starting to," he returned. Then he got up and walked out of the restaurant.

Shortly thereafter, I was transferred to Montana to work at another resort. There I met a man who told me that I would soon meet an Indian man. That he would take me to a sacred place. And that I would be doing work on this Indian land for God. Then he left.

About a month later, I moved to Arizona to help market another property. There I rented a house in Apache Junction. An Indian owned it. He was a medicine man for the Pima Tribe. His father was the chief medicine man.

One day he came over and said, "I have a message for you. But I have to ask you some questions."

"Sure. Go ahead," I replied.

"Are you interested in gold?" he asked. He had seen my maps of superstition mountain. Everyday I went up to the top.

"Sure I'm interested in gold," I answered. "But not the yellow kind. I'm looking for the gold of wisdom and knowledge and the hidden secrets."

"I believe that," he said. Then he pulled something out of his leather pouch. He struck a match and lit it. White smoke filled the room as he chanted a special chant. Then he said, "You are of God, and God has work for you to do."

He invited me to go to a sacred ground where no white man had traveled. We spent three days there. On the third day he told me, "You will be with a great 'gathering of eagles.'"

Months later I received a phone call from a buddy of mine. He invited me to take a position with another resort in central Oregon. I asked, "What's the name of the place?"

"Eagle Crest."

"Uh oh, here we go," I thought. "I'm on my way."

The following week I left for my new marketing post in the great Northwest. And that's where I met my wife.

Linda was described to me, to a tee, by the old Mexican fellow years earlier. "This will be the woman you marry," he told me.

So Linda and I got married. Soon thereafter, we moved into an old cabin in Sandpoint, Idaho, in the Pacific Northwest.

Shortly, we met a group of people—metaphysical and spiritual types. One evening they asked me, "How'd you get here?" And I told them the story, mentioning the "gathering of eagles."

One woman there, Mary Leery, said, "My Lord!" She told me that someone from Missouri had given her a spiral bound book. The man said, "Mary this isn't for you. But you'll know who to give it to." Mary had put the book away. "This morning," she said, "I found it on my car. I hadn't looked at it for months. I never read it, and I didn't put it there. I don't know who did. This book is obviously for you."

"Really?"

She pulled it out of her handbag, then handed it to me. I read the title, *The Gathering of Eagles*.

The book was written by a Canadian man who owned a window washing company. He sold the company to get the money to print the book. He wrote that God had told him to do this. The book predicted that "the eagles will be gathering in the Pacific Northwest, in the panhandle of Idaho." That was exactly where we settled. In the "end times," he wrote, "Jesus will give these eagles guidance." Mary cried when she handed me the book.

About a year later, Mark Hammer, an alleged "channeler of Jesus" with whom most fundamentalist Christians are offended, came to Sandpoint to give a lecture. In the interim I had gotten his book, *The Jeshua Letter*, from my friend John who owns a bookstore in Sandpoint. As I read it, I had this sense that I was there, walking with Jeshua ben Joseph (the Hebrew name for Jesus pronounced *Yah-shoe-ah*). I felt as though Jeshua was a close friend of mine. His book had such an impact on me that I bought ten copies of it, and gave them out to my friends. So when Mark Hammer came to town, several of them called me to get me to attend his lecture. But I didn't want to go.

"That channeling stuff gives me the hebejeebees," I told them, even though I had enjoyed Hammer's book.

Early Monday morning, following the event, one of my friends, Steve, called me and said, "Joey, you should've been there. It was fantastic." After telling me all about it, my friend said, "Hey, you know those business tapes you have. Can you drop them off for me at John's bookstore? Mark Hammer is doing private readings there between eleven and noon, and I'm scheduled for a session. After that, you and I can go to lunch if you want."

"Yeah? What does a private session with Hammer cost?"

"A hundred bucks."

I laughed and sarcastically said, "I can talk to God for free. What are you crazy? Spending that much money? No thanks," I continued. "I'll meet you at my office."

So a little before eleven, I began the twenty mile ride to downtown Sandpoint. Just north of town, I got to the junction of routes 95 and 200. At the traffic light, while stopped, I lit a cigarette, which was my ritual.

This time, when I lit it, something strange happened. I went through the traffic light, and suddenly blacked out. That was the last thing I remember.

Next, not sure of how much time passed, I realized my truck had stopped. I looked up and I was parked with the motor running. I looked at my cigarette and it didn't go down the slightest bit.

"How can this be?" I thought. "I don't even remember going through town. Now I'm parked in front of John's bookstore?"

My heart was pounding wildly as I turned off the engine. "My word! I went through town, time and space and don't even remember it." Trembling, I put my cigarette out and got out of the truck. I had to pee so bad, due to the fright, I needed a bathroom *immediately*. So I went into the bookstore to use the restroom.

When I came out, Mark Hammer was in the corner of the bookstore doing a reading with some lady. Just then, she got up and, with tears running from her eyes she repeated, "How could he know? How could he know?"

Then John said, "Joey, come here. I want you to meet Mark Hammer."

Hesitantly I said, "Okay."

The next moment, I was shaking this guy's hand as his eyeballs rolled back and forth all twisted in his head. It reminded me of Marty Feldman. As he looked at me all weird like that, I thought, "Ewww. This guy's a real freak." So I quickly pulled my hand back, wiped it off on my pants, and said, "Excuse me," not wanting to appear too rude.

Then I left the store for my office, still all shook up. As soon as I got there, Steve was coming out the door. "Here are your tapes," I said and handed them over to him. "Don't bother me about lunch. I need to lie down. I'll talk to you later."

I needed to lie down like never before in my entire life. I didn't care if the phone rang. I was too spooked to speak with anyone. I laid down and tried to figure out what was happening to me. And as I did, I went through a deja vu. Then I fell asleep.

It was a quarter-to-five when I awoke. And the phone was ringing. I thought, "Well maybe it's Linda?" So I picked up the phone.

"Hello. It's John at the bookstore. Mark Hammer wants to talk to you Joey. He says he received a message for you from Jesus."

"Oh really now. That's cool. Put him on the phone," I replied. Proudly I thought, "Hey, I get a call from Jesus. This is amazing."

"It don't work that way, Joey. You've got to come down here."

I said, "Yeah? Cool."

So I called Linda, told her I would be late for dinner; told her, "You're not gonna believe what I've been through today, but I'll tell you later." Then I hesitantly drove to the store.

As I arrived, I saw a big limousine parked in front of John's place. A large group of inquisitive people gathered around it. And when I walked up to the door, John came out and told me, "Mark was scheduled to go to Spokane; then fly off to do a major event. But Jesus told him he must relay a message to you. So he just cancelled everything to spend time with you."

I went inside the store, and waited for Mark to get ready. Sitting there I thought, "I don't want to do this. He might know all the crap I did in my life. All the dirty tricks." Realizing this likelihood, and the aversion I, a Christian, maintained towards "channeling," I suddenly got up and headed for the door. "I'm not going to go through with this," I thought.

John called after me, "Joey! Where are you going?"

"I'm leaving."

"You're not leaving! He cancelled everything to be with you. You're not going anywhere."

Realizing my departure would be rude, and that maybe Jesus *was* trying to reach me, for even God uses devildoers when desired, I broke into a cold sweat and returned to my seat.

A minute later Mark Hammer sat down across from me at a table with a tape recorder. "We're going to tape this 'cause Jeshua wants you to play it anytime you need to."

Next Hammer said a prayer to bring on what he said was "a pinpoint of light" in which he allegedly saw Jeshua's image in his mind's eye. Then, I now believe, he began to receive Jeshua's message:

"Blessed be unto you my Holy brother, Holy child of God. Thank you for coming. It is by no accident that you were led to where you are at this time and place. Don't worry that I will judge you on your past, I only choose to look at the love that abides in your heart now." With that I felt better.

"It was by no accident that you repeatedly received my messengers who foretold of your mission here," he continued.

"You will soon find a place where there will be a gathering of people—a 'gathering of eagles.' There will be much healing that occurs there," he said. Tears began to roll down my face. "I'll speak with you again soon."

A few months later, again through synchronicity, I met Ken Page, a hypnotherapist who my friends highly recommended. I told them, "Hell no. I ain't going. No nonsense. No hocus pocus. No psychotherapy!" But again, through a bizarre series of events, I ended up going to see Mr. Page.

He told me that the chronic pain in my neck had stemmed from the time that I had shared the pain of Jesus' crucifixion.

During Page's session, although he hypnotized me, I remained aware of my surroundings. I couldn't open my eyes, but I could hear Page's instructions. Once in this "trance," I personally identified with *Joseph of Aramethea*, the uncle, teacher, and confidant of the beloved Jesus. In my mind's eye, he had long hair, wore a robe, and walked with Jeshua to his death.

"Where are you?" Page asked.

"I'm here with Jesus in the garden," I replied.

"What are you doing?"

"I'm crying," I said. "Because Joseph's power, money, nor access to the Sanhedrin and the Roman officials, could not stop the crucifixion and mass murders. The people wanted this murder stopped, but Jesus said to Joseph, 'You can't stop it.'"

"Why not?"

"Because an angel said it must happen. . . . You have never let me down, but you have to let me do this now," Jesus said to Joseph. "I know you raised me . . ."

"Yes," Joseph interrupted, "but now I see you've been raised for the slaughter. I can't live with that!"

I intensely identified with Joseph's feelings, particularly guilt. This stress seemed to manifest in a pain in my neck and shoulder. The same place it had bothered me for years. I seemed to be holding that horrible incident in that part of my body.

Jeshua confirmed this diagnosis and then said, "Now we must attend to some unfinished business."

Page then asked, "Joey, are you ready to go to the time and place of the crucifixion?"

"Yes," I replied.

"May I come with you?" he asked.

"Sure."

Moments later I saw myself kneeling at the cross, looking at Jeshua, with tears streaming down my face as he spoke to me.

"What did he say?" Page asked.

"He said 'I forgive you all.'"

"No," Page directed. "What did he say to you personally?"

"He said to me, 'You have served me well.'"

"That's right," Page affirmed. "What do you see now?" he prodded me to continue.

I looked to my right and there was a little hand holding onto my hand. It was a little boy kneeling with me below the cross. The head on the little boy became clear as he turned toward me. He had Ken Page's younger face. And before I said anything at all to describe what I was seeing, Page said, "Do you see that little boy on your right holding your hand?"

"Yes," I said, stunned that he saw what I was seeing.

"That's me," he said. "I'm with you. That's why Jesus and the angels directed me to you."

Then he broke the hypnotic trance ending the session.

We both laid down on the floor for awhile and cried. Page was so moved he cancelled all of his appointments for the rest of the day. He walked out of the store, crossed the street, and laid down on a park bench. That was the last time I saw him.

I thought a lot about that experience in the following days and weeks. "All of this is hard to believe," I realized. Especially given my attitude, and life-long misconduct, that I would feel so close to Jesus. Later, when I told Mark Hammer this consideration he said, "You always had a good heart."

Despite the fact that Ken Page and Mark Hammer did not know each other, they both told me virtually the same thing: That I always served Jeshua well.

Months later, during my second session with Hammer, Jeshua ended the session reminding me of the "gathering of eagles." "This meeting will unfold as I send the eagles your way. They will gather around you. You have never let me down, and you will not now."

I offered to pay both Page and Hammer for their time with me. Both refused any money. "Normally I charge for my consultations," Mark Hammer said, "but when Jesus asks to speak to you, I can't charge."

As a result of these experiences, I maintained a very close connection to Jeshua who directed me to the sacred Indian ground where I now reside and work. Here, with blessings from Native American tribes, whose medicine men awarded me a special bear tooth necklace in honor of my having saved the life of one of their most beloved elders, I established myself as a naturopathic doctor and spiritual healer. All of this has come about with Jeshua's constant support. The Indians also told me their wise men said I walk with the "Pale Prophet"—their name for Jesus.

One Sunday I was entertaining several friends when two truck loads of Indians—Lakota Sioux—drove up to our house. They were dressed in full ceremonial attire. I had been warned that they would come. One of their elders told me he knew I would be doing important work here. "Work like an eagle, at a 'gathering of eagles,'" he said. Then he added. "We have to do a ceremony to protect you and the property. It's an ancient ceremonial ground. There is a vortex here and a sacred altar in the mountains above the land."

The Indians jumped out of their trucks, dusted everyone with feathers, and lit incense. They sang songs and beat their drums. They tied tobacco leaves all around the house and property.

After that, I started getting visions. Bible codes started coming to me for decoding and healing. What follows is the story and result of these gifts. It is vitally important, at this critical time in history, for world healing.

My wife Linda, for example, was recently diagnosed with cancer—a malignant melanoma. She was given four months to live by her oncologist. By applying the knowledge given us in this book, we beat the melanoma in three-and-a-half weeks.

What follows mostly is a book about faith. The bits of information we provide are like facets of a beautiful gem. Each facet holds a special truth. We hope, when all is said and done, that a most magnificent jewel will emerge from the totality of this truth.

Peace be unto you.

Dr. Joseph "Joey" Puleo

*Healing Codes for the Biological Apocalypse*

# Chapter 1.
# The "Gathering of Eagles"

"Having the glory of God: and her light
was like unto a stone most precious, even
like a jasper stone, clear as crystal. . . ."
Revelation 21:11, *King James Bible*

Not long after Joey's Indian visitation and blessing, extraordinary events began to occur for him. During social gatherings, for example, friends and family would ask him questions regarding spirituality and healing. Their questions would often compel him to drift into receptive states of consciousness from where their answers came.

"All of a sudden this white light would appear just as it did for Mark Hammer," he recalled. "Then I was able to answer all the questions people posed to me. Linda scrambled for our tape recorder, and we often recorded the messages I received.

"But I felt uncomfortable about this. I didn't want to be just another human telephone. People told me to hold counseling sessions and charge $50 per hour. But that didn't appeal to me at all. That felt as though I would be exploiting God.

"So one evening, alone in our hot tub, I began praying. 'I don't want to do this,' I told God. 'I don't want to be another telephone.' Then I got angry, looked up at the stars, and prayed, 'I'm not going to do this. I'm not going to be anyone's telephone.'

"Suddenly this angel appeared before me. Whether or not I was hallucinating or imagining it, or whether it was real, I can't be sure. But I told the angel, 'I'm not going to do this' and the angel replied, 'Your beloved Jesus and God has spoken. The gift is yours. But since you surrender it, because of your reasons, your wish is granted. You will have another way to serve God consciously. You will remain conscious as the spirit comes to you.'

Later Joey reflected on this and replayed the recording Mark Hammer made during their session. 'You will be communicating with me. First in the way of thought. Then as an energy feeling. You will come to know me well.' And since that time, this has happened.

"When I do research, I begin with a prayer," Joey explained. "Then these intuitive insights come to me. I can often see things.

"While working with people the same thing happens. I pray, the clarity comes, and then I see what their problem is. I see their internal illnesses. I hear things that are inaudible. Occasionally I perceive people's entire lifetimes in a flash. I understand it all. I can tell them dates and times when they were molested or hurt. This has become a main tool in my healthcare practice."

## Numbers on the Windshield

One misty fall evening, while driving home from his office, Joey and Linda were listening to music when all of a sudden something appeared on the windshield before him. He could see the road, but on the glass two columns of numbers appeared. At the top of the first column, on the left side, the number ten initially appeared. To the right, adjacent that column and number, the number eleven suddenly appeared. Then below, on the left, came twelve. Then thirteen on the right. This pattern continued until two numbered columns filled the windshield. Joey noticed that all even numbers appeared on the left, and all odd numbers on the right. A similar pattern is depicted in figure 1.1.

"Joey, what are you looking at?" Linda asked, noticing him looking oddly at the road ahead.

"Do you see those numbers?"

"What numbers?"

"The numbers on the windshield," Joey replied.

She could not.

The next day, while waiting to see a physician friend, Dr. Peter Metcalf, Joey became entranced in the doctor's waiting room. He took

## Fig. 1.1. EVEN and "OD" Number Column

| EVEN/LEFT COLUMN / "OD" or Even Result... | "OD"/RIGHT COLUMN / EVEN or "OD" Result... |
|---|---|
| 1 0 – 1 + 0 = 1 | 1 1 – 1 + 1 = 2 |
| 1 2 – 1 + 2 = 3 | 1 3 – 1 + 3 = 4 |
| 1 4 – 1 + 4 = 5 | 1 5 – 1 + 5 = 6 |
| 1 6 – 1 + 6 = 7 | 1 7 – 1 + 7 = 8 |
| 1 8 – 1 + 8 = 9 | 1 9 – 1 + 9 = 1 0 |
| | |
| 2 0 – 2 + 0 = 2 | 2 1 – 2 + 1 = 3 |
| 2 2 – 2 + 2 = 4 | 2 3 – 2 + 3 = 5 |
| 2 4 – 2 + 4 = 6 | 2 5 – 2 + 5 = 7 |
| 2 6 – 2 + 6 = 8 | 2 7 – 2 + 7 = 9 |
| 2 8 – 2 + 8 = 1 0 | 2 9 – 2 + 9 = 1 1 |
| | |
| 3 0 – 3 + 0 = 3 | 3 1 – 3 + 1 = 4 |
| 3 2 – 3 + 2 = 5 | 3 3 – 3 + 3 = 6 |
| 3 4 – 3 + 4 = 7 | 3 5 – 3 + 5 = 8 |
| 3 6 – 3 + 6 = 9 | 3 7 – 3 + 7 = 1 0 |
| 3 8 – 3 + 8 = 1 1 | 3 9 – 3 + 9 = 1 2 |
| | |
| 4 0 – 4 + 0 = 4 | 4 1 – 4 + 1 = 5 |
| 4 2 – 4 + 2 = 6 | 4 3 – 4 + 3 = 7 |
| 4 4 – 4 + 4 = 8 | 4 5 – 4 + 5 = 9 |
| 4 6 – 4 + 6 = 1 0 | 4 7 – 4 + 7 = 1 1 |
| 4 8 – 4 + 8 = 1 2 | 4 9 – 4 + 9 = 1 3 |

The first set of numbers that appeared on Dr. Puleo's car window that initiated his search for the Pythagorean skein. He later learned his information related to the importance of mathematics in the development of left and right brain balance. It also related to spiritual evolution and physical creation.

out a legal pad, and began to decipher the numbers he had seen the night before.

He noticed that the odd numbers he deciphered added together to produce even numbers up to 19. The even numbers he added produced odd ones up to 18.

After deciphering several pages of numbers this way, Dr. Metcalf entered the waiting room. "What's that you're working on?" he asked.

"These numbers just came to me," Joey replied as he handed the doctor the pages of data.

"Gee. That almost looks like an eyechart I use with my patients, Joey. Do you know how to spell odd?"

"Sure I do," Joey replied. "O-D-D."

"Then why did you spell it 'OD'?" Metcalf asked.

"Well, that's the way it came through," Joey explained.

"OD stands for 'opthalmic diopter.' It has to do with the eyes," the physician noted. "Perhaps it has to do with the left eye and the right eye."

"Well that make sense," Joey said, "but what would that have to do with the numbers?"

The doctor did not know.

This baffled Joey for awhile. Finally he realized that more than left eye and right eye, the issue related to left brain and right brain. That is, the left hemisphere of the brain, more commonly associated with rational thinking, processes information differently than the right hemisphere, more often linked to intuition. It had to do with what Joey termed "matrices of thought." And since mathematics has its own language, the numbers came to him divided, left from right, and even from "OD," for a very important reason. It provided a glimpse into the development of language. Numbers and language, Joey considered, can affect thought processes and consciousness.

Initially, for instance, Hebrew and Sanskrit were read right to left. Now, modern languages read left to right. Could this transposition have impacted spirituality? Very likely and dramatically Joey later learned. David John Oates's research in "Reverse Speech™" showed that English speech backwards is commonly encrypted with far more "honest" expressions, and even appears to "reflect peoples' repressed souls."[1]

Shortly, all of this will become clearer. You will soon see how this was also a preparatory lesson to help Joey decipher some of the most important spiritually empowering Bible codes.

## Points of Reference

"You see," Joey explained, "we are all taught conceptual thinking from the cradle to the grave. As the saying goes, 'Know ye of God,' we all know of God. But 'God ye not know.' Because most of us only have a concept, rather than an experience of God—what other people tell us about him. What friends and family members tell us about God. What ministers, priests, and preachers teach us about God. The concept, for example, that God's wrath will be poured down upon us if we misbehave in certain ways. These are all concepts that we have developed that can have a profound affect on our spirituality and lives.

"This frightened me," Joey continued, "'Vengeance is mine, sayeth the Lord.' It scared me." Earnestly he questioned, "Who wants to serve someone that wants to scare you? I observed Christians killing Muslims, Muslims killing Jews, Jews killing Arabs, Whites killing Blacks and visa versa. All commonly done in the name of God? I had to think that there was something better and that Jeshua was far more loving and sensible than that."

So as he searched for a kinder God, his search also became one for truth. Then the numbers became necessary. Through his experience with these numbers, the truth about conceptual thinking fell upon him.

"We were only taught *concepts* about everything," Joey realized. From religion to medicine and from marriage to children. What's right. What's wrong. Good and bad. Such conceptual thinking applied certain constraints on human experience for better or worse. In either case, conceptual thinking blocked people's easy access to spirituality—to God.

Alternatively, higher matrices of thought connected people to universal knowledge and God's love, which is omnipresent. Some of the world's greatest scientists, inventors, artists, and musicians, including

Einstein, Tesla, Keely, Rife, and Beethoven, got their information and creative insights from this higher matrix of thought. They were more closely connected to the spiritual realm because of it.

Unbeknownst to Joey, by doing the mathematical exercises he had received, he further integrated his left and right brain to function more holistically. The whole brain function is greater than the sum of its left and right brain parts. So in the process of writing down these equations, and doing the math, he further attuned himself to receive spiritual messages. And this, he advanced, is available to everyone who goes through the process individually. (Figure 1.2 has been added for you to fill in the blanks so that you may have this unique experience yourself.)

The goal is to become closer to God. As Joey experienced, this mathematical exercise helped him transcend conceptual thinking, and go beyond his "points of reference" including his concept of God. As a result he felt closer to Jeshua than ever before.

When you look up the word "God" in the dictionary, he explained, it says "the concept of a deity with some control over humanity." That implies that God only has "some control" when in fact God has absolute control.

As a *concept*, however, God only has *some* control. That's why people argue about God and end up fearing, hating, and killing one another. All in God's name which is used thereby in vain.

In other words, to experience the full glory and power of God, and the brotherly and sisterly love consistent with his grace, you must go beyond divisive "points of reference" — beyond thinking ego-centered, fear-based concepts; into integrated whole brain function and absolute truth. To do this, it helps to do the mathematical exercise provided in figure 1.2.

Jeshua told Joey that people who search for spiritual experiences generally acquire them. But the masses who do not remain limited by conceptual religious beliefs. Religion is not "bad" per se, he continued, but the fact that religions have, for instance, prostituted Jesus'

## Fig. 1.2. Pythagorean Skein Fill In The Blank Exercise

| EVEN/LEFT COLUMN / "OD" or Even Result... | "OD"/RIGHT COLUMN / EVEN or "OD" Result... |
|---|---|
| $1\ 0 - 1 + 0 = \square$ | $1\ 1 - 1 + 1 = \square$ |
| $1\ 2 - \square + 2 = 3$ | $1\ 3 - 1 + \square = 4$ |
| $1\ 4 - 1 + 4 = \square$ | $1\ 5 - 1 + 5 = \square$ |
| $1\ 6 - 1 + \square = 7$ | $1\ 7 - \square + 7 = 8$ |
| $1\ 8 - 1 + 8 = \square$ | $1\ 9 - 1 + 9 = \square$ |
| | |
| $2\ 0 - \square + 0 = 2$ | $2\ 1 - 2 + \square = 3$ |
| $2\ 2 - 2 + 2 = \square$ | $2\ 3 - 2 + 3 = \square$ |
| $2\ 4 - 2 + \square = 6$ | $2\ 5 - \square + 5 = 7$ |
| $2\ 6 - 2 + 6 = \square$ | $2\ 7 - 2 + 7 = \square$ |
| $2\ 8 - \square + 8 = 1\ 0$ | $2\ 9 - \square + 9 = 1\ 1$ |
| | |
| $3\ 0 - 3 + 0 = \square$ | $3\ 1 - 3 + 1 = \square$ |
| $3\ 2 - \square + 2 = 5$ | $3\ 3 - 3 + \square = 6$ |
| $3\ 4 - 3 + 4 = \square$ | $3\ 5 - 3 + 5 = \square$ |
| $3\ 6 - 3 + \square = 9$ | $3\ 7 - \square + 7 = 1\ 0$ |
| $3\ 8 - 3 + 8 = \square$ | $3\ 9 - 3 + 9 = \square$ |
| | |
| $4\ 0 - 4 + 0 = \square$ | $4\ 1 - 4 + 1 = \square$ |
| $4\ 2 - \square + 2 = 6$ | $4\ 3 - 4 + \square = 7$ |
| $4\ 4 - 4 + 4 = \square$ | $4\ 5 - 4 + 5 = \square$ |
| $4\ 6 - 4 + \square = 1\ 0$ | $4\ 7 - \square + 7 = 1\ 1$ |
| $4\ 8 - 4 + 8 = \square$ | $4\ 9 - 4 + 9 = \square$ |

A self-development exercise using the numbers associated with the Pythagorean skein. This information relates to the importance of mathematics in the development of left and right brain balance. It also relates to spiritual evolution and physical creation as you will increasingly learn in the coming chapters.

name, is ample cause to refer to him as Jeshua instead of Jesus. "Then people may know me and my father, instead of merely knowing *of* me and my father.

"The truth," Jeshua explained to Joey, "shall set you free. That's the primary reason they crucified me. I exposed the lies. My exposures made those implicated angry. So they put a contract on my head and nailed me to a cross.

"Now we're going to finish the work we began, and you're going to help me as you did before," Jeshua told Joey.

A fundamental lie that needs to be exposed now, more than ever, is the truth about points of reference and conceptual versus integrative thinking. The religious and spiritual elite—the ancient rabbis and clergy—were allowed this information. They kept it from the masses for reasons of control. Spiritually endowed people could not be controlled if they knew the truth and maintained a direct connection to God.

"In truth," Jeshua told Joey, "if you believe in God, and if you believe him to be your father, *the* Father, *the* Creator, then you therefore must be *His* child. Correct?

"That means you must be a holy child of God. And if you are a holy child of God, you must, therefore, be a spiritual being. And if you are a *spiritual being* then you are far more than a human being."

Joey was then directed to reread Matthew 16:23, where Jesus said to Peter "Thou, Satan, get thee behind me. For thou savorest not the ways of God, but the ways of man."

"If you look up the word 'Satan' in *Strong's Concordance* where the derivations of every word in the Bible are explained," Joey said, "the word Satan is defined as 'to dispel, rebuke, or go against' such as an adversary. There is no evil entity described.

"If you abide by the ways of God," he continued, "then you are a spiritual being who rebukes Satan. And if you abide by the ways of man, then you are a human being who embraces Satan. Both are in flesh. It only depends on your points of reference. Are you referencing from mankind or from Godkind? 'Know ye of God? or God ye not know.'

"You've got to discover the truth about who you're not," Joey concluded. "I said this to my wife, Linda, one day. She said, 'Can't you ever be human?' I replied, 'Are you crazy? They lie, they cheat, they steal. You want me to be like that?'

"Of course when you lie, cheat and steal, in the spiritually integrated sense, you're lying, cheating and stealing from yourself as well as from others."

The fundamental issue, and greatest problem, is that mankind's spiritual endowment has been stolen, or at least hidden. Recovering this truth, and the truth about who you are, is the most important message this book holds and the Bible delivers.

For people who ask, "Who am I?" The answer is "You are a holy child of God."

People who seek spiritual experiences and don't find them might be surprised to learn the reason why. "You can't find something you already are," Joey professed. "Stop looking beyond yourself and you might find your true nature in spirit and in God. Learn to shift your points of reference, and your focus, and ye will know God. We are spiritual beings having a human experience. If we all knew this truth, then we would quit lying to ourselves and to each other. "

## Exercise in Trust, Faith and God

Jeshua instructed Joey to learn how mathematics, the most exact language, speaks the truth to the subconscious. He was told to take the alphabet, from A to Z, as seen in figure 1.3, and number each letter. For example, A=1, B=2, C=3 and so on to Z=26. Figure 1.4 is provided for you to do this exercise.

Later, Joey was instructed to take the words "TRUST," "FAITH," and "GOD," and perform a mathematical translation on them.

For "TRUST" T=20 + R=18 + U=21, + S=19 and T=20 totals 98. As seen in figure 1.3, Jeshua directed Joey to reduce each number to a single digit. So 9+8=17; then finally, 1+7=8.

## Fig. 1.3. Derivation of English Letter Number Values

| Letter & Number | Pythagorean Skein Equivalent | Key Word Number Derivations |
|---|---|---|
| A 1 | 1 | T 20–2 + 0 = 2 |
| B 2 | 2 | R 18–1 + 8 = 9 |
| C 3 | 3 | U 21–2 + 1 = 3 |
| D 4 | 4 | S 19–1 + 9 = 1 |
| E 5 | 5 | T 20–2 + 0 = 2 |
| F 6 | 6 | 98=8            17=8 |
| G 7 | 7 | |
| H 8 | 8 | |
| I 9 | 9 | F 6–6 + 0 = 6 |
| J 10 | 1 + 0 = 1 | A 1–1 + 0 = 1 |
| K 11 | 1 + 1 = 2 | I 9–9 + 0 = 9 |
| L 12 | 1 + 2 = 3 | T 20–2 + 0 = 2 |
| M 13 | 1 + 3 = 4 | H 8–8 + 0 = 8 |
| N 14 | 1 + 4 = 5 | 44=8            26=8 |
| O 15 | 1 + 5 = 6 | |
| P 16 | 1 + 6 = 7 | G 7–7 + 0 = 7 |
| Q 17 | 1 + 7 = 8 | O 15–1 + 5 = 6 |
| R 18 | 1 + 8 = 9 | D 4–4 + 0 = 4 |
| S 19 | 1 + 9 = 10 | 26=8            17=8 |
| T 20 | 2 + 0 = 2 | |
| U 21 | 2 + 1 = 3 | The number 8 |
| V 22 | 2 + 2 = 4 | represents infinity. |
| W 23 | 2 + 3 = 5 | 9 represents |
| X 24 | 2 + 4 = 6 | completion |
| Y 25 | 2 + 5 = 7 | |
| Z 26 | 2 + 6 = 8 | |

Table shows the English alphabet and its equivalent numbers. Two or more digit numbers can be reduced to single digit numbers to employ the Pythagorean skein and determine the mathematical "truth." Notice that numbers one through nine repeat; and the number 8, the universal sign for "infinity," is also the total for "Trust," "Faith" and "God." The number nine (9) represents completion.

For "FAITH" F=6, A=1, I=9, T=20, and H=8 totals 44. And 4+4=8. For "GOD," G=7, O=15 and D=4 totals 26. And again 2+6=8.

Eight, Jeshua explained to Joey, is the sign of infinity.

Next, to prove that mathematics was an exact and correct language and science, Jeshua led Joey to the Pythagorean skein. This analysis had been "lost" for more than two thousand years. "The time has come to bring it back to the world," Jeshua told Joey.

If you read these numbers across, you will get the same result. That is if T=20 and 2+0 = 2; R=18 and 1+8=9; U=21 and 2+1=3; S=19 and 1+9=10 and 1+0=1, and finally T=20 again, where 2+0=2, these numbers added together total 17. Again 1+7=8, the number for infinity!

This can be similarly demonstrated when deciphering the mathematical values of the words "FAITH" and "God." Reading them across their letters add up to 8.

These, along with many other revelations, convinced Joey that language was integrated with mathematics and encoded with numbers, that potentially relayed spiritual information and transmitted revealing messages.

"Ultimately I learned that you can't take mathematics, or even science, out of God, or God out of science, because that leaves you with only half the picture," Joey said.

## Pythagorean Mathematics

Referring to Manley P. Hall's book, *Secret Teachings of All Ages,* his section titled, "Pythagorean Mathematics" further elucidated the point of this previously known and currently concealed premise. He wrote:

Concerning the secret significance of numbers, there has been much speculation. Though many significant discoveries have been made, it may be safely said that with the death of Pythagoras, the great *key* to this science was lost for nearly 2,500 years. Philosophers of all nations have attempted to unravel the Pythagorean skein, but apparently none have been successful. Notwithstanding attempts to obliterate all records of the teachings of Pythagoras, fragments have survived which give clues to

## Fig. 1.4. Exercise in the Derivation of English Letters

| Letter & Number | Pythagoreus Skein Equivalent | Key Word Number Derivations |
|---|---|---|
| A 1 | 1 | T $20-2 + 0 = 2$ |
| B 2 | 1 | R $18-1 + \square = 9$ |
| C $\square$ | 3 | U $21-2 + 1 = \square$ |
| D 4 | 9 | S $19-\square + 9 = 1$ |
| E 5 | 5 | T $20-2 + 0 = \square$ |
| F $\square$ | 6 | $98 = \underline{8}$  $26 = \underline{8}$ |
| G 7 | $\square$ | |
| H 8 | 8 | |
| I $\square$ | 9 | F $6-6 + 0 = 6$ |
| J 10 | $1 + \square = 1$ | A $1-1 + \square = 1$ |
| K 11 | $1 + 1 = \square$ | I $9-\square + 0 = 9$ |
| L $\square$ | $1 + 2 = 3$ | T $20-2 + \square = 2$ |
| M 13 | $1 + \square = 4$  1 | H $8-8 + 0 = 8$ |
| N $\square$ | $1 + 4 = 5$ | $44 = \underline{8}$  $26 = \underline{8}$ |
| O 15 | $1 + 5 = \square$  9 | |
| P $\square$ | $1 + 6 = 7$ | G $7-7 + \square = 7$ |
| Q 17 | $1 + \square = 8$ | O $15-1 + 5 = 6$ |
| R $\square$ | $1 + 8 = 9$ | D $4-4 + 0 = \square$ |
| S 19 | $\square + 9 = 10$ | $26 = \underline{8}$  $17 = \underline{8}$ |
| T 20 | $2 + \square = 2$ | |
| U $\square$ | $2 + 1 = 3$  1 | **The number 8** |
| V 22 | $\square + 2 = 4$ | **represents infinity.** |
| W 23 | $2 + \square = 5$  8 | **9 represents** |
| X 24 | $\square + 4 = 6$ | **completion** |
| Y $\square$ | $2 + 5 = 7$ | |
| Z 26 | $2 + \square = \underline{8}$ | |

A self-development exercise in the use of the Pythagorean skein and the English alphabet's equivalent numbers. Fill in the blanks with the deleted digits to employ the Pythagorean skein and access the mathematical "truth." Notice the repeating one-through-nine digits; wherein the number 8, the universal sign for "infinity," is also the total for "Trust," "Faith" and "God." The number nine (9) represents completion.

some of the simpler parts of his philosophy. The major secrets were never committed to writing, but were communicated only to a few chosen disciples. These apparently dared not to divulge their secrets to the profane. The result being that when death sealed their lips, the arcana died with them.

Certain of the secret schools of today are perpetuations of the ancient mysteries. And although it is quite possible that they may possess some of the original numerical formulae, there is no evidence in their voluminous writings which have issued from these groups during the last five hundred years. These writings, while frequently discussing Pythagoras, show no indication of a more complete knowledge of his intricate doctrines than the post-Pythagorean Greek speculators had who talked much, wrote little, knew less, and concealed their ignorance under a series of mysterious hints and promises.

Here and there among the literary products of early writers are found the enigmatic statements which they made no effort to interpret. The following example is quoted from Plutarch: "The Pythagoreans indeed go farther than this, and honor even numbers and geometrical diagrams with the names and titles of gods. . . . For [example] . . . the power of the triangle is expressive of the nature of Pluto, Bacchus, and Mars; and the properties of the square of Rhea, Venus, Ceres, Vesta, and Juno."

Plutarch did not pretend to explain the inner significance of the symbols, but believed that the relationship which Pythagoras established between the geometrical solids and the gods was the result of images the great sage had seen in the Egyptian temples.[2]

From this Hall concluded: "It is unwise to make definite statements founded on the indefinite and fragmentary information available concerning the Pythagorean system of mathematical philosophy." Then he went on to discuss the "method of securing the numerical power of words" thusly:

The first step in obtaining the numerical value of a word is to resolve it back into its original tongue. Only words of Greek or Hebrew derivation can be successfully analyzed by this method, and *all words must be spelled in their most ancient and complete forms*. Old Testament words and names, therefore, must be translated back into the early Hebrew characters and New Testament words into the Greek. . . .

The *Demiurges* of the Jews is called in English Jehovah, but when seeking the numerical value of the name *Jehovah* [meaning "God'] it is necessary to resolve the name into its Hebrew letters. It becomes יהוה and is read from right to left. The Hebrew letters are: ה, He; ו , Vau; ה, He; י , Yod; and when reversed into the English order from left to right read: *Yod–He–Vau–He*. By consulting the table of letters [shown in figure 1.5 that remained from Pythagoras's work] it is found that the four characters of this sacred name have the following numerical significance [in agreement with the ancient arcana]: *Yod* equals 10, *He* equals 5, *Vau* equals 6, and the second *He* equals 5. Therefore, 10+5+6+5=26, a synonym of Jehovah. If the English letters were used, the answer obviously would not be correct.

But Joey realized that 26 *was* identical to the English numerical value for *God* according to the skein Jeshua had given him. He tested this method again and again, and each time it provided numbers consistent with the English and Hebrew derivations. Thus, he concluded, this channel of numbers must be part of Pythagoras's lost knowledge. Information that he felt was vitally important and ripe for modern revelation.

"This previously secret information," Joey advanced, "is critical for all seekers of God and truth." With its recovery, everyone may now use these mathematical derivations and letter values to *cause their matrix of thought to change*. "Users can experience a higher matrix of thought associated with advanced spirituality and expanded intuition," he proclaimed. "We call it ascended thought. That's where the 'magic' comes from."

Joey had spent days writing down and adding pages of numbers, all the while unconsciously purging "matrices of concepts" and "unlocking" and "integrating higher matrices of thought."

Pythagoras understood the power within his discovery, his skein, and that's why he hid it. If people were to learn the arcanum—the mysterious knowledge—and the power, having seen what people were capable of, he worried they would use it for destructive and coercive means. That's why it died with him and his disciples.

Thus, hidden for more than 2,500 years, Joey became one of the first people to rediscover the secret mathematics. Couple this with the

## Fig. 1.5. Numerical Values of the Hebrew, Greek, and English Alphabets Based on Pythagorus's Work

| 1 | 2 | 3 | 4 | 5 | 6 | 7 | 8 |
|---|---|---|---|---|---|---|---|
| Aleph | [illegible] | א | 1 | Α α | • | Alpha | A |
| Beth | [illegible] | ב | 2 | Β β | • | Beta | B |
| Gimel | [illegible] | ג | 3 | Γ γ | • | Gamma | G |
| Daleth | [illegible] | ד | 4 | Δ δ | • | Delta | D |
| He | [illegible] | ה | 5 | Ε ε | • | Epsilon | E |
| Vau | [illegible] | ו | 6 | Ϝ | • | Digamma | Fv |
| Zain | [illegible] | ז | 7 | Ζ ζ | | Zeta | |
| Heth | [illegible] | ח | 8 | Η η | | Eta | |
| Teth | [illegible] | ט | 9 | Θ ϑ θ | | Theta | |
| Jod | [illegible] | י | 10 | Ι ι | • | Iota | I |
| Caph | [illegible] | כ | 20 | Κ κ | • | Kappa | C |
| Lamed | [illegible] | ל | 30 | Λ λ | • | Lambda | L |
| Mem | [illegible] | מ | 40 | Μ μ | • | Mu | M |
| Nun | [illegible] | נ | 50 | Ν ν | • | 'Nu | N |
| Samech | [illegible] | ס | 60 | Ξ ξ | | Xi | |
| Oin | [illegible] | ע | 70 | Ο ο | • | Omicron | O |
| Pe | [illegible] | פ | 80 | Π π | • | Pi | P |
| Tzadi | [illegible] | צ | 90 | ϛ | | Episemon bau | |
| Kopth | [illegible] | ק | 100 | | | επισημον βαυ | |
| | | | 100 | Ρ ρ | • | Rho | R |
| Resh | [illegible] | ר | 200 | | | | |
| | | | 200 | Σ σ | • | Sigma | S |
| Shin | [illegible] | ש | 300 | | | | |
| | | | 300 | Τ τ | • | Tau | T |
| Tau | [illegible] | ת | 400 | | | | |
| | | | 400 | Υ υ | • | Upsilon | U |
| | | | 500 | Φ φ | | Phi | |
| | | | 600 | Χ χ | | Chi | |
| | | | 700 | Ψ ψ | | Psi | |
| | | | 800 | Ω ω | | Omega | |
| | | | 900 | ϡ | | Sanpi | |

The above chart, referenced by Hill and published by Higgins in the book *Celtic Druids*, provides the names and letters of the Hebrew alphabet in columns 1 and 3, the Greek letters in column 7, and an incomplete list of the English letters in column 8.

fact that his important healing work had been prophesied at the "gathering of eagles," and his story took on expanded importance.

"This work," he offered, was "a labor of love for God. Perhaps it is time for everyone to open up to the correct matrices of thought, or the correct points of reference, to who we really are. Not who we think we are, but who God endowed and intended us to be."

"The 'gathering of eagles' is a gathering God's children who volunteered to come to Northern Idaho during the 'End Times,' not so much to learn, but to rescue souls. How do you rescue souls?" Joey asked rhetorically. "By giving people the truth and telling them who they are not.

"And as people, one by one, awaken to the holy children of God that they are, the madness on earth that we have experienced for millenniums will cease. The institutionalized deception and false limited identity with which people have identified will stop. The beating, starving, and manipulation of humanity will end. It must. It is our destiny.

"Two-thousand years have come and gone since Christ blessed this planet. We can put rockets into space and men on the moon while it's more dangerous to walk the streets than it has ever been; we have more plagues and infectious agents, more greed and mass manipulation, more rage and insanity; we have more Bibles printed today with more people than ever before capable of reading them. *Something is wrong with this picture* because people just don't know the truth."

In the following chapters you will learn the astonishing truth, and examine stunning documentation encoded in the Bible. Lastly, you will realize there is a great deal of vitally important work to be done with this newly recovered knowledge.

## References:

1. For additional information on Reverse Speech™ contact David John Oates's website http://www.reversespeech.com/

2. Hall M. *Secret Teachings of All Ages.* Los Angeles, CA: Philosophical Research Society, Inc. (3910 Los Feliz Blvd. Los Angeles, CA. 90027), 1989, pp. LXIX.

# Chapter 2.
# New Bible Codes

What many people do not know about Pythagoras, besides the fact that he was murdered and his school was burned, is that he was an astrologer. If you wanted to attend his school you first needed to learn astrology. This had to do with the radionics of spheres—the comparative vibratory rates of bodies in space.

Pythagoras was also a great physician besides a mathematician. Radionics and mathematics, sound and light, he taught, were intimately connected. They were of utmost importance in healing and the practice of spiritual medicine.

If you research the Bible and refer to *Strong's Concordance* to look up the words "magic" or "magi," "Assean," and "Chaldean," you will find that these words mean "astrologer." Many Bible-believing Christians consider astrology to be a Satanic practice. This seems odd since the great magis of King David and King Solomon's time, and those that hailed and honored Jesus as king of the Jews were the high Levi priests for the royal bloodline.

Likewise, all of the great soothsayers and seers throughout time and most of the world's powerful leaders, including the evil and destructive ones like Hitler, used astrology to help arrange their schedules and, to some extent, gauge the future. Even today astrology is an important practice for many world leaders. One need only recall Nancy Reagan's White House visit with an astrologer to see that this practice continues. In addition to its political applications, astrology is used today by business leaders and healers throughout the world.

Like any science or technology, astrology has been used and abused by good people and bad people, with good intentions and bad intentions, to help bring about positive results or negative results.

Astrology as well as geometry, Pythagoras taught, was based on mathematics. Without an appreciation for pure and simple mathematics, geometry and astrology could not be learned or applied. He taught his students that "magic" in astrology could be demystified and the science more easily understood when the underlying mathematics were examined. In other words, rather than focusing on illusions, he taught them to focus on the math—the numbers.

One evening, not long after Joey became aware of this information, an angel appeared before him. "Are you ready to take your next step?" he asked.

"Yes," Joey replied.

"Well, what have you been studying?"

"Points of references."

"Yes, but what kinds of points of references?"

"Numbers."

"Correct. And 'TRUST,' 'FAITH,' and 'GOD' was what number?"

"Eight," Joey answered.

"Good. Now I'm going to teach you how to find the truth. If you have faith and trust, I will take you to the truth of God," the angel promised. Then he asked, "Can mathematics lie?"

"No," Joey replied. "Because two plus two equals four, and four plus four equals eight, it can never be anything else. Mathematics is a language unto itself. It is pure, clean and can never lie unless someone makes a mistake or falsely applies it."

"Right," the angel affirmed. Then he instructed Joey to make a column of eights, as depicted in figure 2.1, and decipher their multiples.

He began 1X8=8; 2X8=16; 3X8=24; 4X8=32; 5X8=40 and so on until he came to 8X8=64. At this point the angel stopped him. "Notice that 64 is an important *cardinal number*," he said. "That 6+4=10 which equals 1 using the Pythagorean skein.

"Furthermore, 8 is the first cardinal number that multiplied times itself equals one (1) using the Pythagorean skein. It is no 'coincidence' that sixty-four (64) is the number of squares on a chess board that Egyptians invented," he continued. "There are eight octaves in music. And 88 keys on a standard regulation size piano."

## Fig. 2.1. Column Showing Multiples of Eights (8)

| Multiple of Eights | Reverse Alphabet | Alphabet w/ Numbers | Sum of Two Alphabet #s |
|---|---|---|---|
| 1 X 8 = 8 ——— 8 Z | | A 1 | 9 |
| 2 X 8 = 1 6 ——— 7 Y | | B 2 | 9 |
| 3 X 8 = 2 4 ——— 6 X | | C 3 | 9 |
| 4 X 8 = 3 2 ——— 5 W | | D 4 | 9 |
| 5 X 8 = 4 0 ——— 4 V | | E 5 | 9 |
| 6 X 8 = 4 8 ——— 3 U | | F 6 | 9 |
| 7 X 8 = 5 6 ——— 2 T | | G 7 | 9 |
| 8 X 8 = 6 4 ——— 1 S | | H 8 | 9 |
| 9 X 8 = 7 2 ——— 9 R | | I 9 | 9 |
| 1 0 X 8 = 8 0 ——— 8 Q | | J 1 | 9 |
| 1 1 X 8 = 8 8 ——— 7 P | | K 2 | 9 |
| 1 2 X 8 = 9 6 ——— 6 O | | L 3 | 9 |
| 1 3 X 8 = 1 0 4 ——— 5 N | | M 4 | 9 |
| 1 4 X 8 = 1 1 2 ——— 4 M | | N 5 | 9 |
| 1 5 X 8 = 1 2 0 ——— 3 L | | O 6 | 9 |
| 1 6 X 8 = 1 2 8 ——— 2 K | | P 7 | 9 |
| 1 7 X 8 = 1 3 6 ——— 1 J | | Q 8 | 9 |
| 1 8 X 8 = 1 4 4 ——— 9 I | | R 9 | 9 |
| 1 9 X 8 = 1 5 2 ——— 8 H | | S 1 | 9 |
| 2 0 X 8 = 1 6 0 ——— 7 G | | T 2 | 9 |
| 2 1 X 8 = 1 6 8 ——— 6 F | | U 3 | 9 |
| 2 2 X 8 = 1 7 6 ——— 5 E | | V 4 | 9 |
| 2 3 X 8 = 1 8 4 ——— 4 D | | W 5 | 9 |
| 2 4 X 8 = 1 9 2 ——— 3 C | | X 6 | 9 |
| 2 5 X 8 = 2 0 0 ——— 2 B | | Y 7 | 9 |
| 2 6 X 8 = 2 0 8 ——— 1 A | | Z 8 | 9 |

Column of multiples of eights (8) deciphered according to the Pythagorean skein in which all integers are reduced to single digits using addition of each digit in the whole number. Example: 208=2+0+8=10; then 10=1+0=1. This number is associated with the letter A. When A=1 is added to the reverse alphabet letter Z=8, the sum is 9. The number nine (9) implies completion and results everytime the numerical equivalents to letters are similarly added.

## The Math Behind Language

Next the angel showed Joey the unique "reverse alphabet countdown pattern" he produced in figure 2.1 using multiples of 8 and the Pythagorean skein. Try it for yourself. Eight (8) is the only number that produces this unique countdown when multiplied by itself. The countdown repeats 8–1, 9–1 and 9–1. This is the direct opposite to the pattern of number equivalents for the English alphabet. All other single digit numbers including 2, 3, 4, 5, 6, 7, and 9 *do not produce this effect* as shown in figure 2.2. Here the multiples of three (3), six (6), and nine (9) are used as examples.

This is where the "magic" began for Joey in discovering the ancient Bible codes. He recalled that using the Pythagorean skein wherein two or more digit numbers were added to reduce them to a single digit, the pattern of numbers 1 through 9 repeated beginning with the letter "J." This produced the alphabetical numerical pattern of 1 through 9, 1 through 9, and 1 through 8 seen in figure 2.1.

Moreover, Joey saw that when he applied the Pythagorean skein to this column of eight's multiples, *the entire alphabetical and numerical pattern reversed itself perfectly* as well. (See also Figure 2.1.)

This, the angel explained, was why the English and Hebrew alphabets can be equally deciphered, and why you can read from left to right in English and right to left in Hebrew without altering the mathematical result. The angel explained that if people knew these numerical and letter codes, they could translate the original Bible scriptures from either language into the other *mathematically.* Joey later learned that this also worked for other languages as well.

The simple fact is that language—first called "Babel" as in the "Tower of Babel"—was invented, at least partially, to express the Godly perfection of mathematics. The word Babel evolved from the Hebrew word *Bábhel,* which interestingly came from the early Semitic Mesopotamian language called Akkadian. It literally means "gate to God."

Unfortunately today, language no longer does justice to the perfection of mathematics. Over the past two millenniums, during the pro-

## Fig. 2.2. Columns Showing Multiples of Three (3), Six (6), and Nine (9) Using the Pythagorean Skein (PS)

| | Multiples of 3 | Multiples of 6 | Multiples of 9 |
|---|---|---|---|
| A 1 | 1 X 3 = 3 | 1 X 6 = 6 | 1 X 9 = 9 |
| B 2 | 2 X 3 = 6 | 2 X 6 = 12 – 3 | 2 X 9 = 18 – 9 |
| C 3 | 3 X 3 = 9 | 3 X 6 = 18 – 9 | 3 X 9 = 27 – 9 |
| D 4 | 4 X 3 = 12 – 3 | 4 X 6 = 24 – 6 | 4 X 9 = 36 – 9 |
| E 5 | 5 X 3 = 15 – 6 | 5 X 6 = 30 – 3 | 5 X 9 = 45 – 9 |
| F 6 | 6 X 3 = 18 – 9 | 6 X 6 = 36 – 9 | 6 X 9 = 54 – 9 |
| G 7 | 7 X 3 = 21 – 3 | 7 X 6 = 42 – 6 | 7 X 9 = 63 – 9 |
| H 8 | 8 X 3 = 24 – 6 | 8 X 6 = 48 – 3 | 8 X 9 = 72 – 9 |
| I 9 | 9 X 3 = 27 – 9 | 9 X 6 = 54 – 9 | 9 X 9 = 81 – 9 |
| J 1 | 10X3=30 – 3 | 10X6=60 – 6 | 10X9=90 – 9 |
| K 2 | 11X3=33 – 6 | 11X6=66 – 3 | 11X9=99 – 9 |
| L 3 | 12X3=36 – 9 | 12X6=72 – 9 | 12X9=108 – 9 |
| M 4 | 13X3=39 – 3 | 13X6=78 – 6 | 13X9=117 – 9 |
| N 5 | 14X3=42 – 6 | 14X6=84 – 3 | 14X9=126 – 9 |
| O 6 | 15X3=45 – 9 | 15X6=90 – 9 | 15X9=135 – 9 |
| P 7 | 16X3=48 – 3 | 16X6=96 – 6 | 16X9=144 – 9 |
| Q 8 | 17X3=51 – 6 | 17X6=102 – 3 | 17X9=153 – 9 |
| R 9 | 18X3=54 – 9 | 18X6=108 – 9 | 18X9=162 – 9 |
| S 1 | 19X3=57 – 3 | 19X6=114 – 6 | 19X9=171 – 9 |
| T 2 | 20X3=60 – 6 | 20X6=120 – 3 | 20X9=180 – 9 |
| U 3 | 21X3=63 – 9 | 21X6=126 – 9 | 21X9=189 – 9 |
| V 4 | 22X3=66 – 3 | 22X6=132 – 6 | 22X9=198 – 9 |
| W 5 | 23X3=69 – 6 | 23X6=138 – 3 | 23X9=207 – 9 |
| X 6 | 24X3=72 – 9 | 24X6=144 – 9 | 24X9=216 – 9 |
| Y 7 | 25X3=75 – 3 | 25X6=150 – 6 | 25X9=225 – 9 |
| Z 8 | 26X3=78 – 6 | 26X6=156 – 3 | 26X9=234 – 9 |
| | 126 = 9 | 153 = 9 | 153 = 9 | 234 = 9 |

Columns show the numbers resulting from multiples of three, six and nine using the Pythagorean skein. Notice the resulting single digit numbers repeat forming patterns such as "3, 9, and 6" for the 6s column. Multiples of nine, the highest integer in the Pythagorean skein, consistently produces a "9" as does the addition of numbers associated with the forward and backward letters of the English alphabet as shown in Fig. 2.1. Multiples of four, five, and seven produce no readily observable pattern aside from their integral sums that total nine as well.

cess of translating from perfect math into language, much precision and truth was compromised. Some languages, or parts of them, appear to have been intentionally developed to circumvent math—to hide the "gate to God"—or conceal the truth about the spiritual nature of communication and humanity.[1]

Specifically, each sound or syllable, especially in Hebrew, emits a special frequency when spoken or sung—frequencies of spiritual value. The fact is, sounds generate electromagnetic frequencies. These form the basis for today's computerized language translation and word processing programs. They can actually print out the Hebrew or English characters and words in response to the sound or wave frequency recognitions or vibrational reconnaissance.[1]

Another strange thing is that there are twenty-two characters in the Hebrew alphabet. There are twenty-two degrees between Fa and So on the music scale. And there is a twenty-two-year sun cycle wherein every eleven years it reverses its polarity from north to south.

More than chance occurrences, these patterns indicate the underlying influence of mathematics on matter, energy, and the universe at large. Joey was being directed to discover the mathematics that made everything tick.

One evening, not long after all of this became apparent, Jeshua reappeared to Joey to guide his next step. "What were you working with?" Jesus asked his confused friend.

Joey replied, "Eights?"

"No. What else *were* you working with?"

"Well, the alphabet."

"So go to the Hebrew alphabet," Jeshua directed.

For the next three days Joey traveled tirelessly around northern Idaho to find a book containing the Hebrew alphabet. Unfortunately none could be found north of Spokane. Anxious to complete the assignment, Jesus returned to Joey on the third day and said, "Joey, just go into my book—Psalm 119. There you will find the Hebrew alphabet."

## Fig. 2.3. PSALM 119 From The King James Bible

PSALM 119
*Psalm* of *Meditation on the*
Law
*ALEPH*

1 BLESSED are the undefiled in the way, who walk in the law of the LORD.

2 Blessed are they that keep his testimonies, *and that* seek him with the whole heart.

3 They also do no iniquity: they walk in his ways.

4 Thou hast commanded us to keep thy precepts diligently.

5 O that my ways were directed to keep thy statutes!

6 Then shall I not be ashamed, when I have respect unto all thy commandments.

7 I will praise thee with uprightness of heart, when I shall have learned thy righteous judgments.

8 I will keep thy statutes: O forsake me not utterly.

*BETH*

9 WHEREWITHAL shall a young man cleanse his way? by taking heed thereto according to thy word.

10 With my whole heart have I sought thee: O let me not wander from thy commandments.

11 Thy word have I hid in mine heart, that I might not sin against thee.

12 Blessed art thou, O LORD: teach me thy statutes.

13 With my lips have I declared all the judgments of thy mouth.

14 I have rejoiced in the way of thy testimonies, as *much as* in all riches.

15 I will meditate in thy precepts, and have respect unto thy ways.

16 I will delight myself in thy statutes: I will not forget thy word.

*GIMEL*

17 DEAL bountifully with thy servant, *that* I may live, and keep thy word.

18 Open thou mine eyes, that I may behold wondrous things out of thy law.

19 I am a stranger in the earth: hide not thy commandments from me.

20 My soul breaketh for the longing *that it hath* unto thy judgments at all times.

21 Thou hast rebuked the proud *that are* cursed, which do err from thy commandments.

22 Remove from me reproach and contempt; for I have kept thy testimonies.

23 Princes also did sit and speak against me: but thy servant did meditate in thy statutes.

24 Thy testimonies also are my delight and my counsellors.

*DALETH*

25 MY soul cleaveth unto the dust: quicken thou me according to thy word.

26 I have declared my ways, and thou heardest me: teach me thy statutes.

27 Make me to understand the way of thy precepts: so shall I talk of thy wondrous works.

28 My soul melteth for heaviness: strengthen thou me according unto thy word.

29 Remove from me the way of lying: and grant me thy law graciously.

30 I have chosen the way of truth:

thy judgments have I laid *before me.*

31 I have stuck unto thy testimonies: O LORD, put me not to shame.

32 I will run the way of thy commandments, when thou shalt enlarge my heart.

*HE*

33 TEACH me, O LORD, the way of thy statutes; and I shall keep it unto the end.

34 Give me understanding, and I shall keep thy law; yea, I shall observe it with my whole heart.

35 Make me to go in the path of thy commandments; for therein do I delight.

36 Incline my heart unto thy testimonies, and not to covetousness.

37 Turn away mine eyes from beholding vanity; and quicken thou me in thy way.

38 Stablish thy word unto thy servant, who *is devoted* to thy fear.

39 Turn away my reproach which I fear: for thy judgments are good.

40 Behold, I have longed after thy precepts: quicken me in thy righteousness.

*VAU*

41 LET thy mercies come also unto me, O LORD, even thy salvation, according to thy word.

42 So shall I have wherewith to answer him that reproacheth me: for I trust in thy word.

43 And take not the word of truth utterly out of my mouth: for I have hoped in thy judgments.

44 So shall I keep thy law continually for ever and ever.

45 And I will walk at liberty: for I seek thy precepts.

46 I will speak of thy testimonies also before kings, and will not be ashamed.

47 And I will delight myself in thy commandments, which I have loved.

48 My hands also will I lift up unto thy commandments, which I have loved; and I will meditate in thy statutes.

*ZAIN*

49 REMEMBER the word unto thy servant, upon which thou hast caused me to hope.

50 This is my comfort in my affliction: for thy word hath quickened me.

51 The proud have had me greatly in derision: yet have I not declined from thy law.

52 I remembered thy judgments of old, O LORD; and have comforted myself.

53 Horror hath taken hold upon me because of the wicked that forsake thy law.

54 Thy statutes have been my songs in the house of my pilgrimage.

55 I have remembered thy name, O LORD, in the night, and have kept thy law.

56 This I had, because I kept thy precepts.

*CHETH*

57 *THOU art* my portion, O LORD: I have said that I would keep thy words.

58 I entreated thy favour with my whole heart: be merciful unto me according to thy word.

59 I thought on my ways, and turned my feet unto thy testimonies.

60 I made haste, and delayed not to keep thy commandments.

61 The bands of the wicked have

robbed me: but I have not forgotten thy law.

62 At midnight I will rise to give thanks unto thee because of thy righteous judgments.

63 I am a companion of all *them* that fear thee, and of them that keep thy precepts.

64 The earth, O LORD, is full of thy mercy: teach me thy statutes.

### TETH

65 THOU hast dealt well with thy servant, O LORD, according unto thy word.

66 Teach me good judgment and knowledge: for I have believed thy commandments.

67 Before I was afflicted I went astray: but now have I kept thy word.

68 Thou art good, and doest good; teach me thy statutes.

69 The proud have forged a lie against me: but I will keep thy precepts with my whole heart.

70 Their heart is as fat as grease; *but* I delight in thy law.

71 *It is* good for me that I have been afflicted; that I might learn thy statutes.

72 The law of thy mouth is better unto me than thousands of gold and silver.

### JOD

73 THY hands have made me and fashioned me: give me understanding, that I may learn thy commandments.

74 They that fear thee will be glad when they see me; because I have hoped in thy word.

75 I know, O LORD, that thy judgments are right, and *that* thou in faithfulness hast afflicted me.

76 Let, I pray thee, thy merciful kindness be for my comfort, according to thy word unto thy servant.

77 Let thy tender mercies come unto me, that I may live: for thy law *is* my delight.

78 Let the proud be ashamed; for they dealt perversely with me without a cause: but I will meditate in thy precepts.

79 Let those that fear thee turn unto me, and those that have known thy testimonies.

80 Let my heart be sound in thy statutes; that I be not ashamed.

### CAPH

81 MY soul fainteth for thy salvation: but I hope in thy word.

82 Mine eyes fail for thy word, saying, when wilt thou comfort me?

83 For I am become like a bottle in the smoke; yet do I not forget thy statutes.

84 How many are the days of thy servant? when wilt thou execute judgment on them that persecute me?

85 The proud have digged pits for me, which are not after thy law.

86 All thy commandments are faithful: they persecute me wrongfully; help thou me.

87 They had almost consumed me upon earth; but I forsook not thy precepts.

88 Quicken me after thy loving kindness; so shall I keep the testimony of thy mouth.

### LAMED

89 FOREVER, O LORD, thy word is settled in heaven.

90 Thy faithfulness is unto all generations: thou hast established the earth, and it abideth.

91 They continue this day accord-

ing to thine ordinances: for all *are* thy servants.

92 Unless thy law *had been* my delights, I should then have perished in mine affliction.

93 I will never forget thy precepts: for with them thou hast quickened me.

94 I am thine, save me; for I have sought thy precepts.

95 The wicked have waited for me to destroy me: but I will consider thy testimonies.

96 I have seen an end of all perfection: but thy commandment is exceeding broad.

### MEM

97 O how love I thy law! it *is* my meditation all the day.

98 Thou through thy commandments hast made me wiser than mine enemies: for they are ever with me.

99 I have more understanding than all my teachers: for thy testimonies are my meditation.

100 I understand more than the ancients, because I keep thy precepts.

101 I have refrained my feet from every evil way, that I might keep thy word.

102 I have not departed from thy judgments: for thou hast taught me.

103 How sweet are thy words unto my taste! *yea, sweeter* than honey to my mouth!

104 Through thy precepts I get understanding: therefore I hate every false way.

### NUN

105 THY word *is* a lamp unto my feet, and a light unto my path.

106 I have sworn, and I will perform it, that I will keep thy righteous judgments.

107 I am afflicted very much: quicken me, O LORD, according unto thy word.

108 Accept, I beseech thee, the freewill offerings of my mouth, O LORD, and teach me thy judgments.

109 My soul is continually in my hand: yet do I not forget thy law.

110 The wicked have laid a snare for me: yet I erred not from thy precepts.

111 Thy testimonies have I taken as an heritage for ever: for they are the rejoicing of my heart.

112 I have inclined mine heart to perform thy statutes alway, *even unto* the end.

### SAMECH

113 I hate vain thoughts: but thy law do I love.

114 Thou art my hiding place and my shield: I hope in thy word.

115 Depart from me, ye evildoers: for I will keep the commandments of my God.

116 Uphold me according unto thy word, that I may live: and let me not be ashamed of my hope.

117 Hold thou me up, and I shall be safe: and I will have respect unto thy statutes continually.

118 Thou hast trodden down all them that err from thy statutes: for their deceit is falsehood.

119 Thou puttesty away all of the wicked of the earth like dross: therefore I love thy testimonies.

120 My flesh trembleth for fear of thee; and I am afraid of thy judgments.

### AIN

121 I have done judgment and justice: leave me not to mine oppressors.

122 Be surety for thy servant for good: let not the proud oppress me.

123 Mine eyes fail for thy salvation, and for the word of thy righteousness.

124 Deal with thy servant according unto thy mercy, and teach me thy statutes.

125 I am thy servant; give me understanding, that I may know thy testimonies.

126 *It is* time for *thee,* LORD, to work: for they have made void thy law.

127 Therefore I love thy commandments above gold; yea, above fine gold.

128 Therefore I esteem all *thy* precepts *concerning all things to be* right, *and* I hate every false way.

### PE

129 Thy testimonies are wonderful: therefore doth my soul keep them.

130 The entrance of thy words giveth light; it giveth understanding unto the simple.

131 I opened my mouth, and panted: for I longed for thy commandments.

132 Look thou upon me, and be merciful unto me, as thou usest to do unto those that love thy name.

133 Order my steps in thy word: and let not any iniquity have dominion over me.

134 Deliver me from the oppression of man: so will I keep thy precepts.

135 Make thy face to shine upon thy servant; and teach me thy statutes.

136 Rivers of waters run down mine eyes, because they keep not thy law.

### TZADDI

137 RIGHTEOUS art thou, O LORD, and upright are thy judgments.

138 Thy testimonies that thou hast commanded are righteous and very faithful.

139 My zeal hath consumed me, because mine enemies have forgotten thy words.

140 Thy word is very pure: therefore thy servant loveth it.

141 I am small and despised: yet do not I forget thy precepts.

142 Thy righteousness is an everlasting righteousness, and thy law *is* the truth.

143 Trouble and anguish have taken hold on me: yet thy commandments are my delights.

144 The righteousness of thy testimonies is everlasting: give me understanding, and I shall live.

### KOPH

145 I cried with my whole heart; hear me, O LORD: I will keep thy statutes.

146 I cried unto thee; save me, and I shall keep thy testimonies.

147 I prevented the dawning of the morning, and cried: I hoped in thy word.

148 Mine eyes prevent the *night* watches, that I might meditate in thy word.

149 Hear my voice according unto thy loving kindness: O LORD,

quicken me according to thy judgment.

150  They draw nigh that follow after mischief : they are far from thy law.

151 Thou art near, O LORD; and all thy commandments are truth.

152 Concerning thy testimonies, I have known of old that thou hast founded them forever.

### RESH

153 CONSIDER mine affliction, and deliver me: for I do not forget thy law.

154 Plead my cause, and deliver me: quicken me according to thy word.

155  Salvation is far from the wicked for they seek not thy statutes.

156  Great are thy tender mercies, O LORD: quicken me according to thy judgments.

157  Many are my persecutors and mine enemies; yet do I not decline from thy testimonies.

158  I beheld the transgressors, and was grieved; because they kept not thy word.

159 Consider how I love thy precepts: quicken me, O LORD, according to thy loving kindness.

160 Thy word is true from the beginning: and every one of thy righteous judgments endureth for ever.

### SCHIN

161 PRINCES have persecuted me without a cause: but my heart standeth in awe of thy word.

162  I rejoice at thy word, as one that findeth great spoil.

163  I hate and abhor lying: but thy law do I love.

164 Seven times a day do I praise thee because of thy righteous judgments.

165  Great peace have they which love thy law: and nothing shall offend them.

166  LORD, I have hoped for thy salvation, and done thy commandments.

167  My soul hath kept thy testimonies; and I love them exceedingly.

168  I have kept thy precepts and thy testimonies: for all my ways are before thee.

### TAU

169  LET my cry come near before thee, O LORD: give me understanding according to thy word.

170 Let my supplication come before thee: deliver me according to thy word.

171  My lips shall utter praise, when thou hast shown me thy statutes.

172 My tongue shall speak of thy word: for all thy commandments *are* righteousness.

173  Let thine hand help me; for I have chosen thy precepts.

174  I have longed for thy salvation, O LORD; and thy law *is* my delight.

175  Let my soul live and it shall praise thee; and let thy judgments help me.

176  I have gone astray like a lost sheep; seek thy servant; for I do not forget thy commandments.

Sure enough Psalm 119 began with the letter "ALEPH" and continued to provide all the letters of the Hebrew alphabet as seen in figures 1.5 and 2.3.

## The Hidden Code in Psalm 119

Given the history provided in the next chapter, it is far easier to understand why King James VI of Scotland/James I of England, a member of the Scottish Rite, Knights Templar, and Freemasons, decided to commission the writing of a new encoded English Bible. It insured the special arcana *numbers*, that Jeshua had directed Joey to recover, would never be lost to the "illumined."

Many Christians who believe that every word in the King James Bible is God's may have trouble with the concept that King James knew about these codes. This must be the case since the "Book of Numbers," that draws attention to the importance of *numbers*, was originally called "In The Wilderness" in the Torah.

However, King James's complete motives remain unclear. Given the scrutiny of the Roman Catholic Church and the political upheaval associated with all spiritual writings at the time, including Martin Luther's "heretical" works and the suppressed books of the Bible known as the Protestant Apocrypha that the Romans and Catholic Church demanded be censured, King James either: 1) encoded the English Bible, as the Hebrews, Greeks, and Romans had done with previous editions, in an effort to keep the masses ignorant of the knowledge considered most important to royalty and others in power; 2) tried to hide powerful knowledge in Bible codes in an effort to protect it from the Catholic Church. Or, as you will learn in Chapter 3, King James may have 3) worked like a "double agent" with the Vatican—sharing secrets with both Catholic and Protestant political and religious leaders.

In any case, these and many other Bible codes have remained hidden from the masses for a long time. You can now begin to identify them by following the directions below:

Beginning with the first verse in Psalm 119, where it says "ALEPH" write "1" there, because it is verse one.

What is the numbered verse following the next Hebrew letter "BETH"? "9" is the answer. Circle the number "9" in verse nine.

Now, go to the next Hebrew letter "GIMEL," which is followed by verse "17."

But, what did you learn from Pythagoras about double digit numbers? You resolve them to single digits. So 1+7=8. Therefore, write "8" to the left of "GIMEL" adjacent the designated verse number "17," and circle it.

Now you are beginning to crack the code and gain an important point of reference.

The next Hebrew letter is "DALETH" above verse "25." Again add 2+5=7. Write the number "7" adjacent the number "25" to the left of the word "DALETH" and circle it.

Go to the next letter of the Hebrew alphabet, which is "HE" above verse "33" and decipher 3+3=6. Place a "6" adjacent the number "33" in Psalm 119 and circle it.

Next find the Hebrew letter "VAU" and the verse "41" below it. Change the double digit again to its single digit Pythagorean skein number "5." Place this number adjacent the "41" and circle it.

Are you getting the pattern?

Complete this exercise by continuing to determine the single digit numbers beside each of the remaining Hebrew letters found in Psalm 119. When finished, you should have recorded on the pages under figure 2.3 the following numbers:

1,9,8,7,6,5,4,3,2,1,9,8,7,6,5,4,3,2,1,9,8,7,6,5 . . .

Notice that this is the same pattern we developed in figure 2.1. Recall that 8 was the only multiple that originated this pattern.

Now count the number of verses between each Hebrew letter in Psalm 119. How many are there? Consistently there are 8!

"So the King James Bible is encoded with the Pythagorean skein and the truth," Joey advanced. "Anyone who reached the highest degrees of Freemasonry were given this knowledge to spiritually acquire higher matrices of thought and the spiritual power inherent in it."

These numbers and patterns hold tremendous power. As you will soon see, they can be positively employed for healing, developing powerful therapeutic formulas, applying reconstructive vibrations, and other areas related to hyperdimensional physics. Unfortunately for the ignorant masses, they may also be used to control or kill people.

## A Second Code in Psalm 119

You will now be guided to discover the second code within Psalm 119 that Jeshua showed Joey. It has to do with the sequence of use of the repeating words "law" and "word." Beginning with the first verse—"Blessed *are* the undefiled in the way, who walk in the law of the Lord." Find the word "law" in the first verse of Psalm 119 (in figure 2.3) and for the purpose of this exercise, underline it.

Next, go to verse number 9 under the Hebrew letter BETH. It reads: "Wherewithal shall a young man cleanse his way? by taking heed *thereto* according to thy word." Underline the word "word."

Go next to verse number 17 under GIMEL. It reads: "Deal bountifully with thy servant, *that* I may live, and keep thy word." Underline the word "word" again.

Proceed to DALETH and verse number 25. It reads: "My soul cleaveth unto the dust: quicken thou me according to thy word." Once again, underline the word "word."

Next, under HE, verse number 33 reads: "Teach me, O Lord, the way of thy statutes; and I shall keep it *unto* the end." Here, underline the word "statutes."

Next, move down to VAU and in verse number 41, underline the word "word" once again.

Move down to verse number 49 under ZAIN and underline the word "word" again.

Continue this exercise on the next page, under CHETH, and in verse number 57 underline the word "words."

Next, under TETH, in verse number 65, underline the word "<u>word</u>" once again.

Under JOD, in verse number 73, underline the word "<u>commandments</u>."

Under CAPH, read verse number 81 and underline the word "<u>word</u>."

Under LAMED, read verse number 89 and underline the word "<u>word</u>."

Under MEM, read verse number 97 and underline the word "<u>law</u>."

Under NUN, read verse number 105 and underline the word "<u>word</u>."

Under SAMECH, read verse number 113 and underline the word "<u>law</u>."

Under AIN, read verse number 121 and underline the word "<u>justice</u>."

Under PE, read verse number 129 and underline the word "<u>testimonies</u>."

Under TZADDI, read verse number 137 and underline the word "<u>judgments</u>."

Under KOPH, read verse number 145 and underline the word "<u>statutes</u>."

Under RESH, read verse number 153 and underline the word "<u>law</u>."

Under SCHIN, read verse number 161 and underline the word "<u>word</u>."

And finally, under TAU, read verse number 169 and underline the word "<u>word</u>."

Now, count the number of verses cited above in which you underlined the word "word." There should be twelve (12), out of twenty-two (22), which is the number of apostles. The twelve apostles spoke *His* word.

In the remaining ten verses, you underlined "law," "statutes," "testimonies," and "commandments." These all refer to the Ten Commandments. These presented *His* laws.

Now count the number of verses cited above in which you underlined the word "statutes." There should be two (2). Jesus said that the Ten Commandments would be kept if you obeyed just the *two* most important—to love the Lord thy God with all your might and to love thy neighbor as thyself.

Notice also the words "testimonies" and "judgments" are each used once with the latter following the former in verses 129 and 137. God provided the only true testimony. (The first definition in *Webster's Dictionary* of the word "testimony" is "the tablets inscribed with the Mosaic law . . . the ark containing the tablets . . . a divine decree attested in the Scriptures.") And only God, the Holy *One*, could lay judgement upon mankind.

So twelve apostles spoke His "word"—the Ten Commandments, that presented His "law" of which two were most relevant. Only one source originated this truth and could judge humanity for its transgressions.

## The Column of Sixes

After the above was revealed to Joey, Jeshua returned and directed him to decipher the columns of 9s and 6s as seen in figure 2.2.

Joey noted that using the Pythagorean skein, all multiples of nine (9) produced itself. This made sense since 9 was the last and highest number allowed using the Pythagorean skein, and thus it represented completion as the figure shows.

As seen in the 6's column, 1x6=6; 2x6=12; 3x6=18 and so on to the bottom of the alphabet and column. Notice that the pattern produced by the sums of the multiples was repeatedly 6,3,9,6,3,9,6,3,9, etc. to infinity. Notice also that the sum of each sequence in this column, as well as the sum total of the entire column equaled 9. Plus, when he added the sum total of the English alphabet, it also equaled 9!

Struck with this inexplicable mathematical phenomena, Joey prayed to Jeshua for additional direction and clarity.

## Revealing the Numbers in NUMBERS

Later that night, Joey experienced another enlightening phenomenon. While attempting to fall asleep he suddenly found himself being able to see through his eyelids to the end of his bed as though his eyes were open.

He thought he was dreaming. So to make sure, he ran his fingers over his eyes to be certain both were closed. Indeed they were. Yet, he could see clearly through them to witness a large angel standing beside Jesus at the foot of his bed. Both were smiling.

"There was a violet smoky aura around them," Joey recalled.

"So I opened my eyes thinking I'd wake up and I saw the same thing! I didn't panic though because I'd been working with this sort of thing for awhile and I love God and Jesus. So I wasn't scared. It just startled me. So I thought, 'Well let me view this a little bit here.' Then it sunk in that there was one big hunk'n angel standing there. And in the angel's hands was a huge Bible. I could see it said 'Holy Bible' on the front. Then the angel opened the Bible and everything became blurry.

"The angel then said to me, 'You have your challenge. You're working for God, but not everything is given.'

"'I'm going to ask you some questions,' the angel continued. "If you can answer the questions and unlock the key, you will have the information you seek."

So the angel asked Joey, "How many days are there in a week?"

"Well that's pretty easy," Joey replied. "Seven."

"How many colors in a rainbow are visible?"

"Seven," Joey returned.

"What about the verse in the Bible: the something son of the something son?"

"Well it's the seventh son of the seventh son."

"That's correct," the angel said. "Now how many musical notes are there?"

"Seven," Joey said.

"Correct again."

Suddenly Joey saw that the fuzzyness surrounding the angel and the Bible began to clear.

"Now how many months in a year are there?" the angel continued.

"Twelve."

"How many signs in the zodiac?"

"Twelve."

"How many apostles are there?"

"Twelve."

"That is correct. And what are we working with?" the angel challenged.

"Numbers," Joey said.

"That's correct. And what is the fourth book of the Bible called?"

"Numbers."

Instantly all the haze around the angel, Jesus and the Bible cleared. The page of the Bible to which the angel had opened suddenly illuminated. "Remember our lesson," the angel said to Joey. Then he and Jesus suddenly vanished.

Joey sat up, jumped out of bed, ran to his office, and opened a Bible that he had been marking up. He opened it to "The Fourth Book of Moses, called Numbers."

Then he recalled the first answers he gave the angel was the number seven (7). Knowing what he knew about the Bible codes in Psalm 119, he went to the seventh chapter in the book of Numbers.

He recalled the second series of answers he gave the angel was the number twelve (12). So he went directly to verse 12 in Chapter 7 and began to read. (See figure 2.4)

Part way through the chapter he already noticed a pattern. Verse 12 started: "And he that offered his offering the first day was Nah'shon the son of Am-min'a-dab, of the tribe of Judah:"

"Why would anybody put that in the Bible?" Joey asked himself. "Who gives a heck about Nah'shon the son of Am-min'a-dab, of the

## Fig. 2.4. A King James Bible Code Hidden in NUMBERS, Chapter 7, Beginning With Verse Twelve

**CHAPTER 7**

*Offerings of the Princes at the Dedication*

12 And he that offered his offering the first day was Nahshon the son of Amminadab of the tribe of Judah:

13 And his offering *was* one silver charger, the weight thereof *was an* hundred and thirty *shekels,* one silver bowl of seventy shekels, after the shekel of the sanctuary; both of them *were* full of fine flour mingled with oil for a meat offering:

14 One spoon of ten *shekels* of gold, full of incense:

15 One young bullock, one ram, one lamb of the first year, for a burnt offering:

16 One kid of the goats for a sin offering:

17 And for a sacrifice of peace offerings, two oxen, five rams, five he goats, five lambs of the first year: this *was* the offering of Nahshon the son of Amminadab.

18 On the second day Nethaneel the son of Zuar, prince of Issachar did offer:

19 He offered for his offering one silver charger, the weight whereof *was* an hundred and thirty shekels, one silver bowl of seventy shekels, after the shekel of the sanctuary; both of them full of fine flour mingled with oil for a meat offering:

20 One spoon of gold of ten *shekels,* full of incense:

21 One young bullock, one ram, one lamb of the first year, for a burnt offering:

22 One kid of the goats for a sin offering:

23 And for a sacrifice of peace offerings, two oxen, five rams, five he goats, five lambs of the first year: this *was* the offering of Nethaneel the son of Zuar.

24 On the third day Eliab the son of Helon, prince of the children of Zebulun, *did offer:*

25 His offering *was* one silver charger, the weight whereof *was* an hundred and thirty *shekels,* one silver bowl of seventy shekels, after the shekel of the sanctuary; both of them full of fine flour mingled with oil for a meat offering:

26 One golden spoon of ten *shekels,* full of incense:

27 One young bullock, one ram, one lamb of the first year, for a burnt offering:

28 One kid of the goats for a sin offering:

29 And for a sacrifice of peace offerings, two oxen, five rams, five he goats, five lambs of the first year: this *was* the offering of Eliab the son of Helon.

30 On the fourth day Elizur the son of Shedeur, prince of the children of Reuben, *did offer:*

31 His offering *was* one silver charger of the weight of an hundred and thirty *shekels,* one silver bowl of seventy shekels, after the shekel of the sanctuary; both of

them full of fine flour mingled with oil for a meat offering:

32 One golden spoon of ten *shekels*, full of incense:

33 One young bullock, one ram, one lamb of the first year, for a burnt offering:

34 One kid of the goats for a sin offering:

35 And for a sacrifice of peace offerings, two oxen, five rams, five he goats, five lambs of the first year: this *was* the offering of Elizur the son of Shedeur.

36 On the fifth day Shelumiel the son of Zurishaddai, prince of the children of Simeon, *did offer:*

37 His offering *was* one silver charger, the weight whereof *was an* hundred and thirty *shekels*, one silver bowl of seventy shekels, after the shekel of the sanctuary; both of them full of fine flour mingled with oil for a meat offering:

38 One golden spoon of ten *shekels*, full of incense:

39 One young bullock, one ram, one lamb of the first year, for a burnt offering:

40 One kid of the goats for a sin offering:

41 And for a sacrifice of peace Offerings, two oxen, five rams, five he goats, five lambs of the first year: this *was* the offering of Shelumiel the son of Zurishaddai.

42 On the sixth day Eliasaph the son of Deuel, prince of the children of Gad, *offered:*

43 His offering *was* one silver charger of the weight of an hundred and thirty *shekels*, a silver bowl

of seventy shekels, after the shekel of the sanctuary; both of them full of fine flour mingled with oil for a meat offering:

44 One golden spoon of ten *shekels*, full of incense:

45 One young bullock, one ram, one lamb of the first year, for a burnt offering:

46 One kid of the goats for a sin offering:

47 And for a sacrifice of peace offerings, two oxen, five rams, five he goats, five lambs of the first year: this *was* the offering of Eliasaph the son of Deuel.

48 On the seventh day Elishama the son of Ammihud, prince of the children of Ephriam, offered:

49 His offering *was* one silver charger, the weight whereof *was an* hundred and thirty *shekels*, one silver bowl of seventy shekels, after the shekel of the sanctuary; both of them full of fine flour mingled with oil for a meat offering:

50 One golden spoon of ten *shekels*, full of incense:

51 One young bullock, one ram, one lamb of the first year, for a burnt offering:

52 One kid of the goats for a sin offering:

53 And for a sacrifice of peace offerings, two oxen, five rams, five he goats, five lambs of the first year: this *was* the offering of Elishama the son of Ammihud.

54 On the eighth day offered Gamaliel the son of Pedahzur, prince of the children of Manaseh:

55 His offering *was* one silver charger of the weight of an hun-

dred and thirty *shekels,* one silver bowl of seventy shekels, after the shekel of the sanctuary; both of them full of fine flour mingled with oil for a meat offering:

56 One golden spoon of ten *shekels,* full of incense:

57 One young bullock, one ram, one lamb of the first year, for a burnt offering:

58 One kid of the goats for a sin offering:

59 And for a sacrifice of peace offerings, two oxen, five rams, five he goats, five lambs of the first year: this *was* the offering of Gamaliel the son of Pedhazur.

60 On the ninth day Abidan the son of Gideoni, prince of the children of Benjamin offered:

61 His offering *was* one silver charger, the weight whereof *was an* hundred and thirty *shekels,* one silver bowl of seventy shekels, after the shekel of the sanctuary; both of them full of fine flour mingled with oil for a meat offering:

62 One golden spoon of ten *shekels,* full of incense:

63 One young bullock, one ram, one lamb of the first year, for a burnt offering:

64 One kid of the goats for a sin offering:

65 And for a sacrifice of peace offerings, two oxen, five rams, five he goats, five lambs of the first year: this *was* the offering of Abidan the son of Gideoni.

66 On the tenth day Ahiezer the son of Ammishaddai, prince of the children of Dan, *offered:*

67 His offering *was* one silver charger, the weight whereof *was an* hundred and thirty *shekels,* one silver bowl of seventy shekels, after the shekel of the sanctuary; both of them full of fine flour mingled with oil for a meat offering:

68 One golden spoon of ten *shekels,* full of incense:

69 One young bullock, one ram, one lamb of the first year, for a burnt offering:

70 One kid of the goats for a sin offering:

71 And for a sacrifice of peace offerings, two oxen, five rams, five he goats, five lambs of the first year: this *was* the offering of Ahiezer the son of Amishaddai.

72 On the eleventh day Pagiel the son of Ocran, prince of the children of Asher offered:

73 His offering *was* one silver charger, the weight whereof *was an* hundred and thirty *shekels,* one silver bowl of seventy shekels, after the shekel of the sanctuary; both of them full of fine flour mingled with oil for a meat offering:

74 One golden spoon of ten *shekels,* fall of incense:

75 One young bullock, one ram, one lamb of the first year, for a burnt offering

76 One kid of the goats for a sin offering:

77 And for a sacrifice of peace offerings, two oxen, five rams, five he goats, five lambs of the first year: this *was* the offering of Pagiel the son of Ocran.

78 On the twelfth day Ahira the son of Enan, prince of the children

of Naptha, *offered:*

79 His offering *was* one silver charger, the weight whereof *was an* hundred and thirty *shekels,* one silver bowl of seventy shekels, after the shekel of the sanctuary; both of them full of fine flour mingled with oil for a meat offering:

80 One golden spoon of ten *shekels,* full of incense:

81 One young bullock, one ram, one lamb of the first year, for a burnt offering:

82 One kid of the goats for a sin offering:

83 And for a sacrifice of peace offerings, two oxen, five rams, five he goats, five lambs of the first year: this *was* the offering of Ahira the son of Enan.

84 This *was* the dedication of the altar, in the day when it was anointed, by the princes of Israel: twelve chargers of silver, twelve silver bowls, twelve spoons of gold:

85 Each charger of silver *weighing* an hundred and thirty *shekels,* each bowl seventy: all the silver vessels *weighed* two thousand and four hundred *shekels,* after the shekel of the sanctuary:

86 The golden spoons *were* twelve, full of incense, *weighing ten shekels* apiece, after the shekel of the sanctuary: all the gold of the spoons *was* an hundred and twenty *shekels.*

87 All the oxen for the burnt offering *were* twelve bullocks, the rams twelve, the lambs of the first year twelve, with their meat offering: and the kids of the goats for sin offering twelve.

88 And all the oxen for the sacrifice of the peace offerings *were* twenty and four bullocks, the rams sixty, the he goats sixty, the lambs of the first year sixty. This *was* the dedication of the altar, after that it was anointed.

89 And when Moses was gone into the tabernacle of the congregation to speak with him, then he heard the voice of one speaking unto him from off the mercy seat that *was* upon the ark of testimony, from between the two cherubims: and he spake unto him.

tribe of Judah? What religious difference would it make to anyone reading this today, tomorrow, or yesterday?"

Joey continued to read verse 13 that said, "And his offering *was* one silver charger, the weight thereof *was* an hundred and thirty *shekels*, one silver bowl of seventy shekels, after the shekel of the sanctuary; both of them *were* full of fine flour mingled with oil for a meat offering."

"More inane text," he thought. As he read, he noticed this seemingly nonsensical text repeated throughout the chapter. *Every six verses!* "Why would they do this?" he thought. "Maybe all this repeating nonsense is here just to cover the *critical verses*. People would read this and think 'I don't understand or want anything to do with that.' Meanwhile, therein lie the keys."

"The keys must begin with the *first day*," Joey reasoned.

Now it's recommended that you do what he did next. He went through the rest of the chapter underlining the second through twelfth days cited progressively in the text, each day was *precisely six verses apart*.

He recalled that it was confusion regarding the repeating numerical pattern in the *column of 6s* that initiated his request for Jeshua's assistance.

Joey then underlined each of the days and their associated verse numbers. Then using the Pythagorean skein on each underlined verse number he realized they provided the same 3,9,6,3,9,6,3,9,6 etc. repeating pattern he saw in his original figure 2.2. In other words, for verse 12, 1+2=3; for verse 18, 1+8=9; for verse 24, 2+4=6 and so on.

## The Missing Solfeggio

Once having discovered this repeating pattern in the Bible, Joey recalled his earlier investigation of Gregorian chants in a book written by Professor Emeritus Willi Apel.[2,3] The professor argued that the chants being used today were totally incorrect and undermined the true *spirit* of the Catholic faith. He wrote:

No true admirer of Gregorian chant can help looking with dismay at present trends . . . This practice, although ostensibly
meant to promote the chant, is actually bound to destroy it. To
what extent it has dulled the minds of "those that should hear"
became clear to me . . . Invariably it will sound like "something"
other than what it really is and what it should be. Moreover, the
very variety of possibilities inherent in this practice is bound to
weaken the catholicity of one of the most precious possessions of
the Catholic Church.

Moreover, Professor Apel reported that one-hundred fifty-two
chants were apparently missing. The Catholic Church presumably
"lost" these original chants. The chants were based on the ancient
original scale of *six* musical notes called the Solfeggio. These are
shown in figure 2.5.

Apel wrote:

The origin of what is now called Solfeggio . . . arose from a
Mediaeval hymn to John the Baptist which had this peculiarity
that the first six lines of the music commenced respectively on
the first six successive notes of the scale, and thus the first syllable of each line was sung to a note *one degree higher* than the
first syllable of the line that preceded it.

By *degrees* these syllables [seen in Fig.2.5] became associated
and identified with their respective notes and as each syllable
ended with a vowel they were found to be peculiarly adapted for
vocal use. Hence Ut was artificially replaced by "Do." Guido of
Arezzo was the first to adopt them in the 11th century, and Le
Marie, a French musician of the 17th century, added "Si" for the
seventh note of the scale, in order to complete the series. It might
have been formed from the initial letter of the two words in this
line, S and I*. . . . (Emphasis added.)

Thus *nature and grace illustrate each other*, and reveal the great
fact that there is a secret ear, more delicate than any "organs of
Corti," that can detect sounds invisible as well as inaudible to the
senses, and which enables those who possess it to say:

**"Sweeter sounds than music knows**
**Charm me in Emanuel's name;**
**All her hopes my spirit owes**
**To his birth, and cross, and shame."**

## Fig. 2.5. Evolution of the Gregorian Musical "Solfeggio" (Scale) From Initially Six (6) Notes

**The Original Solfeggio**
1. Ut – queant laxis
2. Re – sonare fibris
3. Mi – ra gestorum
4. Fa – muli tuorum
5. Sol – ve polluti
6. La – biireatum

**The Earlier Modified Solfeggio**
1. Ut – queant laxis
2. Re – sonare fibris
3. Mi – ra gestorum
4. Fa – muli tuorum
5. Sol – ve polluti
6. La – biireatum
7. SI – Sancto Iohannes

### The Current Modified Solfeggio
1. Do – queant laxis
2. Re – sonare fibris
3. Mi – ra gestorum
4. Fa – muli tuorum
5. Sol – ve polluti
6. La – biireatum
7. TI – Sancto Iohannes

| C | D | E | F | G | A | B | C |
|---|---|---|---|---|---|---|---|
| Do | Re | Mi | Fa | Sol | La | Si | Do |

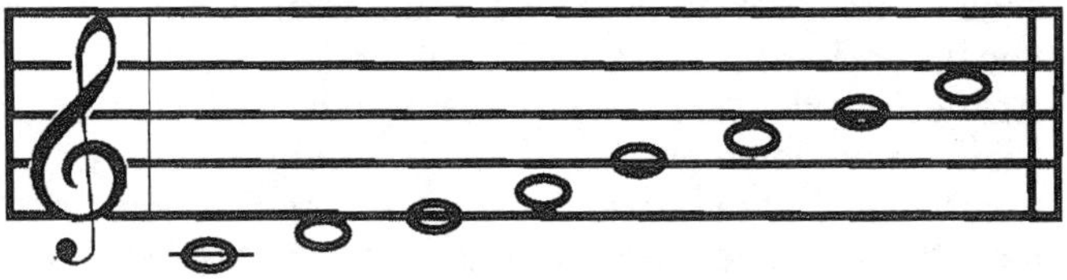

In other words, "nature and grace"—the physical and the spiritual—reflect each other, and reveal "the great fact" that there is a secret tone scale—or set of sounds—that vibrates at the exact frequencies required to transform spirit to matter or matter to spirit.

Emanuel, the spiritual name given to Christ, means, according to the Bible (Matthew 1:23), "God with us." The number value for the name, according to the Pythagorean skein, is eight (8)—the same as GOD.

## A Song of Degrees

Before becoming aware of the six note Solfeggio and the six verse repeating code in Numbers (beginning in Chapter 7, verse 12), Jeshua had directed Joey to discover two stanzas of music encoded in Psalms 120 through 134.

Psalm 120 is titled, "A Song of degrees." As seen in figure 2.6, each successive verse from 120 through 134 is *"one degree" higher* than the one preceding it.

Again, Professor Apel documented that "the origin of what is now called [the] Solfeggio . . . arose from a Mediaeval hymn to John the Baptist which had this peculiarity that *the first six lines of the music commenced respectively on the first six successive notes of the scale*," the scale being "Ut, Re, Mi, Fa, Sol, La. " Thus, "the first syllable of each line was sung to a note *one degree higher* than the first syllable of the line that preceded it." (Emphasis added.)

Long after the Solfeggio was developed, the first note—"Ut"— was changed to "Do." Pope Johannes later became a saint—Sancto Iohannes—and then the scale was changed. The seventh note "Si" was added from his name. "Si" later became "Ti." These changes significantly altered the frequencies sung by *the masses*. The alterations also weakened the spiritual impact of the Church's hymns. Because the music held mathematical resonance, frequencies capable of spiritually inspiring humankind to be more "Godkind," the changes effected alterations in conceptual thought as well, further distancing humanity from God.

In other words, whenever you sing a Psalm, it is music to the ears. But it was originally intended to be music for the soul as well, or the "secret ear." Thus, by changing the notes, higher matrices of thought, and to a great extent well being, was squelched.

Now it is time to recover these missing notes.

So go to figure 2.6 that displays Psalms 120 through 134, and underline or highlight each phrase listed below:

## Fig. 2.6. Numerical Musical Pattern Encoded in King James Bible From PSALM 120 Through 134

### PSALM 120
#### *A Song of degrees*

IN my distress I cried unto the LORD, and he heard me.

2 Deliver my soul, O LORD, from lying lips, and from a deceitful tongue.

3 What shall be given unto thee? or what shall be done unto thee, thou false tongue?

4 Sharp arrows of the mighty, with coals of juniper.

5 Woe is me, that I sojourn in Mesech, that I dwell in the tents of Kedar.

6 My soul hath long dwelt with him that hateth peace.

7 I *am for* peace: but when I speak, they are for war.

### PSALM 121
#### *A Song of degrees*

I WILL lift up mine eyes unto the hills, from whence cometh my help.

2 My help cometh from the LORD, which made heaven and earth.

3 He will not suffer thy foot to be moved: he that keepeth thee will not slumber.

4 Behold, he that keepeth Israel shall neither slumber nor sleep.

5 The LORD is thy keeper: the LORD *is* thy shade upon thy right hand.

6 The sun shall not smite thee by day, nor the moon by night.

7 The LORD shall preserve thee from all evil: he shall preserve thy soul.

8 The LORD shall preserve thy going out and thy coming in from this time forth, and even for evermore.

### PSALM 122
#### *A Song of degrees of David*

I WAS glad when they said unto me, Let us go into the house of the LORD.

2 Our feet shall stand within thy gates, O Jerusalem.

3 Jerusalem is builded as a city that is compact together:

4 Whither the tribes go up, the tribes of the LORD, unto the testimony of Israel, to give thanks unto the name of the LORD.

5 For there are set thrones of judgment, the thrones of the house of David.

6 Pray for the peace of Jerusalem: they shall prosper that love thee.

7 Peace be within thy walls, and prosperity within thy palaces.

8 For my brethren and companions sakes, I will now say, Peace be within thee.

9   Because of the house of the LORD our God I will seek thy good.

### PSALM 123
#### *A Song of degrees*

UNTO thee lift I up mine eyes, O thou that dwellest in the heavens.

2 Behold, as the eyes of servants look unto the hand of their mas-ters, and as the eyes of a maiden unto the hand of her mistress; so our eyes *wait* upon the LORD our God, until that he have mercy upon us.

3   Have mercy upon us, O LORD, have mercy upon us: for we are exceedingly filled with con-tempt.

4   Our soul is exceedingly filled with the scorning of those that are at ease and with the contempt of the proud.

### PSALM 124
#### *A Song of degrees of David*

IF *it had not been* the LORD who was on our side, now may Israel say;

2   If *it had not been* the LORD who was on our side, when men rose up against us:

3   Then they had swallowed us up quick, when their wrath was kindled against us:

4   Then the waters had over-whelmed us, the stream had gone over our soul:

5   Then the proud waters had gone over our soul.

6   Blessed be the LORD, who hath not given us *as* a prey to their teeth.

7   Our soul is escaped as a bird out of the snare of the fowlers: the snare is broken, and we are escaped.

8   Our help *is* in the name of the LORD, who made heaven and earth.

### PSALM 125
#### *A Song of degrees*

THEY that trust in the LORD *shall* be as Mount Zion *which* cannot b removed, *but*abideth forever.

2 As the mountains *are* round about Jerusalem, so the LORD is round about his people from henceforth even for ever.

3   For the rod of the wicked shall not rest upon the lot of the righteous; lest the righteous put forth their hands unto iniquity.

4   Do good, O LORD, unto *those that* be good, and to *them that are* upright in their hearts.

5   As for such as turn aside unto their crooked ways, the LORD shall lead them forth with the workers of iniquity: but peace *shall be* upon Is-rael.

### PSALM 126
#### *A Song of degrees*

WHEN the LORD turned again the captivity of Zion, we were like them that dream.

2   Then was our mouth filled with laughter, and our tongue with singing: then said they

among the heathen, the LORD hath done great things for them.

3 The LORD hath done great thing for us; *whereof* we are glad.

4 Turn again our captivity, O LORD, as the streams in the south.

5 They that sow in tears shall reap m Joy.

6 He that goeth forth and weepeth, bearing precious seed, shall doubtless come again with rejoicing, bringing his sheaves *with him.*

## PSALM 127
### *A Song of degrees for Solomon*
EXCEPT the LORD build the house, they labour in vain that build it: except the LORD keep the city, the watchman waketh but in vain.

2 *It is* vain for you to rise up early, to sit up late, to eat the bread of sorrows: for so he giveth his beloved sleep.

3 Lo, children are an heritage of the LORD: and the fruit of the womb is his reward.

4 As arrows are in the hand of a mighty man; so are children of the youth.

5 Happy is the man that hath his quiver full of them: they shall not be ashamed, but they shall speak with the enemies in the gate.

## PSALM 128
### *A Song of degrees*
BLESSED is every one that feareth the LORD; that walketh in his ways.

2 For thou shalt eat the labour of thine hands: happy *shalt* thou be, and *it shall be* well with thee.

3 Thy wife *shall be* as a fruitful vine by the sides of thine house: thy children like olive plants round about thy table.

4 Behold, that thus shall the man be blessed that feareth the LORD.

5 The LORD shall bless thee out of Zion: and thou shalt see the good of Jerusalem all the days of thy life.

6 Yea, thou shalt see thy children's children, and peace upon Israel.

## PSALM 129
### *A Song of degrees*
MANY a time have they afflicted me from my youth, may Israel now say:

2 Many a time have they afflicted me from my youth: yet they have not prevailed against me.

3 The plowers plowed upon my back: they made long their furrows.

4 The LORD is righteous: he hath cut asunder the cords of the wicked.

5 Let them all be confounded and turned back that hate Zion.

6 Let them be as the grass upon the house tops, which withereth afore it groweth up:

7 Wherewith the mower filleth not his hand; nor he that bindeth sheaves his bosom.

8 Neither do they which go by

say, The blessing of the LORD be upon you: we bless you in the name of the LORD.

## PSALM 130
### *A Song of degrees*

OUT of the depths have I cried unto thee, O LORD.

2  Lord, hear my voice: let thine ears be attentive to the voice of my supplications.

3  If thou, LORD, shouldest mark iniquities, O Lord, who shall stand?

4  But *there is* forgiveness with thee, that thou mayest be feared.

5  I wait for the LORD, my soul doth wait, and in his word do I hope.

6  My soul *waiteth* for the Lord more than they that watch for the morning: *I say, more than* they that watch for the morning.

7  Let Israel hope in the LORD: for with the LORD *there is* mercy, and with him is plenteous redemption.

8  And he shall redeem Israel from all his iniquities.

## PSALM 131
### *A Song of degrees of David*

LORD, my heart is not haughty, nor mine eyes lofty: neither do I exercise myself in great matters, or in things too high for me.

2  Surely I have behaved and quieted myself, as a child that is weaned of his mother: my soul is even as a weaned child.

3   Let Israel hope in the LORD from henceforth and for ever.

## PSALM 132
### *A Song of degrees*

LORD, remember David, and all his afflictions:

2  How he sware unto the LORD, and vowed unto the mighty *God* of Jacob;

3  Surely I will not come into the tabernacle of my house, nor go up into my bed;

4  I will not give sleep to mine eyes, or slumber to mine eyelids,

5  Until I find out a place for the LORD, an habitation for the mighty *God* of Jacob.

6  Lo, we heard of it at Ephratah: we found it in the fields of the wood.

7  We will go into his tabernacles: we will worship at his footstool.

8  Arise, O LORD, into thy rest; thou, and the ark of thy strength.

9  Let thy priests be clothed with righteousness; and let thy saints shout for joy.

10  For thy servant David's sake turn not away the face of thine anointed.

11  The LORD hath sworn in truth unto David; he will not turn from it; Of the fruit of thy body will I set upon thy throne.

12   If thy children will keep my

covenant and my testimony that I shall teach

them, their children shall also sit upon thy throne for evermore.

13  For the LORD hath chosen Zion; he hath desired it for his habitation.

14  This *is* my rest for ever: here will I dwell; for I have desired it.

15  I will abundantly bless her provision: I will satisfy her poor with bread.

16  I will also clothe her priests with salvation: and her saints shall shout aloud for joy.

17  There will I make the horn of David to bud: I have ordained a lamp for mine anointed.

18  His enemies will I clothe with shame: but upon himself shall his crown flourish.

### PSALM 133

#### *A Song of degrees of David*

BEHOLD, how good and how pleasant *it is* for brethren to dwell together in unity!

2  *It is* like the precious ointment upon the head, that ran down upon the beard, even Aaron's beard: that went down to the skirts of his garments;

3  As the dew of Hermon *and as the dew* that descended upon the mountains of Zion: for there the LORD commanded the blessing, *even* life for evermore.

### PSALM 134

#### *A Song of degrees*

BEHOLD, bless ye the LORD, all *ye* servants of the LORD, which by night stand in the house of the LORD.

2  Lift up your hands in the sanctuary, and bless the LORD.

3  The LORD that made heaven and earth bless thee out of Zion.

In Psalm 120 underline —"A Song of degrees"
In Psalm 121 underline —"A Song of degrees"
Under Ps. 122—"A Song of degrees of David." Then circle "David." (5)
In Psalm 123 underline —"A Song of degrees"
Under Ps. 124—"A Song of degrees of David." Then circle "David." (7)
In Psalm 125 underline —"A Song of degrees"
In Psalm 126 underline —"A Song of degrees"
Under Psalm 127—"A Song of degrees for Solomon." Then circle
"Solomon."
In Psalm 128 underline —"A Song of degrees"
In Psalm 129 underline —"A Song of degrees"
In Psalm 130 underline —"A Song of degrees"
Under Ps. 131—"A Song of degrees of David." Then circle "David." (5)
In Psalm 132 underline —"A Song of degrees"
Under Ps. 133—"A Song of degrees of David." Then circle "David." (7)
In Psalm 134 underline —"A Song of degrees"

Observe that "A Song of degrees" changes to "A Song of degrees of David" in Psalm 122 (or 5 using the Pythagorean skein), 124 (or 7), 131 (or 5) and 133 (or 7). Then in Psalm 127 (or 1), the stanza is broken with a "A Song of degrees of Solomon." This yields seven Psalms before and seven Psalms after the stanza break. If you deduct one "Song of degrees of David" from either side of the break, due to the repeat, then you get six degrees above and six degrees below "A Song of degrees for [King] Solomon."

Generally speaking, in the Bible, when you see such a pattern change, there is a hidden code being revealed to you.

Moreover, Joey learned that additional information regarding what a "tone" meant was referenced in Leviticus beginning with Chapter 23:26. These verses dealt with "atonement" or what "a-tone-ment." The numerical encryption here undoubtedly related to music. (See appendix section for more information on "atonement" and what "a tone meant.")

## Beethoven's Musical Mathematics

Beethoven, whose best friend was a mathematician, studied the Bible avidly and understood the spiritual power behind the tones or notes in the Solfeggio. Though totally deaf, he used his "secret ear" to "hear" the music.

Although he knew many clergymen, Beethoven was not an avid church goer. Rather, "he sought God through eastern mysticism and in a Persian book of religion found texts that he copied and kept framed upon his desk," wrote his biographer Eric Blom. "God was the source of his music, and he the agent chosen to spread the divine message. . . . To him the human and spiritual issues enunciated by the text of the Mass [the Bible] would be a call upon all the resources of imagination and *craft* within the range of his art."[4] (Emphasis added.)

Beethoven's most cherished teacher was Franz Joseph Haydn who was born in 1732 and became a "staunch Catholic." In 1785, he became a Freemason "to please his friend Mozart," wrote biographer William J. Finn in *The Catholic Encyclopedia.* [5]

Mozart "openly acknowledged [to Haydn and others] the role played by the [Masonic] Craft in his life." Considered the "supreme musical genius of the Enlightenment," Mozart "saw Freemasonry as an essential part of his life in Vienna. Indeed, it may be argued that for the last—and most productive—seven years of his short career, the Craft was the pivot around which his social and cultural life revolved."[6]

Mozart's "Masonic enthusiasm" is reflected most dramatically in his opera *The Magic Flute* which he performed shortly before his death in 1791.[6]

Haydn, highly influenced by Mozart, became "the first great symphonic composer," but was "equally famous for his masses, chamber music, and the two oratorios, *The Creation* and *The Seasons.*[6]

Finn reported that "the reform of Church music instituted by Pope Pius X . . . equivalently debarred" Haydn's very popular "Masses . . . from use at liturgical services, in some instances on account of the alterations and repetitions effected in the text, and in others [allegedly] because . . . the operatic character of the music itself" was said to be 'scandalously gay.'"[5]

It was far more likely Haydn's work was barred from the Masses because of its mathematical and spiritual impartations and implications.

Haydn had also been heavily influenced by Emanuel Bach, son of Johann Sebastion Bach, who had also influenced Beethoven.[5]

It is well documented that Bach's canons included "numerological symbols." One such example he called the "canon on the ground Fa Mi for seven voices with separation of a double bar." Another composition, written for an organist named Walter, was shown to contain notes that totaled 82 — the sum of W+A+L+T+E+R. The work also contained "the number of pitches in the canon and twice the sum of J+S+B+A+C+H. Written in score there are 14 (B+A+C+H) measures."[7]

Thus, Beethoven, like his Masonic mentors, most likely created his masterpieces transposing the mathematics encoded in the Bible, and elsewhere, into musical scores.

Likewise today, many musicians and composers may be listening with their "secret ear" without knowing they are tapping into this spiritual channel communicated by way of mathematical frequency vibrations.

### In Search of John the Baptist's Secret Poem

The primary "secret" not revealed in Professor Apel's or Dr. Bullinger's books is *the hymn for John the Baptist*. Joey discovered the missing hymn, again through a series of serendipitous events. Beginning with his investigation of Latin texts in search of the poem, he ultimately made contact with a history professor at Yale University's Mediaeval Department. (The man requested anonymity.) Joey exchanged a certain mathematical equation he discovered in the Bible for the poem along with testimony that Yale's Mediaeval Department has been generously funded by the Vatican since its inception. Yale is the home of the infamous "Skull and Bones" fraternity. As you will later learn, this is important.

On a side note, additionally foreshadowing the later chapters of this book, Yale's virology department is considered the world's leading repository of deadly viruses. It has remained heavily funded by the Rockefeller Foundation, and in recent years, has heavily promoted the "Rockefeller plan" to establish "fifteen disease surveillance clinics" on the fringes of tropical rain forests.[8] These clinics will, for all practical purposes, track the mass of predicted deaths from plagues like AIDS and Creutzfeld-Jakob Disease, that is CJD, or "mad cow disease" in humans. Such "plagues" were also prophesied in the Bible. Thus, as you will increasingly learn, in light of these current and coming plagues, Joey's Bible code discoveries are especially important as they provide powerful therapeutic and preventive applications at a most critical time in history.

Having entered a zone of restricted access, Joey relayed the following story of his exclusion from Mediaeval Latin history as he searched for John the Baptist's poem:

"I got a Latin book," he recalled. "And none of these things—Ut, Re, Mi, Fa, Sol, La—were in the Latin book. So I brought the book back to the library and asked the librarian if she knew why not."

"Because it's not a Mediaeval Latin text," she said.

"Can you get me one?" Joey asked.

"I'll see what I can do." With that she took off only to return a few minutes later to report, "I can't get you one. They're all packed away in the archives under glass in churches and museums because they're so old. Some universities might have a few, but we can't help you."

So Joey asked around for leads. Soon a friend directed him to a university, in Spokane, WA, where a monsignor became his contact. The clergyman was head of the Mediaeval department. "He knew all about the 'organs of Corti,' Solfeggio, Guido of Arezzo, and the whole thing," Joey recalled.

Following twenty minutes on the telephone with the man, he asked Joey, "It's wonderful to speak to you, my son, but what exactly is it that I can do for you?"

"Can you decipher Mediaeval Latin, Monsignor?"

"Absolutely!"

"And you know the musical scale and everything?"

"Absolutely!"

"Well then could you tell me what 'Ut – queant laxis' means?"

After a brief pause the Monsignor quipped, "It's none of your business." Then he hung up.

Weeks later, the Spokane librarian who had done the search for Joey called him back. "I didn't forget you," she said. "I tried to find out more on the subject. Some people I contacted told me to drop it; to just forget it!"

"Are you serious?"

"Yes," she replied. "I'm very serious."

So, Joey went back to the Bible and the references he already had. He reread Dr. Bullinger's book wherein he reported under "Sound & Music":

Sound is the impression produced on the ear by the vibrations of air. The Pitch of the musical note is higher or lower accordingly as these vibrations are faster or slower. When they are too slow, or not sufficiently regular and continuous to make a musical sound, we call it noise.

Experiments have long been completed which fix the number of vibrations for each musical note; by which, of course, we may easily calculate the difference between the number of vibrations between each note. . . .[3]

The scale of "Do" shown in figure 2.5 is described by Bullinger as follows. In terms of the number of vibrations per second under each note and the differences between them Bullinger reported:

The numbers of vibrations in a second, for each note, is a multiple of eleven and the difference in the number of vibrations between each note is also a multiple of eleven. . . .[3]

71

"A multiple of eleven," Joey considered. "There is an eleven-year single-polarity sun cycle, and it takes twenty-two years to complete the bipolar cycle." Then he continued reading:

> These differences are not always the same. We speak of tones and semitones, as though all tones were alike, and all semitones were alike; but this is not the case. The difference between the semitone Mi and Fa is 22; while between the other semitone, Si and Do, it is 33. So with the tones: the difference between the tone Do and Re, for example, is 33; while between Fa and Sol it is 22; Between Sol and La it is 44; and between La and Si it is 55. . . .[3]

They are all multiples of eleven, Joey realized, then thought, "I wonder if the original Solfeggio is related to the solar cycles or even light frequencies?"

Dr. Bullinger continued:

> There are vibrations which the ear cannot detect, so slow as to make no audible sound, but there are contrivances by which they can be made visible to the eye. When sand is thrown upon a thin metal disc, to which a chord is attached and caused to vibrate, the sand will immediately arrange itself in a perfect geometrical pattern. The pattern will vary with the number of the vibrations. These are called "Chladni's figures." Moist plaster on glass or mist water-colour on rigid surfaces will vibrate at the sound, say, of the human voice, or of a cornet, and will assume forms of various kinds—geometrical, vegetable, floral; some resembling ferns, others resembling leaves and shells, according to the pitch of the note.[3] (More discussion on "Chladni's figures" is presented in Chapter 10, figure 10.2.)

In other words, specific vibrations could create special forms in physical matter. Musical sound vibrations that transmit spiritual energies can thus impact, if not become, physical matter. "Sound energy impacting matter," Joey considered. *"The First Book of Moses, Genesis,* when God *spoke* and said, 'Let there be light, and there was light' attests to this as well. God must have created heaven and earth, and all that lives, by saying or singing it so."

The fall of the wall of Jericho by "seven priests bearing the seven trumpets," was another example. The major destructive force must have occurred through similar vibrations during the first *six* days the priests were directed to circle the city and blow their horns. On the seventh day, when they finally allowed the people to come, scream, shout and participate, the wall fell. But it had already been shattered by the sixth day. *"The destructive forces must therefore be in sounds and vibrations as well,"* Joey realized.

How might this be explained?

John Keely, an expert in electromagnetic technologies, wrote that the vibrations of "thirds, sixths, and ninths," were extraordinarily powerful. In fact, he proved the "vibratory antagonistic thirds" was "thousands of times" more forceful in separating hydrogen from oxygen in water than heat! In his "Formula of Aqueous Disintegration" he wrote that, "In all molecular dissociation or disintegration of both simple and compound elements, whether gaseous or solid, a stream of vibratory antagonistic thirds, sixths, or ninths, on their chord mass will compel progressive subdivisions. In the disintegration of water the instrument is set on thirds, sixths, and ninths, to get the best effects."[9]

Other scientists, including the geniuses Nikola Tesla and Royal Raymond Rife, who will both be discussed later, as well as others including Haydn, Mozart, Beethoven, and Chladni, all must have known about, and used, this too—the inherent power of threes, sixes, and nines.

Then, a sobering thought tempered Joey's consideration—"The people who have been controlling the world, manipulating the masses, and suppressing this knowledge, must be using this too."

## References:

1. The definition of Akkadian, meaning "an extinct Semitic language of ancient Mesopotamia" that held the "gate to God," is found in *Merriam Webster's Collegiate Dictionary: Tenth Edition.* Springfield, MA: Merriam-Webster, Inc., 1994, pp. 26 and 83. The tower of Babel, that is, the effort to elevate man's consciousness into the heavens, or bring mankind up to "Godkind," was halted because of "the confusion of tongues" or sounds.

This confusion in language, and underlying mathematics, was intentionally done, several authors have advanced, so that only those holding the sacred knowledge would be uniquely empowered.

It should also be noted that those who selfishly tricked the masses this way, according to author David Icke, worshipped the sun as "a multidimensional consciousness" as it emitted unseen electromagnetic frequencies. The sun, Icke noted, is 864,000 miles in diameter and contains "99% of the matter in the solar system." Notice that $8+6+4 = 18$, as does $9 + 9$. These deciphered to the Pythagorean single digit equals 9 or completion. See: Icke D. *The Biggest Secret*. Scottsdale, Arizona: Bridge of Love, 1999, p 55.

Also, David John Oates's work in "Reverse Speech™" appears to offer a "gateway to God." English speech, he argues, played backwards commonly relays subconscious "truths" reflecting the "soul" or a human being's more divine nature. See: http://www.reversespeech.com/

2. Apel W. *Gregorian Chant*. Bloomington, IN: Indiana University Press, 1990.

3 Bullinger, E.W. *Number in Scripture, First Edition*, England: Kregel Publications, 1894, pp. 15-18.

4. Blom E. *Grove's Dictionary of Music and Musicians, Fifth Edition*. London: Macmillan & Co. Ltd., 1954, pp. 556-57.

5. Mason D. *Beethoven and his Forerunners* (1904) and Finn, WJ. Franz Joseph Haydn (1913). In: Finn, WJ. *Catholic Encyclopedia*. The Encyclopedia Press, 1913. Electronic version by New Advent, Inc. 1997. URL# http://www.knight.org/advent/

6. Hamill J and Gilvert R. *Freemasonry: A Celebration of the Craft*. London: Greenwich Editions, 1993, pp. 170-171; 234.

7. Smith TA. *Honorific Canons*. Phoenix, AZ: Arizona University, 1997. Website. URL#: www.2.nau.edu/

8. Garrett L. *The Coming Plague*. New York: Penguin Books, 1994, pp. 33, 56, 595, 602, and 729.

9. Pond D, Keely J, Tesla N and Cayce E, et al. *Universal Laws Never Before Revealed: Keely's Secrets*. Sante Fe, NM: The Message Company, (RR2 Box 307 MM, Sante Fe, NM 87505 (505) 474-0998) 1990, p. 80.

# Chapter 3.
# King James, The Bible,
# and the Secret Societies

It might be asked, "Why, with so many other good Bibles available at the time of Martin Luther, did King James commission another Bible to be written that most Christian fundamentalists prescribe to this very day?"

Well if you study history, you will learn that King James was not only King of Scotland, but was also simultaneously King of England as well. His royalty helped to unite England and Scotland against France, Italy, and according to many authors, the Vatican.[1]

How was it that King James VI of Scotland (who was later crowned King James I of England) came to this high level of authority in both England and Scotland? The answer lies in the Knights Templar—a secret society believed to have formed during the early twelfth century. The Knights had sought refuge in Scotland which was largely controlled by their allies, the Freemasons.

Templar history is both fascinating and controversial. In *The Hiram Key*, Masonic Order members Christopher Knight and Robert Lomas reviewed "the development of modern Freemasonry and its impact on the world." Their text provided far more insight than many other books intended to promote Freemasonry as an entirely benign, largely humanitarian, spiritual fraternity.

According to Knight and Lomas, "From the completion of Rosslyn Chapel [in southern Scotland in 1486], to the official opening of the Grand Lodge of England on 24 June 1717," the Freemasons evolved from the Templar Order. "For reasons of self preservation the organization remained hidden from general view until the power of the Vatican began to slide rapidly in the sixteenth century."[1]

This "slide" in Roman Catholic Church authority, more commonly called "The Reformation," began on October 31st—the day we now celebrate Halloween—1517. Then, Martin Luther, an Augustinian professor at the University of Wittenberg, with suspicious ties to the German Rosicrucian Order, issued ninety-five theses considered heretical by the papacy. Luther, generally considered anti-Semitic, sexist, but otherwise supportive to Jesus' Naazrean theology, wrote three famous treatises distributed in 1520: *An Open Letter to the Christian Nobility of the German Nation Governing the Reform of the Christian Estate*; *The Babylonian Captivity of the Church*, and *On the Freedom of a Christian*. These works won him tremendous popular support as they strongly professed Luther's conviction that forgiveness of sins and human salvation was God's free gift of grace extended to everyone—a position that left the papacy out of the divine pecking order. This enraged the pope who subsequently directed Luther's excommunication in 1521.[1]

Soon thereafter, King Henry VIII began to have marital problems with his first wife, Catherine of Aragon, and sought resolution from the Vatican. The pope refused. Thus began England's separation from the Catholic Church. In 1533, Thomas Cromwell, King Henry's chief minister, ushered the "Act in Restraint of Appeals" through Parliament. Likewise, the following year, he passed the "Act of Supremacy" which authorized full control of the church by the king. To facilitate the jihad, the Archbishop of Canterbury, Thomas Cranmer, authorized the first English translation of the Bible.[1]

Thus, the Church of England usurped the power of the Roman Catholic Church for a time, though not without contest. One brief reversal occurred during the reign of Henry VIII's daughter, Queen Mary I. Partly because her royalty was feigned by Henry, once in power, the queen began to restore Catholicism, earning her the epithet "Bloody Mary" for her role in executing hundreds of Protestants. "In 1554, she married King Philip II of Spain, son of Holy Roman Emperor Charles V," recalled the authors of *The Hiram Key*. "The event sparked several rebellions which were harshly put down and afterwards 300 Protestants were burned at the stake for their beliefs. Under her successor, Queen Elizabeth I, England grew into a strong and Protestant nation."[1]

King James was reared during this bloody time in English history. Born on June 19, 1566, the only child of Mary Queen of Scots, James was "only fifteen months old when he succeeded his Catholic mother to the Scottish throne, but did not begin his personal rule of Scotland until 1583."[1]

A bright young king, James was intellectually reared by one of the greatest Latin scholars of his age—the late Renaissance poet and leading humanist George Buchanan. Under Buchanan's tutelage, "James successfully asserted his position as head of Church and State in Scotland, outwitting the nobles who conspired against him. Being eager to succeed the childless Elizabeth I to the English throne," Knight and Lomas chronicled that James merely made "a mild protest when his mother was executed for treason against Elizabeth in 1587."[1]

The authors continued to recant King James's evolution into dual royalty and Freemasonry positions this way:

> At the age of thirty-seven, two years after becoming a Freemason, James became the first Stuart king of England, and he devoted himself largely to English affairs thereafter. Although raised as a Presbyterian, he immediately antagonized the rising Puritan movement by rejecting a petition for reform of the Church of England at the Hampton Court Conference in 1604. Roman Catholic hostility to a Protestant monarch was widespread, and in 1605 a Catholic plot, led by Guy Fawkes, failed in an attempt to blow up both king and Parliament. Despite this assassination plot, there was suspicion in England that *James was secretly rather pro-Catholic because he had concluded peace with Spain in 1604.* [2][Emphasis added.]

"That makes sense," Joey thought. "James was apparently a highly intelligent political mover and shaker. Anyone who could disregard his own mother's execution for royal advancement would not likely feign a mutually beneficial proposal from the Catholic Church. This was evidenced by his alliance with Spain."

That knowledge placed a new light on the alleged and perceived "division" between the English and Catholic churches. Joey questioned, "I wonder if this is part of the buried knowledge and great deception of the masses?" His thoughts raced with new possibilities.

"Much like today," he speculated, "shadow governors expertly devise ways to 'divide the "sheeple" to conquer the flock.' They separate rich from poor, black from white, Jew from gentile, Christian from Muslim, liberal from conservative, all while the oligarchy that controls the military–industrial complex makes money manipulating people with fear, directing them into bloody conflicts, and thus reducing, when desired, unwanted populations. Just like the James Bond myth—the British and Americans suspect the Russians; the Russians suspect the Americans, meanwhile 'SPECTRE' is really the lethal instigators," Joey thought. "'SPECTRE,' I wonder what that word means? I'll have to look it up sometime."[2]

Knight and Lomas continued their historic analyses of King James's biblical scholarship:

> James was a speculative mason and also wrote books about king-ship, theology, witchcraft, and even tobacco; significantly he also commissioned a new 'Authorised' version of the Bible which is called after him—the King James Bible (it is the version that omits the two anti-Nazarean Books of Maccabees). The introduction that still appears in the front of this Protestant Bible reveals no Catholic sympathies; one section reads:

> ". . . So that if, on the one side, we shall be traduced by Popish Persons at home or abroad, who therefore will malign us because we are poor instruments to make God's holy Truth to be yet more and more known unto the people, whom they desire still to keep in ignorance and darkness . . ."[1]

*The Hiram Key* authors, much like other modern Masonic testimonials, added that "Modern Freemasonry is nonsectarian and it boasts that it always has been so." Yet, because of this alleged "period of anti-Catholicism," Knight and Lomas reported that "the circumstances of the early seventeenth century provided the perfect conditions for the secret society of masons to emerge into the public arena."

They then went on to explain King James's leadership in the burgeoning Masonic movement:

With the king a speculative [white collar] mason himself and the power of the Pope blocked for all time in Scotland, the need for utter secrecy was suddenly gone. King James was a thinker and a reformer and he must have felt that the structure of the growing Masonic movement needed to be formalized, so fifteen years after he had taken active control of his Scottish kingdom, two years before being accepted as a Freemason and five years before becoming the English monarch, he ordered that the existing Masonic structure be given leadership and organization. He made a leading Mason by the name of William Schaw his General Warden of the Craft and instructed him to improve the entire structure of Masonry. Schaw started this major project on 28 December, 1598 when he issued "The statutes and ordinances to be observed by all the master maissouns within this realme," signing himself as "the General Warden of the said craft" . . .

Two years after Schaw's work began, King James appointed himself Grand Master of the "Shaw Lodges" of Freemasons. Thereafter, the previously secret Lodges of Scotland began listing the names of their members and keeping minutes of their meetings. They still did not broadcast their existence but we can easily identify them today. The geographical location of the first registered Lodges show how the rituals cemented at Rosslyn by William Schaw became a major movement during the reign of James VI.[1]

"It was the regulation of both operative and speculative masonry by William Schaw," Knight and Lomas concluded, "that formalised the ritual into what we now know as the *three degrees* of Craft Freemasonry. . . . [A] speculative mason was distinguished from an operative mason by the title 'Freemason.'. . . From this point onwards, Freemasonry had a Lodge structure which would soon spread to England, and eventually the entire Western world."[1] (Emphasis added.)

"Interesting," Joey considered, "how knowledge of the power of threes, sixes, and nines—3x3 and 'a song of degrees' might have translated into the Masonic hierarchy. The 33rd level of Freemasonry is the most famous, or rather infamous, *degree*."

## The Birth of Modern Science

When King James VI of Scotland, in 1603, acquired his English kingdom, one of his first acts was to confer knighthood on Francis Bacon—one of the King's favorite intellectuals as well as brother Freemason. Bacon was then rapidly promoted from "Solicitor-General to the Crown," to "Attorney General," to "Lord Keeper of the Great Seal," and finally to "Lord Chancellor" in 1618.

Considered among history's leading philosophers, brother Bacon sought to rid the human mind of "idols," that is, "tendencies to error." He planned the *Instauratio Magna*, or "Great Restoration," in an effort to restore human mastery over nature. It contained the following *six* parts as detailed in *The Hiram Key*:

1. a classification of sciences.
2. a new inductive logic.
3. a gathering of empirical and experimental facts.
4. examples to show the efficacy of his new approach.
5. generalisations derivable from natural history.
6. a new philosophy that would be a complete science of nature.[1]

Bacon's work expressed "an inductive philosophy of nature" over which man, not God, demonstrated control. A century later, Voltaire and Diderot, the famous French philosophers, described Bacon as "the father of modern science."

Bacon, in fact, intermingled his mystical Masonic knowledge with his political aspirations in his book *The New Atlantis*. In it, he advanced his intention to rebuild King Solomon's Temple in the spiritual sense. The purpose of this work was to develop "a temple of science" and great "palace of invention." His vision included a new state in which the pursuit of knowledge was organized much like science is today. From this early intellectual seed, modern science, as well as the United States Constitution, later germinated.

Given this background, it is understandable that James would have selected Bacon, above anyone, to coordinate the authorized King James Bible writing project.[3]

## The Knights Templar's Power

To understand why King James authorized a Bible which, as you will increasingly learn, encoded Masonic secrets requires further discussion. Particularly the persecution of the Templars by the Roman Catholic Church leaders should be entertained.

What is believed to have been the central source of discord between the two groups is the great power and wealth the esoteric knowledge provided those who possessed the arcana.[2] According to many authors, the Templars were said to have discovered many of the ancient scrolls and much of the Sion booty that the Romans had originally lifted from King Soloman's Temple in the Holy Land in 70 A.D. Some say the Freemasons found the treasures themselves in Solomon's Temple while they were guarding the Holy Land at a later date. Researchers also speculate that this ancient treasure of knowledge and wealth "repeatedly changed hands through the centuries—passing perhaps from the temple of Jerusalem, to the Romans, to the Visigoths, eventually to the Cathars [who were persecuted and then mass murdered in France] and/or the Knights Templar."[4]

According to Lawrence Gardner, "the appointed historian and sovereign genealogist to *thirty-three* royal families" (emphasis added) and "Britain's Grand Prior of the Sacred Kindred of St. Columba—the Royal Ecclesiastical Seat of the Celtic Church," who had access to Celtic Church records dating back to 37 A.D. and Templar documents removed from Europe in 1128 A.D., the Templars became "a specific target of the Inquisition in 1307 [A.D.] when the armies of Pope Clement V and King Philip IV of France were sent in their direction. Not only had the Knights returned from the Holy Land with important, first-century documentation, but they had also returned with incredible wealth and treasure. They were not only in a position to dismantle the church structure with their knowledge [of royal bloodline genealogy], but the [Templar] order was financially far richer than the Vatican itself and, therefore, posed a significant threat. In fact, the Templars at that stage were the richest single order that the world has ever known. The whole of our international banking network, that we all use today in our clearing houses, was all established by the Knights Templars in that era when they funded every European court."[5]

Gardner continued during a speech at Yale University in 1994, "The papal armies scoured Europe for the Templar documents and the treasure. But like the other Cathar inheritants, nothing was found. Many Knights were tortured, executed in the process, and their companions were banished to regions outside the papal domain. But the Templar hoard, although not found, was never lost. Its day-by-day existence is recorded, and all the time they were searching for it in Southern France, it was locked away in the treasury vaults of Paris.[5]

"One night it was loaded onto eighteen galleys at the Port of LaRochelle, and the fleet set sail for Scotland. There the Templars were welcomed by King Robert the Bruce along with the whole Scottish nation. . . . The Templars and their treasure from that moment in time, apart from an offshoot order in Portugal, remained in Scotland. The Templar treasure today remains in Scotland."[5]

Additional background on this important historic period was written by Baigent, Leigh, and Lincoln in their work, *Holy Blood Holy Grail*. At dawn on Friday the 13th, 1307, King Philippe IV of France and Pope Clement V (who Philippe IV had installed by conspiring with his ministers to kill Pope Bonifact VIII and Pope Benedict XI), rounded up the all the Knights including their grand master, Jacques de Molay. The pope wanted their empowering scrolls; the king their great wealth. The scrolls, again, contained the arcana—the mysterious knowledge that only Templar initiates were taught. It also contained the spiritually important numbers that were believed to facilitate God's magic.[2,4]

To escape capture and death, many of the Knights Templar fled to Scotland in the flotilla described by Gardner. Thus, the lion's share of the Templar's treasure escaped the French King and Pope. The Templar fleet sailed to Scotland where the treasures and survivors were believed to have just disappeared.

King Robert the Bruce of Scotland welcomed the Knights who built a temple there that still stands today. Amazingly it is built to the *exact* ratio and proportion to King Soloman's Temple in the Holy Land. Many believe the arcana remains buried there. Others believe remnants may still lurk in France.

The flags that the Knights Templar flew on their voyage to Scotland was the "skull and bones." They were not pirates. That was their colors. Today we have the "Skull and Bones" secret college fraternity, headquartered at Yale, to which many of the world's wealthiest most powerful leaders—men like past Central Intelligence Agency (CIA) director and past president, George Bush, belonged.

That Gardner presented his most famous "Bloodlines of the Holy Grail" lecture at Yale University, the home of the Templar's "skull and bones," and the Vatican-funded Mediaeval Department, seemed suspicious to Joey. That Gardner stated "thirty-three" as the number of royal families he served in compiling the evidence for his books and theses seemed uniquely "coincidental" to the "thirty-third degree"—the highest peak to which Masons aspire. Not to mention the 3x11 or 33 vibrations per second Dr. Bullinger wrote was associated with the note "MI" on the Solfeggio scale. Yet, "what could all this mean?" Joey questioned.

That Gardner was "Britain's Grand Prior of the Sacred Kindred of St. Columba—the Royal Ecclesiastical Seat of the Celtic Church," and had direct access to ancient sacred Celtic Church records, further fueled suspicions of Masonic loyalty. As will be discussed later, key arguments in Gardner's testimony are difficult to reconcile, particularly his witnessing of Templar goodwill in spreading Christianity according to Jesus, that is, in the strict Nazarene sense.

Moreover, as you will soon see, far more is implied by "MI" and its vibrational rate of six (6) as it relates to thirty-three (or 3+3) in Pythagorean sense.

## Jesus' Life and Death?

Aside from these suspicions, Gardner presented a riveting and controversial thesis. He alleged that Jesus had not died on the cross, but went on to extend his Davidian bloodline. This knowledge, considered heresy to Christians, was also the source of great ecumenical discontent in King James's time and long before. Gardner said that this knowledge, allegedly based on royal documents, was the principle cause of the Catholic Church's brutal inquisition—when church leaders sought to supersede legitimate royal rule.

"The King of the Jews" growing popularity, knowledge of Christ's royal bloodline, and the long-term threat posed by his messianic lineage, Gardner advanced, was the primary reason for Jesus' three day crucifixion. This was said to be merely a symbolic dethroning of Christ from his royalty.

Moreover, Jesus' "rising," Gardner stated, was the modern interpretation of Christ's living body being carried up and over the hill, away from the crucifixion site, by Joseph. (See appendix for further discussion.)

Gardner further proposed that Christ continued to live with Mary Magdalene and raise children. His holy bloodline continued to threaten the Catholic Church at the time of the Templars as Gardner explained thusly:

> . . . [T]hey continued to be a high threat to the great church and the figurehead monarchs and governments empowered by that church. They were the very reason for the implementation of the brutal inquisition because they upheld a moral and social code that was quite contrary to church requirements. This was especially apparent during the age of chivalry which embraced a respect for womanhood. This was exemplified by the early Knights Templars whose constitutional oath supported the veneration for the great grail mother Queen Mary Magdalene.

Undaunted by the inquisition, the Nazarene movement pursued its own course. And the story of the bloodline [that Gardner said evolved from Jesus' royal offspring] was perpetuated in literature—romantic literature now, such as *The Grandsome Grail,* and *The High History of the Holy Grail.* These writings were largely sponsored by the grail courts of France themselves—the Courts of Champagne, Anjou, and others, and also by the Knights Templar and directly by the dispossinic houses. And it was at that stage that Arthurian romance suddenly emerged in the late Middle Ages as a popular vehicle for the grail tradition.[5]

Gardner went on to record that King Arthur and his Knights of the Round Table later became central figures in the grail story. "Arthur was absolutely unique in a particular stage of the bloodline heritage— he held a dual heritage in the messianic line. King Arthur was by no means mythical as so many have supposed and surmised," he said and then continued.

"Arthur was born in 559 [A.D.] and he died in battle in 603. And his mother was a Gurner d' Lac—the daughter of Queen Vivian of Avalon in direct descent, in the female matriarchial line, from Mary Magdalene. His father was high King Aden of Del Reyada—the western highlands of Scotland, which are now called Argyle. . . . Aden at that time was the British Pen Dragon, the head dragon, the *king* of kings in a direct Nazarene descent from Jesus' brother James."[5]

## The Modern Templars

According to *Holy Blood Holy Grail,* by the 1700s, many secret and semisecret fraternities hailed the Templars as both their "precursors and mystical initiates." Many Freemasons at the time "appropriated the Templars as their own antecedents." Some Masonic "rites" or "observances" were to have come from the order. Arcane secrets were considered inherited. The evolution of the modern Templars was described as follows:

By 1789 the legends surrounding the Templars had attained positively mythic proportions and their historical reality was obscured by an aura of obfuscation and romance. Knights Templar were regarded as occult adepts, illumined alchemists, magi and sages, master masons, and high initiates—veritable supermen endowed with an awesome arsenal of arcane power and knowledge. They were also regarded as heroes and martyrs, harbingers of the anticlerical spirit of the age . . .

Since the French Revolution the aura surrounding the Templars has not diminished. At least three contemporary organizations today call themselves Templars, claiming to possess a pedigree from 1314, and characters whose authenticity has never been established. Certain Masonic lodges have adopted the grade of "Templar" as well as rituals and appellations supposedly descended from the original order. Toward the end of the nineteenth century a sinister Order of the New Templars was established in Germany and Austria, employing the swastika as one of its emblems. [See figure 3.1] Figures like H. P. Blavatsky, founder of Theosophy, and Rudolf Steiner, founder of Anthroposophy, spoke of an esoteric "wisdom tradition" running back through the Rosicrucians to the Cathars and Templars—who were purportedly repositories of more ancient secrets still. In the United States teenage boys are admitted into the De Molay Society, without either their or their mentors' having much notion whence the name derives. In Britain as well as elsewhere in the West, recondite rotary clubs dignify themselves with the name "Templar" and include eminent public figures.[2]

## The Knights Templar of Malta and the Nazis

During their investigation of the Knights Templar and their affiliated agents and organizations, *Holy Blood Holy Grail* authors Baigent, Leigh, and Lincoln identified a "secret order behind the Knights Templar, which created the Templars as its military and administrative arm." This had been most often referred to as the Prieuré de Sion (PdS), or Priory of Sion. Although the volume of supporting evidence for this was "copious," these authors provided a detailed summary of their findings especially relevant to the later chapters of this book, that is, those dealing with organized conspiracy and methods of deceiving, controlling, and even killing large populations.

In fact, this was not their original intent. The authors feverishly set about to dismiss any conspiracy theory involving the PdS. They did so "with a cynical, almost derisory skepticism, fully convinced the out-

## Fig. 3.1. Cover of Oriental Templars Constitution

˒ I ˛ N ˛ R ˛ I ˛

CONSTITUTION

of the

𝕬ncient

𝕺rder of 𝕺riental 𝕿emplars

. O . T . O .

Ordo Templi Orientis.

With an Introduction
and a Synopsis of the Degrees
of the O. T. O.

Cover of the *Ordo Templi Orientis*, or Order of the Temple of the East, showing a small swastika. The order was formed by defrocked Cistercian Monk Jorg Lanz von Liebenfels, a personal friend and confidant of Adolf Hitler. Lanz is believed to have helped lead Hitler into homosexual, occult, racist, and sexist practices and ideologies. He modeled the O.T.O. based on the Teutonic Knights and Knights Templars—militaristic monastic orders. (See: Lively S and Abrams K. *The Pink Swastika: Homosexuality in the Nazi Party, Third Edition.* Keiser, OR: Founders Publishing Co., 1997, pp. 69-71.)

landish claims would wither under even cursory investigation." In the final analysis, they were "greatly surprised" by what they unearthed. The following is a smattering of what the authors stated are "indisputable historical facts."

The Prieuré de Sion, still operating today, "has been directed by a sequence of grand masters whose names are among the most illustrious in Western history and culture." The list of these men is shown in figure 3.2. "Acting in the shadows," and "behind the scenes," the PdS has orchestrated certain of the critical events in Western history. Currently, the secret society is highly "influential and plays a role in high-level international affairs as well as in the domestic affairs" of leading developed nations. *"To some extent it is responsible for the body of information disseminated since 1956."*⁶ (Emphasis added.)

The investigators offered several insightful sections detailing the lives and activities of many of the PdS's most famous, or infamous, grand masters. Among them was Robert Fludd, "among the most eloquent and influential exponents of Rosicrucian thought," who presided as the sixteenth grand master of the PdS. The Rosicrucians's secret "invisible" fraternity of German and French "initiates" promised that human knowledge, and subsequently the world, would be transformed in accordance with esoteric principles. The goal included a new epoch of spiritual expression in which human liberation would release the hitherto dormant "secrets of nature." Man would govern his and nature's destiny in accordance with all-pervading cosmic laws. Concurrently, Rosicrucian manifestos believed to have been written by Johann Valentin Anrea, the seventeenth PdS grand master, attacked the Catholic Church and the Holy Roman Empire for stifling such human potential.⁶

Later on in Paris, in 1802, PdS grand master Charles Nodier revealed his affections for a secret society that combined "Biblical and Pythagorean" elements.⁶

A review of modern Templar history would be incomplete without mention of the now documented connections between Hitler's Third

## Fig. 3.2. Grand Masters of the Prieuré de Sion

| | |
|---|---|
| Jean de Gisors | 1188–1220 |
| Marie de Saint-Clair | 1220–1266 |
| Guillaume de Gisors | 1266–1307 |
| Edouard de Bar | 1307–1336 |
| Jeanne de Bar | 1336–1351 |
| Jean de Saint-Clair | 1351–1366 |
| Blanche d'Evreux | 1366–1398 |
| Nicolas Flamel | 1398–1418 |
| René d' Anjou | 1418–1480 |
| Iolande de Bar | 1480–1483 |
| Sandro Filipepi | 1483–1510 |
| Leonardo da Vinci | 1510–1519 |
| Connétable de Bourbon | 1519–1527 |
| Ferdinand de Gonzague | 1527–1575 |
| Louis de Nevers | 1575–1595 |
| Robert Fludd | 1595–1637 |
| J. Valentin Andrea | 1637–1654 |
| Robert Boyle | 1654–1691 |
| Isaac Newton | 1691–1727 |
| Charles Radclyffe | 1727–1746 |
| Charles de Lorraine | 1746–1780 |
| Maximilian de Lorraine | 1780–1801 |
| Charles Nodier | 1801–1844 |
| Victor Hugo | 1844–1885 |
| Claude Debussy | 1885–1918 |
| Jean Cocteau | 1918–* |

* List appeared in the *Dossiers secrets* by Henri Lobineau of planche no. 4., of the Ordre de Sion. These individuals were referred to as the *Nautonniers*—the old French word that meant "navigator" or "helmsman." From: Baigent M, Leigh R, and Lincoln H. *Holy Blood Holy Grail*. New York: Dell, 1983, p. 131.

Reich and: 1) a Templar evolved group called the Soverign Military Order of Malta, or SMOM, 2) the Vatican, 3) Rockefeller oil and banking, and 4) American intelligence.

In *The Secret War Against the Jews*,[7] authors John Loftus and Mark Aarons summarized these ties and related events thusly:

> In 1936 the Rockefellers entered into partnership with Dulles's Nazi front, the Schröder Bank of New York, which . . . was the key institution in the Fascist economic "miracle." In 1939 the Rockefeller-controlled Chase National Bank secured $25 million for Nazi Germany and supplied Berlin with information on ten thousand Nazi sympathizers in the United States. Except for a few months' interruption, the Rockefeller-owned Standard Oil of New Jersey company shipped oil to the Nazis through Spain all throughout the war. The roster of the Rockefeller's known pro-Nazi behavior is horrendous. . . . [I]n 1942 Senator Harry Truman described the behavior of the Rockefellers' company as treasonous. . . . [In a related court case, Judge Clark ruled] "Standard Oil can be considered an enemy national in view of its relationships with I. G. Farben after the United States and Germany had become active enemies. . . Despite the fact that Rockefeller sat on the Proclaimed List Committee and was in charge of Latin American intelligence, he turned a blind eye to Standard's shipments of South American oil to Hitler. . . .
>
> By 1947 the Rockefeller publicity machine had things under control, notwithstanding what Judge Clark might have said. Then the Jew[ish intelligence network leaders] arrived with their dossier. They had [Nelson Rockefeller's] . . . Swiss bank records with the Nazis, his signature on correspondence setting up the German cartel in South America, transcripts of his conversations with Nazi agents during the war, and, finally, evidence of his complicity in helping Allen Dulles smuggle Nazi war criminals and money from the Vatican to Argentina.[7]

According to other reputable investigators, and published documents, the exfiltration of Nazis began as a way to protect the German intelligence networks—the Gehlen Org and Merk Net—from being captured or exposed. The Central Intelligence Agency (CIA) was subsequently established from the U.S. military's Office of Strategic Services, the OSS, as a cover organization for these powerful groups. This program was initially called "Operation Sunshine" and then "Project: Paperclip."[8]

Loftus and Aarons added:

> By 1947 the Vatican "Ratline," as it was called by U.S. intelligence, was the single largest smuggling route for Nazi war criminals. Nearly all the major war criminals, from Adolf Eichmann to Pavelic, ended up following Dulles's money route from the Vatican to Argentina. The lower-level Nazis wound up in a variety of countries, including Syria, Egypt, the United States, Britain, Canada, and Australia, although several big-time criminals emigrated to those countries too. For years Angleton and Dulles worked to hide the massive smuggling network at Draganovic's headquarters, San Girolamo, in Rome . . . Draganovic's wartime boss was Ante Pavelic, the Fascist leader of Croatia and one of the most wanted war criminals of World War II. In 1946 the CIC [U.S. Counterintelligence Corp.] began an investigation, code-named "Operation Circle," to explore the murky ties between the Vatican and fugitive Nazis.[7]

Other escapees included Josepf Mengele—the "Angel of Death," Klaus Barbie—the "Butcher of Lyon," and Erich Traub—Hitler's top viral and bacteriological disease specialist "in charge of biological warfare for the Reich Research Institute." Traub was brought to America, paid at least $65,000 annually, plus benefits, to work for the United States Naval Biological Laboratory that later affiliated with the University of California.[9]

## The Templars and the Nazis

How Allen Dulles persuaded President Truman to form the CIA was based on the leverage of Reinhard Gehlen, head of the Gehlen Org and a ranking official in the Sovereign Military Order of Malta (SMOM). Gehlen, and his affiliated organizations, maintained inconceivable financial and political influence.[10]

The SMOM evolved from the Knights Templar following the fall of Jerusalem. Then the Knights of the Order of St. John fled the Holy Land and established themselves on various Mediterranean islands whose names became part of their titles. Author of *Secret Societies and Their Power in the 20th Century*, Jan van Helsing, explained:

They were first called the "Knights of Rhodes," then the "Knights of Malta." They became an amazing military and naval force in the Mediterranean until they were defeated by Napoleon in 1789. In 1834 their headquarters had been transferred to Rome, and today they are known as the SMOM or the "Maltese Cross." Members include: the deceased William Casey (Ex-CIA Director 1981-87), Alexander Haig (former U. S. Secretary of State), Lee Iacocca (Past Chairman of Chrysler Corp.), James Buckley (Radio Free Europe), John McCone (CIA Director under Kennedy), Alexandre de Marenches (Head of the French Secret Service) and Valerie Giscard d'Estaing (former President of France.)[11]

Francoise Hervet, the pseudonym of a researcher who spent many years investigating the SMOM, further revealed:

Representing initially the most powerful and reactionary segments of the European aristocracy, for nearly a thousand years beginning with the early crusades of the Twelfth Century, it has organized, funded, and led military operations against states and ideas deemed threatening to its power. It is probably safe to say that the several thousand Knights of SMOM, principally in Europe, North, Central and South America, comprise the largest most consistently powerful and reactionary membership of any organization in the world today. . . .

To be a Knight, one must not only be from wealthy, aristocratic lineage, one must also have a psychological worldview which is attracted to the "crusader mentality" of these "warrior monks." Participating in SMOM—including its initiation ceremonies and feudal ritual dress—members embrace a certain caste/class mentality; they are sociologically and psychologically predisposed to function as the "shock troops" of Catholic reaction. And this is precisely the historical role the Knights have played in the war against Islam, against the protestant "heresy," and against the Soviet "Evil Empire."

The Catholic Right and the Knights of Malta, in particular Baron Franz von Papan, played a critical role in Hitler's assumption of power and the launching of the Third Reich's Twentieth Century Crusade.[10]

Hervet further explained that the "SMOM's influence in Germany survived World War II intact." On November 17, 1948, Gehlen received the Grand Cross of Merit award, one of the organization's highest honors. Subsequently, he was installed by American intelligence officials as "the first chief of West Germany's equivalent of the CIA, the *Bundesnachtrichtdienst,* under West German Chancellor Adenauer." Adenauer had received "the Magistral Grand Cross personally from SMOM Grand Master Prince Chigi."[10]

Gehlen's brother, in the meantime, "had already been in Rome serving as Secretary to Thun Hohenstein. Conveniently for Reinhard, who was [then] negotiating with American intelligence for the preservation of his Nazi colleagues, Thun Hohenstein was Chairman of one of SMOM's grand magistral charities, the Institute for Associated Emigrations." Hohenstein thus arranged for "two thousand SMOM passports to be printed for political refugees."[10]

Meanwhile, throughout the war, another SMOM member, Joseph J. Larkin, the vice president of the Rockefeller-owned Chase Manhattan Bank, had managed to keep the financial institution open in Nazi-occupied Paris. Larkin "had received the Order of the Grand Cross of the Knights of Malta from Pope Pius XI in 1928. He was an ardent supporter of General Franco and, by extension, Hilter."[10]

## Financial Interests and Intelligence Ties

Financial motives, besides ideological, were at the heart of the SMOM and Nazi–American alliance.

Investigative journalist P. D. Scott critically reviewed two books by authors with wartime intelligence backgrounds—one by Ladislas Farago entitled *Aftermath: Bormann and the Fourth Reich* (New York: Avon Books, 1975) and the other by William Stevenson, *The Bormann Brotherhood* (New York: Harcourt, Brace, Jovanovich, 1973). He gleaned enlightening facts about the financial assets of the Nazi bureaucracy and Martin Bormann, Hitler's deputy and party chief. The books, Scott wrote:

> . . . point to the role of the extensive postwar assets collected or plundered by the SS and Bormann. This came from three sources: the proceeds from the SS forgery of British pound notes ("Operation Bernhard"), the looting of Jews and other Nazi

victims, and, most significantly, the corporate contributions to a special fund set up to guarantee the survival of German multinationals abroad after the impending collapse of Hitler. Soon after the war, OSS found the extensive documentation of a meeting in Strasbourg on August 10, 1944 to establish this fund, between representatives of the SS, Nazi Party, and firms like Krupp, I. G. Farben and Messerschmidt.

But as the Cold War encouraged the U.S. to see the German corporate presence in Latin America in a more friendly light, the role of these firms in providing new careers for war criminals abroad was ignored. In fact, it was the key to the postwar status of the *Kameraden* [the comrades network].[12]

After the war, documented evidence revealed that perhaps as many as 2,000 Nazi officials, many of them doctors and scientists, made their way into corporations operating in Latin America and the United States with the help of American intelligence, assistance from the Vatican, and the SMOM.

Moreover, American intelligence played a major role in funding much of the Nazi escape program by protecting the proceeds of "Operation Bernhard." Western intelligence officials knew enough about the Nazi currency forging operation to protect the postwar British pound. Thus, before the British government recalled the old note and issued new ones, the SS profits were assured in the neighborhood of $300 million which "had been converted to genuine currency."[13] Much of which apparently made its way to the Vatican, and from there into Joseph Larkin's hands at Rockefeller's Chase Bank in Paris.[10]

The man charged with laundering this part of the Nazi war chest was Friederich Schwend. Between 1945 and 1946 Schwend became "an important link in establishing SS escape routes," the main route was through the Vatican.[13]

Further regarding this Vatican–Nazi connection, Nazi-tracking authors Farago and Bower provided the following details:

Indeed the Vatican did have a program underway for the exfiltration of anticommunists. This was the work of Bishop Alois Hudal of the Collegium Teutonicum, a priest close both to Pius XII and the future Paul VI as well as a public admirer of the

Third Reich. After an interview in Rome with former Gestapo Chief Heinrich Müller, Hudal had begun the work of supplying Vatican documentation for such prominent fugitives as Müller, Eichmann, and perhaps Martin Bormann.[14] It was Hudal who gave . . . the necessary introductions to the International Red Cross and other officials who, "for a bribe, could smooth the fugitive's path."[15]

The combined efforts of Hudal and others helped hundreds of leading Nazis to escape.[13,16]

Farago detailed Heinrich Müller's exodus. Driven from Merano, north of Italy, to Rome in Schwend's chauffeured Mercedes, he deposited some of the Nazi war chest at a Croatian seminary and made the historic contact with Bishop Hudal. In 1972, documents found in Schwend's possession reported that:

> The bulk of the money the bishop needed was placed at his disposal by . . . a financier named Friederich "Freddy" Merser, partner of Friederich Schwend in Operation Bernhard. The money came from the hoard Schwend had amassed in Swiss accounts.[17]

By 1948 the vast wealth that the Nazis and their partners had accumulated during the war had been reinvested. As detailed by the reputable CBS News correspondent, Paul Manning, in his book *Martin Bormann: Nazi in Exile*, that is precisely what Bormann did "when he set in motion the 'flight capital' scheme August 10, 1944, in Strasbourg. The treasure, the golden ring, he envisioned for the new Germany was the sophisticated distribution of national and corporate assets to safe havens . . ." Chief among them was the Merck pharmaceutical company.[18]

At the time, Merck's president, George W. Merck, was advising President Roosevelt as America's "biological weapons industry director."[19]

The Merck company received windfall "profits" from the Nazi war chest. This cash transfer, according to Manning's evidence, was specifically arranged to "help actualize Hitler's proclaimed 'vision of a thousand-year Third Reich [and] world empire.' This was outlined with clarity in a document called 'Neuordunung,' or 'New [World] Order,' that was accompanied by a letter of transmittal to the [Bormann-led] Ministry of Economics. It declared that a new order for the chemical [and pharmaceutical] industry of the world should supplement Hitler's New Order. . . ."[20]

In essence, the partners decided that a world chemical and pharmaceutical monopoly was necessary to eliminate undesirable populations, while making money, to most effectively create a "master race." Lucrative drugs and chemicals could be used to control minds, dull the senses, and insidiously eliminate unwanted people.

## The United Nations in the New World Order

Few today have ever heard of the word "eugenics." It is defined as the scientific investigation of genetic differences between the races, including the genetic predisposition for diseases to which the different races are more or less susceptible. Author Anton Chaitkin is perhaps the most authoritative source of information in this regard. In numerous reports he has detailed the intimate links between the Rockefellers and the eugenics movement.[21]

The Rockefeller Foundation, Chaitkin chronicled, became the prime promoter of depopulation activities by the Rockefeller-built United Nations. Moreover, evidence showed, "the foundation and its corporate, medical, and political associates organized the racial mass murder program[s] of Nazi Germany."[21]

More support for the Chaitkin exposés came from authors Loftus and Aarons. They not only detailed the Rockefeller–Nazi connections, but their influence over the United Nations since its inception. How this power was developed and exercised included the following:

In July 1940 [Defense Secretary James] Forrestal had offered Nelson Rockefeller the position of Coordinator of Inter-American Affairs, an intelligence shop, which Nelson himself had proposed should be set up, with himself, naturally, in charge. . . . All through the war, at least while Rockefeller was in charge, everything the Germans wanted in South America they got, from refueling stations to espionage bases. . . . Behind Rockefeller's rhetoric of taking measures in Latin America for the national defense stood a naked grab for profits. Under the cloak of his official position, Rockefeller and his cronies ["the Dulles-Forrestal clique"] would take over Britain's most valuable Latin American properties. If the British resisted, he would effectively block raw materials and food supplies desperately needed for Britain's fight against Hitler. . . . [I]n each country Rockefeller set up coordinating committees composed of reactionary executives from Standard Oil, General Electric, and United Fruit, which promptly bled South America dry. It was just the sort of thing that endeared Rockefeller to the State Department. In November 1944 he was asked to serve as assistant secretary of state for Latin American affairs. . . .

It was all a farce, of course. . . . Most of the South American dictators made a fortune from the Nazis during the war. These were the nations that were later to decide the fate of Israel in the United Nations.

Rockefeller's political and corporate strategy was to use his bloc of fascist nations to "buy" the majority vote at the UN to favor U.S.-sponsored resolutions. It was simple arithmetic. The Latin American bloc represented nineteen votes to Europe's nine. Rockefeller made no apologies for his strong-arm tactics, insisting that unless the United States "operated with a solid group in this hemisphere, we could not do what we wanted in the world front." In June 1945 Rockefeller was invited to attend the first UN conference in San Francisco, where his job was to control the Latin American delegation.

He was particularly effective at this job. The only problem was that Rockefeller was too preoccupied with representing the interests of big business, not the United States. With FDR dead, he acted as if the UN was *his* organization, bought and paid for. He could do whatever he wanted, and did, at least until he pushed President Truman beyond his limit.

For Harry Truman, Rockefeller's behavior over Argentina [and the Latin bloc overall] was the last straw. On August 23, 1945, a stunned Nelson Rockefeller left the White House, telling his friends, "He fired me!" For the next two years Rockefeller went back to making money, something he did extremely well. His partner in money-making just happened to be John Foster Dulles, a trustee of the Rockefeller Foundation and a fellow conspirator in smuggling Axis money to safety.[7]

## The Rockefellers, Nazis, Eugenics and the Freemasons

In 1909, Chaitkin recalled, John D. Rockefeller created the Rockefeller Foundation and, by 1929, had invested "$300 million worth of the family's controlling interest in the Standard Oil Company of New Jersey," now called Exxon, into the foundation's account.

According to Chaitkin, this money created the field of "Psychiatric Genetics," and funded the Kaiser Wilhelm Institute for Psychiatry and the Kaiser Wilhelm Institute for Anthropology, Eugenics and Human Heredity. The Rockefellers' chief executive in charge of these institutions "was the fascist Swiss psychiatrist Ernst Rudin, assisted by his proteges Otmar Verschuer and Franz J. Kallmann."[21]

In 1932, Chaitkin recounted, the British-led eugenics movement designated the Rockefellers' Dr. Rudin as the president of the worldwide Eugenics Federation.

Only a few months later Hitler rose to power and "the Rockefeller-Rudin apparatus became a section of the Nazi state." Rudin then headed the "Racial Hygiene Society."[21]

Rudin and his staff, "as part of the Task Force of Heredity Experts chaired by SS chief Heinrich Himmler, drew up the sterilization law." In the United States, this law was described as a "model law" and was adopted in July, 1933, as published in the September, 1933, *Eugenical News* (USA), with Hitler's signature attached.

Verschuer and his assistant, Auschwitz medical chief, Josef Mengele, jointly authored reports for special courts to reinforce Rudin's "racial purity law against cohabitation of Aryans and non-Aryans." They also produced films to help sell their racial-cleansing ideas.

"Under the Nazis," Chaitkin noted, "the German chemical company I. G. Farben and the Rockefellers' Standard Oil of New Jersey were effectively a single firm, merged in hundreds of cartel arrangements. I. G. Farben was led, up until 1937, by the Warburg family, Rockefeller's partner in banking and in the design of Nazi German eugenics."[21]

During the war, I. G. Farben built a huge factory at Auschwitz to capitalize on Standard–Farben patents to make gasoline from coal with the help of concentration camp slave labor. The SS was then assigned to select and guard the inmates deemed fit for I. G. Farben's work-force. Those judged unfit were killed.

Moreover, Chaitkin reported additional Rockefeller-linked Nazi atrocities:

> In 1936, Rockefeller's Dr. Franz Kallmann interrupted his study of hereditary degeneracy and emigrated to America because he was half-Jewish. Kallmann went to New York and established the Medical Genetics Department of the New York State Psychiatric Institute. The *Scottish Rite of Freemasonry* published Kallman's study of over 1,000 cases of schizophrenia, which tried to prove its hereditary basis. In the book, Kallmann thanked his longtime boss and mentor Rudin. [Emphasis/underline added]

> Kallmann's book, published in 1938 in the USA and Nazi Germany, was used by the T4 unit as a rationalization to begin, in 1939, the murder of mental patients and various "defective" people, perhaps most of them children. Gas and lethal injections were used to kill 250,000 under this program, in which the staffs for a broader murder program were desensitized and trained.[21]

Chaitkin further detailed links between Rockefeller interests and the horrific medical experiments conducted at Auschwitz.

In 1943, Josef Mengele's superior, the director of Rockefeller's Kaiser Wilhelm Institute for Anthropology, Eugenics and Human Heredity in Berlin, Otmar Verschuer, secured funds for genetic experiments from the German Research Council. In a progress report, Verschuer wrote for the Council, he stated, "My co-researcher in this research is my assistant, the anthropologist and physician, Mengele. . . . With the permission of the Reichsfuehrer SS Himmler, anthropological research is being undertaken on the various racial groups in the concentration camps and blood samples will be sent to my laboratory for investigation."

Mengele and Verschuer were especially interested in studying twins during their "special protein" investigations that required daily blood drawings.

Horrific experiments followed. Needles were stabbed into people's eyes for eye color experiments. Others were injected with foreign blood and infectious agents. Limbs and organs were commonly removed, occasionally without anesthetics. Women were sterilized, men were castrated, and sexes were surgically altered. Thousands were butchered and their heads, eyeballs, limbs, and organs were delivered to Mengele, Verschuer, and the other Rockefeller-linked contingent at the Kaiser Wilhelm Institute.

Later, in 1946, Verschuer, according to Chaitkin, requested assistance from the Bureau of Human Heredity in London to keep his "scientific research" going. A year later, the Bureau moved to Copenhagen and its new Danish facility was built, once again, with Rockefeller money. It was here that the first International Congress in Human Genetics convened. A decade later Verschuer became a member of the American Eugenics Society—an organizational clone of the Rockefeller Population Council.

According to Chaitkin, Dr. Kallmann directed the American Eugenics Society from 1954 to 1965. He helped rescue Verschuer by testifying at his denazification hearings. And it was Kallmann who created the American Society of Human Genetics, organizers of the "Human Genome Project"—currently a $3 billion effort to map the genetics of humanity along with each race's specific disease susceptibilities.

During the 1950s, "the Rockefellers reorganized the U.S. eugenics movement in their own family offices, with spin-off population-control and abortion groups," and the Eugenics Society's address changed to the Society for the Study of Social Biology, its current name. Moreover, "with support from the Rockefellers, the Eugenics Society (England) set up a subcommittee called the International Planned Parenthood Federation, which for 12 years had no other address than the Eugenics Society."[21]

In conclusion, Chaitkin observed, "the Rockefeller Foundation had long financed the eugenics movement in England" and the genetics industry in America. A disturbing legacy for "the private international apparatus which," along with substantial support from the Scottish Rite Freemasons, "has set the world up for a global holocaust under the UN flag."

The threat of "global holocaust" to which Chaitkin referred currently includes the genetic (or genocidal) biotechnology that will be addressed later in this book—a form of bioterrorism over which Rockefeller subordinates currently exercise immense control.

## Rockefeller Blood Banking and Freemasonry

It was apparently no random "coincidence" that the Rockefeller family gained so much control over international banking, including blood banking. Laurance Rockefeller, as will be discussed later, assembled the New York City blood council that evolved to largely control the international blood banking industry.[22]

The importance of blood and blood lines is a recurring theme in this book as it is for highest level Freemasons. According to the "Structure of Freemasonry," as seen in figures 3.3 and 3.4, the "Order of the Red Cross" stands third in the top echelon of power just behind the SMOM and the "Order of the Knights Templar." Religious scholars cross their Bibles with red marker ribbons today unaware of the symbolism—the Masonic importance of the pure red blood line.

Beginning with the Ordre de la Rose-Croix Veritas, more commonly known as the Rose-Croix, or Rosicrucians, the red (or rose) cross was adopted as an identifying symbol of the Masonic tradition. According to Baigent *et al.,*[23] this practice began in 1188 when the Prieuré de Sion accepted the ceremonies of Ormus, said to have been an Egyptian sage, mystic, and "a Gnostic 'adept' in Alexandria"—a "hotbed of mystical activity" during the first century A. D. Here Ormus is believed to have exchanged theosophies with Judaic, Zoroastrian, Mithraic, Hermetic, neo-Platonic and *Pythagorean* scholars. The name "Ormus" was synonymous with "the principle of light" in Zoroastrian and Gnostic history.[23] Thus, Ormus was not only the originator of the red cross symbol, but he apparently helped propagate the term "Illuminati."

Over time, "Illuminati" has come to mean the few powerfully illumined, or en-light-ened souls, who are said to draw their power from "Lucifer." Illuminati, in fact, according to *Webster's Dictionary*, is derived from the French word "Lucifer" meaning "light bearing." Webster also cross references Lucifer to the word "light."

According to *Secret Societies* author Jan van Helsing, "Illuminati" came into more common use during the 14th century in Germany, where it applied to the high initiates of the "Brotherhood of the Snake"—a "savant brotherhood that had subscribed to the dissemination of spiritual knowledge and the attainment of spiritual freedom from . . . extraterrestrials" more than 3,000 years before Christ.[24]

The Latin name of "Illuminati" and the biblical term for snake have related origins and definitions. The word snake derives from "nahash," which came from the root word "nhsh" meaning to "discover," or "decipher." In Latin, "illuminare" meant "to illumine," or "to recognize," or "know."

Thus, the snake used by organized medicine today, as seen in figure 3.5, became a symbol of evolving illuminance or intelligence. Looking back at the Templar's symbol in figure 3.1, the snake began and ended with a swastika. Additionally related is the fact that the Rockefellers established a monopoly over American medicine in the 1920s.[22]

Citing van Helsing's research, "One of the main branches of the Illuminati in Germany were the mystical Rosicrucians who were introduced at the beginning of the 9th century by Charlemagne."[24]

# Fig. 3.3. The Structure of Freemasonry of the Scottish and York Rites

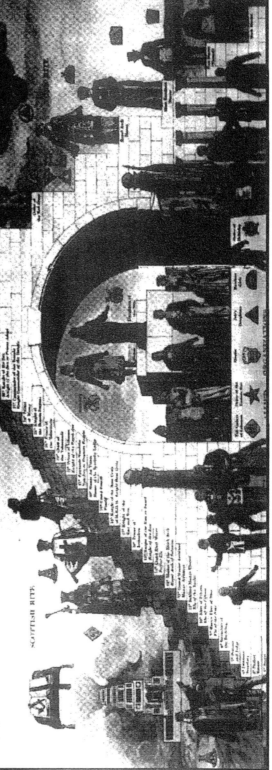

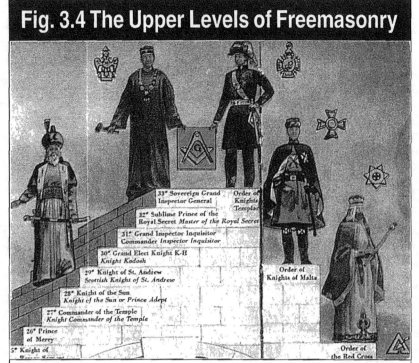

# Fig. 3.4 The Upper Levels of Freemasonry

33° Sovereign Grand Inspector General

Order of Knights Templar

32° Sublime Prince of the Royal Secret *Master of the Royal Secret*

31° Grand Inspector Inquisitor Commander Inspector Inquisitor

30° Grand Elect Knight K-H Knight Kadosh

29° Knight of St. Andrew Scottish Knights of St. Andrew

28° Knight of the Sun Knight of the Sun or Prince Adept

27° Commander of the Temple Knight Commander of the Temple

26° Prince of Mercy

5° Knight of

Order of Knights of Malta

Order of the Red Cross

The upper levels of Freemasonry include the 32°called the "Sublime Prince of the Royal Secret *Master of the Royal Secret*," and the 33° of "Sovereign Grand Inspector General" as seen on the upper left of the Masonic structure. The top three orders shown on the right include: "Order of the Red Cross," "Order of the Knights of Malta," and the highest "Order of Knights Templar." From *Life Magazine*, October 8, 1956.

Several other authors relayed that the Illuminati and the Rosicrucians were the driving force behind the esoteric religious movements of the 17th and 18th centuries. According to *Webster's Dictionary*, "Christian *Rosenkreutz* (NL Rosae Crucis)" was the "reputed 15th cent. founder of the movement (1624) . . . a devotee of esoteric wisdom with emphasis on psychic and spiritual enlightenment. . . ." Their manifestos, fervently supported by the liberal factions of Protestants in Europe, inflamed the leaders of the Catholic Church and the Jesuits. "Among the most eloquent and influential exponents of Rosicrucian thought was Robert Fludd"—the Prieuré de Sion's sixteenth grand master.[23]

The Jesuit and Church backlashes that resulted in the persecution of the Cathars and Templars also helped spark Martin Luther's rebellion. "Martin Luther also had close links to both the Illuminati and the Rosicrucians," wrote van Helsing. Luther's friends recognized the Rosicrucian seal he wore that contained a rose and a cross with his initials. "After Luther's death, his confessional community was supported by Francis Bacon," the highest-ranking Rosicrucian in England, and, as mentioned previously, the general architect of the King James Bible.[3]

## The Red Shield or Rothschild

"Give me control over a nation's currency and I don't care who makes the laws!" asserted Mayer Amschel Rothschild a century later. Rothschild (German meaning "red shield") changed his name from Bauer to more easily relate to royalty, including Prince William IX of Hesse-Hanau, who favored The House of Rothschild for banking his massive wealth. Bauer chose "Rothschild," likely respecting the Freemason symbology he came to know while attending the German order's Masonic Temple with Prince William.[24]

At that time, Francois de Lorraine's Vienna court became, according to *Holy Blood Holy Grail* authors, "Europe's Masonic capital and a center for a broad spectrum of other esoteric interests as well. Francois himself, in fact, was a practicing alchemist with an alchemical laboratory in the imperial palace, the Hofburg."[23] Turning "base metals into gold,"[25] as was de Lorraine's speculative practice, likely piqued the interest of Rothschild who sent his son Salomon to Vienna where he is known to have joined the Freemasons, and opened up a banking branch.[24]

At the same time, Rothschild's four other sons established banking houses throughout Europe. Amshel went to Berlin, Kalman to Naples, Nathan, the eldest son, to London, and Jakob went to Paris where Charles Nodier, the grand master of the Prieuré de Sion, then served.[26]

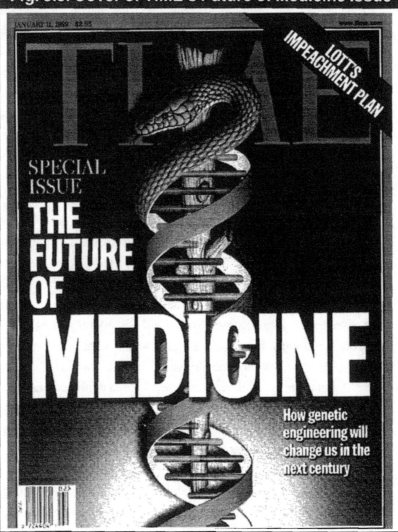

Fig. 3.5. Cover of *TIME*'s Future of Medicine Issue

Cover of the *TIME* magazine, January 11, 1999, "Special Issue" featuring "The Future of Medicine: How genetic engineering will change us in the next century." Graphic displays the use of symbols including the snake, the tree of life, and a strand of double helix DNA.

By the early 1800s, the Rothschild banking dynasty largely controlled European currency markets while Nathan maintained substantial control over English wealth through his Bank of England. Almost a half century had passed since the Rothschilds established and commanded, with the help of Adam Weishaupt, The Secret Order of the Bavarian Illuminati at Ingostadt. Thereafter, the Rothschild family wielded major influence over other important secret lodges including those in America.[24]

A list of the main known organizations of the Illuminati is shown in figure 3.6. The Rothschilds played a commanding role in virtually all of them.

## Cecil Rhodes and His "New World Order" Scholars

On February 5, 1891, several wealthy Englishmen, Lord Rothschild included, joined Cecil Rhodes to found the Committee of 300. The main objective of the group was to promulgate a worldwide British plutocracy. The committee structured itself after the Society of Jesus—the Jesuit Order. Later, Hitler's SS would do the same. In Rhodes's own words, here's what the Committee of 300 intended and why:

> There is a destiny now possible to us—the highest ever set before a nation to be accepted or refused. We are still undegenerate in race; a race mingled of the best northern blood. We are not yet dissolute in temper, but still have the firmness to govern, and the grace to obey. We have been taught a religion of pure mercy, which we must either now betray, or learn to defend by fulfilling. And we are rich in an inheritance of honour, bequeathed to us through a thousand years of noble history, which it should be our daily thirst to increase with splendid avarice, so that Englishmen, if it be a sin to covet honour, should be the most offending souls alive. . . .

> If we had retained America there would be at the present moment many millions more of English living. I contend that we are the finest race in the world and that the more of the world we inhabit the better it is for the human race. Just fancy those parts that are at present inhabited by the most despicable specimen of human beings, what an alteration there would be in them if they were brought under Anglo-Saxon influence. Look again at the extra employment a new country added to our dominion gives. I

contend that every acre added to our territory means, in the future, birth to some more of the English race who otherwise would not be brought into existence.

In Rhodes's first "will and testimony" he gave his purpose more specifics:

The extension of British rule throughout the world, the perfecting of a system of emigration from the United Kingdom and of colonization by British subjects of all lands wherein the means of livelihood are attainable by energy, labour and enterprise, and especially the occupation by British settlers of the entire Continent of Africa, the Holy Land, the valley of the Euphrates, the islands of Cyprus and Candia, the whole of South America, the islands of the Pacific not heretofore possessed by Great Britain, the whole of the Malay Archipelago, the seaboard of China and Japan, the ultimate recovery of the United States of America as an integral part of the British Empire, the consolidation of the whole Empire, the inauguration of a system of Colonial Representation in the Imperial Parliament which may tend to weld together the disjointed members of the Empire, and finally the foundation of so great a power as to hereafter render wars impossible and promote the best interests of humanity.[27]

Much of what is known about Cecil Rhodes also came from eminent scholar and historian, Professor Carroll Quigley—President Clinton's teacher and mentor at Georgetown University during the mid-1960s. During Clinton's acceptance speech before the Democratic Presidential Nominating Convention on July 16, 1992, the Life Member of the Masonic Order of DeMolay for Boys, and Future President of the United States, proclaimed: "As a teenager I heard John Kennedy's summons to citizenship. And then as a student at Georgetown, I heard that call clarified by a professor named Carroll Quigley . . . "[24, 28]

More recently, Professor Quigley's publications were reviewed by Dr. Stanley Monteith, a medical physician who has extensively published on the threat to American life posed by Rhodes's initiatives, which have culminated into what is currently termed the "New World Order." Dr. Monteith pointed out that the Rhodes Scholars—as most American presidents, including Clinton, have been since Rhodes died

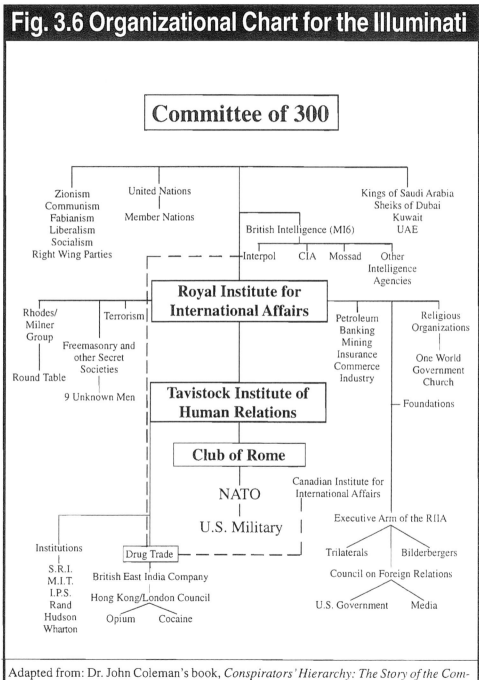

# Fig. 3.6 Organizational Chart for the Illuminati

## Committee of 300

Zionism
Communism
Fabianism
Liberalism
Socialism
Right Wing Parties

United Nations

Member Nations

British Intelligence (MI6)

Interpol    CIA    Mossad

Kings of Saudi Arabia
Sheiks of Dubai
Kuwait
UAE

Other
Intelligence
Agencies

Rhodes/
Milner
Group

Terrorism

Freemasonry and
other Secret
Societies

Round Table

9 Unknown Men

### Royal Institute for International Affairs

Petroleum
Banking
Mining
Insurance
Commerce
Industry

Religious
Organizations

One World
Government
Church

Foundations

### Tavistock Institute of Human Relations

### Club of Rome

NATO

Canadian Institute for
International Affairs

U.S. Military

Executive Arm of the RIIA

Trilaterals    Bilderbergers

Council on Foreign Relations

Institutions

S.R.I.
M.I.T.
I.P.S.
Rand
Hudson
Wharton

Drug Trade

British East India Company

Hong Kong/London Council

Opium    Cocaine

U.S. Government    Media

Adapted from: Dr. John Coleman's book, *Conspirators' Hierarchy: The Story of the Committee of 300*. Carson City, NV: American West Publishers, 1992, p. 265.

and left his vast diamond and gold mining fortune to his plutocratic cause—were part of the British Imperialistic plot.[28] In *The Anglo-American Establishment*, Quigley's revelations provided a sense of continuity between the Freemasonry practice of forming secret societies, including the "Skull and Bones," and the grooming of American presidents and foreign policies:

> The Rhodes Scholarships, established by the terms of Cecil Rhodes's seventh will, are known to everyone. What is not so widely known is that Rhodes in five previous wills left his fortune to form a secret society . . . And what does not seem to be known to anyone is that this secret society was created by Rhodes and his principal trustee, Lord Milner, and continues to exist to this day.[29]

In another work highlighting the evolution of President Clinton's role in Rhodes's scheme to undermine America and place the world again under British control in the "New World Order," Rhodes's letter to his close friend W. T. Stead is revealing. In the autumn of 1890 Rhodes wrote:

> Please remember the key of my idea discussed with you is a Society, copied from the Jesuits as to organization . . . an idea which ultimately [leads] to the *cessation of all wars* and one language throughout the world. . . . The only thing feasible to carry this idea out is a secret [society] one gradually absorbing the wealth of the world to be devoted to such an object. . . . Fancy the charm to young America . . . to share in a scheme to take the government of the whole world![30] [Emphasis added.]

Dr. Dennis Cuddy, the source of the above citation, provided the additional perspective that Rhodes's "universal peace" was scheduled to begin, according to Rhodes, "after one-hundred years." It is interesting, he noted, that in the autumn of 1990 President Bush began to publicly herald his "New World Order" concept for universal peace and cooperation.[30]

Regarding Rhodes's Jesuit reference, it should be recalled that Adam Weishaupt's design for the Rothschild controlled Bavarian Illuminati followed a similar logic and structure. Gary Allen, in *None Dare Call It Conspiracy*, described Weishaupt's efforts in this regard thusly:

It should be noted that the originator of this type of secret society was Adam Weishaupt, the monster who founded the Order of the Bavarian Illuminati on May 1, 1776, for the purpose of conspiracy to control the world. The role of Weishaupt's Illuminists in such horrors as the Reign of Terror is unquestioned, and the techniques of the Bavarian Illuminati have long been recognized as models for Communist methodology. Weishaupt also used the structure of the Society of Jesus (the Jesuits) as his model, and rewrote the Code in Masonic terms.[24]

In his second book *Tragedy and Hope: A History of the World in Our Time*, Professor Quigley revealed that following Rhodes's death, Lord Milner formed an organization in England called The Round Table Group (See figure 3.6.), likely after the legendary Knights of the Round Table, in an effort to actualize Rhodes's will. "Some years later," Dr. Monteith recalled, "The Round Table created a second front in the United States . . . [that] came to be known as the Council of Foreign Relations (CFR)." He documented this from Quigley's writing, "In New York it was known as the Council on Foreign Relations, and was a front for J. P. Morgan . . . in association with the very small American Round Table Group."[31]

## The Rhodes–Rothschild Connection to British Intelligence

As American Secretary to the Rhodes Trustees, Frank Aydelotte recalled that, "In 1888 Rhodes made his third will . . . leaving everything to Lord Rothschild"—his mining enterprise financier.

Later, for strategic reasons, Lord Rothschild's son-in-law, Lord Rosebury, replaced his elder as Rhodes's final heir.

Professor Quigley explained that on behalf of the Rothschild and Rhodes dynasties, the "secret society" inner structures were shielded by successively larger outer circles. The central part of the structure was established by March, 1891, using Rhodes's money. Rothschild trustee Lord Alfred Milner directed the organization—The Round Table—that "worked behind the scenes at the highest levels of British government, influencing foreign policy and England's involvement and conduct of WWI" and later WWII.[24]

According to van Helsing, the British Secret Intelligence Service (MI6) evolved largely from efforts of members of the Committee of 300 and The Round Table. Other sources reported that the MI6 exercises far greater control in the world than virtually anyone realizes. More wiretaps in the United States, for instance, are administered on behalf of the MI6 than the CIA. In this regard, Loftus and Aarons reported that, "for the last fifty years, virtually every Jewish citizen, organization, and charity in the world has been the victim of electronic surveillance by Great Britain, with the knowing and willing assistance of the intelligence services of the United States."[7]

To set the stage for the first World War, The Round Table directors developed the "Royal Institute for International Affairs," or RIIA. It was also known as "Chatham House" and had among its members Lords Albert Grey and Arnold Toynbee. The latter was known as the éminence grise[32] of the MI6. (See figure 3.6.)

*Webster's Dictionary* defines "éminence grise" as the "gray eminence, a nickname of Père Joseph (François du Tremblay) 1638, Fr. monk and diplomat, confidant of Cardinal Richelieu who was known as Éminence Rouge (red eminence)," and "a confidential agent; esp: one *exercising unsuspected or unofficial power.* A related term is "grisaille" defined as a "decoration in tones of a single color and esp. gray designed to produce a three-dimensional effect."

Apparently the Masonic influence in the affairs of the world's leading intelligence organization has been striking and esoteric. Even the name "MI6" reflected knowledge of the ancient mystical arcana as you will soon see.

It was Lord Toynbee of the MI6 who, following "brainstorming" sessions conducted at the Wellington House into ways to condition the public into accepting World War I, delivered the orders from the Committee of 300.[24] Other famous members of the Committee of 300, past and present, are listed in figure 3.7.

Another leading committee member, Lord Rothmere, used his newspapers to test the Wellington House "social conditioning" strategies. Following a six-month test period, it was learned that eighty-seven percent of the public had formed their opinions without using critical or rational judgement—the intended result. Thereafter, the English working class, according to van Helsing, "was subjected to sophisticated propaganda methods to convince them that they had to send their sons by the thousands to their deaths" in WWI.

In response, Teddy Roosevelt, the 26th President of the United States, complained during his 1912 election campaign, "Behind the visible government there is an invisible government upon the throne that owes the people no loyalty and recognizes no responsibility. To destroy this invisible government, to undo the ungodly union between corrupt business and corrupt politics is the task of a statesman."[24]

## Freemasonry and High Finance in America

By the early 1900s, the Masonic-linked "secret societies," including the CFR, held a stranglehold on the principle American social, economic, political, as well as religious institutions.

In fact, the solidification of Freemason power in America began in 1776 around the time Adam Weishaupt was establishing the Order of the Bavarian Illuminati on behest of the Rothschilds. According to van Helsing, the founding of the United States of America was the result of the secret plan carried out by Freemasons beginning in the 17th century. The American War of Independence had been organized by Freemasons. The U.S. Constitution was penned and signed by Freemasons. Almost a third of American presidents have been Freemasons. The Great Seal of the United States with the pyramid and all seeing eye, the bald eagle that replaced the phoenix, the original thirteen states, stars and stripes, were all adopted symbols of Freemasonry. Though they had been put in place by Weishaupt to convey Rothschild wishes, the symbolism dated back to the Masons of ancient Egypt. The Illuminated pyramid on the American dollar bill was the design of Philip Rothschild as Ayn Rand, his lover, divulged in *Atlas Shrugged*.[24]

Following the Revolutionary War, the American Masonic lodges split from the Mother Grand Lodge of England and formed the American Grand Lodge. This composed the York Rite with ten degrees (the tenth is the Templar degree) and the Scottish Rite with thirty-three.[24]

Although early American political leaders Benjamin Franklin and Thomas Jefferson heavily favored private centralized banking, in 1790 Alexander Hamilton was appointed secretary of the treasury, and reformed policy heavily favoring his silent benefactors Mayer Amschel Rothschild and his sons. A year later, Hamilton established the "First National Bank of the United States" fashioned after the "Bank of England." It was controlled by the Rothschilds.[24]

After Mayer Rothschild's death in 1812, Nathan took control over the family fortune and opened the "Nathan Mayer Rothschild & Sons Bank" in London, Vienna, Paris, and Berlin. In America it was represented by J. P. Morgan & Co., August Belmont & Co., and Kuhn Loeb & Company.[24]

During the American Civil War, the Rothschilds financed both sides of the conflict. "The reasons leading to this civil war," van Helsing wrote, "were almost completely due to the actions and provocations of Rothschild agents." One of the troublemakers, founder of the "Knights of the Golden Circle," was George Bickley. Bickley extolled the advantages of succession from the Union by the Confederate States. On the other side, the Rothschild–J. P. Morgan and August Belmont banks financed the Union. In addition, Rothschild's London bank supported the North, while its Paris bank funded the South. It was a glorious business.

President Lincoln finally caught wind of the scam and withheld immense interest payments to the Rothschilds. He then petitioned Congress to print "greenbacks"—dollars over which only the Union held printing power. In response, the furious Rothschilds arranged for his assassination. Lincoln was murdered by John Wilkes Booth on April 14, 1865. Booth was freed from jail due to the efforts of the Knights of

## Fig. 3.7. Famous Members of the "Committee of 300"

Balfour, Arthur
Brandt, Willy
Bulwer-Lytton, Edward
Bundy, McGeorge
Bush, George
Carrington, Lord
Chamberlain, Huston Stewart
Constanti, House of Orange
Delano, Family
Drake, Sir Francis
Du Pont, Family
Forbes, John M.
Frederik IX, King of Denmark
George, Lloyd
Grey, Sir Edward
Haig, Sir Douglas
Harriman, Averill
Hohenzollern, House of
House, Col. Edward Mandell
Inchcape, Lord
Kissinger, Henry
Lever, Sir Harold
Lippmann, Walter
Lackhart, Bruce
Loudon, Sir John
Mazzini, Giuseppe

Mellon, Andrew
Milner, Lord Alfred
Mitterand, Francois
Morgan, J. P.
Norman, Montague
Oppenheimer, Sir Harry
Palme, Olof
Princess Beatrix
Queen Elizabeth II
Queen Juliana
Rainier, Prince
Retinger, Joseph
Rhodes, Cecil
Rockefeller, David
Rothmere, Lord
Rothschild, Baron Edmond de
Shultz, George
Spellman, Cardinal
Thyssen-Bornemisza, Baron
Vanderbilt, Family
von Finck, Baron August
von Habsburg, Otto
von Thurn und Taxis, Max
Warburg, S. G.
Warren, Earl
Young, Owen

Adapted from: Jan van Helsing's *Secret Societies and Their Power in the 20th Century*, Gran Canaria, Spain, Ewertverlag S. L., 1995; and Dr. John Coleman's, *Conspirators' Hierarchy: The Story of the Committee of 300*. Carson City, NV: American West Publishers, 1992.

the Golden Circle. He spent the duration of his days living comfortably in England, funded by the Rothschilds.

In 1913, American banking mogul William Averell Harriman was initiated into the Skull & Bones fraternity. During the "Roaring Twenties" Harriman became the chief Western financier of the Russian government and their Ruskombank—where Max May, a Skull & Bones brother of Harriman, was vice-president. May was simultaneously vice-president of the Guaranty Trust Company controlled by J. P. Morgan and by extension the Nathan Mayer Rothschild Bank. Other Skull & Bones members partnered with J. P. Morgan at that time included Harold Stanley and Thomas Cochran. The capital used to create the Guaranty Trust came from the Harrimans, Rockefellers, Vanderbilts, and Whitneys—all families with blood kin in the Skull & Bones.

Percy Rockefeller represented his family's interest in the Skull & Bones as well as Guaranty Trust which he directed from 1915 to 1930. Rothschild and Bavarian Illuminati representatives helped establish the Rockefeller's European Standard Oil empire as well as Carnegie's steelworks and Harriman's railroad.

The introduction of the "Federal Reserve System" in 1913 enabled the international "banksters" to consolidate their American financial powers. Banking chiefs who were largely supported by the Rothschilds became the chairmen of the first Federal Reserve Bank of New York.

Following passage of "The Federal Reserve Act," Warburg led "the FED," and the U.S. Congress, to pass the 16th Amendment to the Constitution that granted Congress the power to levy personal income taxes on American citizens. The legislation was required since the United States government could no longer print money to finance its operations due to the controlling forces of the international banking cartel.

Opposition to these fiscal policies came, but was grossly inadequate to quell the changing tide. U.S. Congressman Louis McFadden expressed the sentiments of too few when he decried, "We have in this country one of the most corrupt institutions the world has ever known.

I refer to the Federal Reserve Board and the Federal Reserve Bank, hereinafter called the FED. They are not government institutions. They are private monopolies which prey upon the people of these United States for the benefit of themselves and their foreign customers. . . ."[33]

*With No Apologies: The Personal and Political Memoirs of U.S. Senator Barry Goldwater* expressed the insider's view that The Round Table's cover organization, the CFR, tightly controlled the American political scene with Rockefellers at the helm. "I believe the Council on Foreign Relations and its ancillary elitist groups [referring to the other "secret societies" such as the Skull & Bones] are indifferent to communism. They have no ideological anchors. In their pursuit of a new world order they are prepared to deal without prejudice with a communist state, a socialist state, a democratic state, monarchy, oligarchy— it's all the same to them."[34]

Rear Admiral Chester Ward of the U.S. Navy, a sixteen-year veteran of the CFR warned, "The most powerful clique in these elitist groups have one objective in common—they want to bring about the surrender of the sovereignty and the national independence of the United States."[34]

". . . Their rationale rests exclusively on materialism," Senator Goldwater continued. "When a new president comes on board, there is a great turnover in personnel but no change in policy. Example: During the Nixon years Henry Kissinger, CFR member and Nelson Rockefeller's protégé, was in charge of foreign policy. When Jimmy Carter was elected, Kissinger was replaced with Zbigniew Brzezinski, CFR member and David Rockefeller's protégé.[34]

On February 18, 1991, President George Bush, past CIA director, former CFR chief, and a member of the Skull & Bones, Committee of 300 and its offshoot The Bilderbergers, addressed the American people during his State of the Union address. "It is big," he said. "A New World Order, where diverse nations are drawn together in common cause . . . Only the United States has both the moral standing and the means to back it up."[35]

## The *Protocols* of the Prieuré de Sion

On a final note, some authors have alleged that at least part of the most infamous anti-Semitic document in history—*The Protocols of the Elders of Sion*, discussed in greater detail in the next chapter, were reworked during a meeting led in 1773 by Mayer Rothschild, a non-Hebrew Khazar.[24,37] Baigent *et al*[6] provided a harsh reality check regarding the Masonic, not "Jewish," origin of these infamous *Protocols*. Originally a secret document that heralded a deadly totalitarian plot for herding the masses into a "New World Order" run by financial elitists, the document had been turned into an anti-Semitic propaganda piece during the Russian revolution. "By 1919, the *Protocols* were also being circulated by Alfred Rosenberg," who later became the chief racial theoretician and propagandist for the National Socialist Party in Germany. The document was said to have advanced convincing "proof" of an "international Jewish conspiracy." Hitler referred to it in *Mein Kampf* with vicious conviction as to the document's authenticity.

Today, experts generally view the *Protocols* as an insidious forgery. However, following extensive research, *Holy Blood Holy Grail* authors concluded otherwise. The following excerpts relay their discovery that the *Protocols*, likely the world's most infamous document, was a Masonic strategy brief:

> One of the most persuasive testimonials we found to the existence and activities of the Prieuré de Sion dated from the late nineteenth century. . . . [T]here were influential, even powerful esoteric enclaves at the Russian court long before Rasputin. During the 1890s and 1900s one such enclave formed itself around an individual known as Monsieur Philippe and around his mentor, who made periodic visits to the imperial court at Petersburg. . . .the man called Papus—the French esotericist associated with Jules Doinel (founder of the neo-Cathar church in the Languedoc), Péladan (who claimed to have discovered Jesus's tomb), Emma Calvé, and Claude Debussy. In a word, the French occult revival of the late nineteenth century had not only spread to Petersburg, its representatives also enjoyed the privileged status of personal confidants to the czar and czarina. . . .

The *Protocols* propound in outline a blueprint for nothing less than total world domination. On first reading they would seem to be the Machiavellian program—a kind of interoffice memo, so to speak—for a group of individuals determined to impose a new world order, with themselves as supreme despots. The text advocates a many-tentacled hydra-headed conspiracy dedicated to disorder and anarchy, to toppling certain existing regimes, infiltrating Freemasonry and other such organizations, and eventually seizing absolute control of the Western world's social, political, and economic institutions. And the anonymous authors of the *Protocols* declare explicitly that they have "stage managed" whole peoples "according to a political plan which no one has so much as guessed at in the course of many centuries. . . ."[6]

Baigent *et al* continued:

. . . When they were first publicized, however, the *Protocols* were alleged to have been composed at an international Judaic congress that convened in Basle in 1897. This allegation has long since been disproved. . . . Moreover, a copy of the *Protocols* is known to have been in circulation as early as 1884—a full thirteen years before the Basle congress met. The 1884 copy of the *Protocols* surfaced in the hands of a member of a Masonic lodge—the same lodge of which Papus was a member and subsequently Grand Master. Moreover, it was in this same lodge that the tradition of Ormus had first appeared—the legendary Egyptian sage who amalgamated pagan and Christian mysteries and founded the Rose-Croix.

Modern scholars have [allegedly] established . . . that the *Protocols*, in their published form, are based at least in part on a satirical work written and printed in Geneva in 1864. The work was composed as an attack on Napoleon III by a man named Maurice Joly, who was subsequently imprisoned. Joly is said to have been a member of a Rose-Croix order. Whether this is true or not, he was a friend of Victor Hugo; and Hugo, who shared Joly's antipathy to Napoleon III, was a member of a Rose-Croix order [and grand master of the PdS].[6]

These PdS investigators concluded that "no anti-Semitic forger with even a modicum of intelligence would possibly have concocted such references in order to discredit Judaism. . . . the text of the *Protocols* ends with a single statement. 'Signed by the representatives of Sion of the 33rd Degree.'" As discussed previously and seen in figure

3.3—a diagram of "The Structure of Freemasonry" that was published in a 1956 issue of *Life Magazine*—the significant numerical designation of "33rd Degree" in Freemasonry is the so-called "Strict Observance." Thus, if anything, the *Protocols* "would seem to refer to something specifically Masonic."

The *Protocols* contained numerous "cryptic" statements that Baigent and his colleagues felt smacked of Masonic influence. For example, the text repeatedly hailed the birth of a "Masonic kingdom" and "King of the blood of Sion" who would rule over this domain. Not only was this reminiscent of grail history, but several Masonic orders included the word Sion in their titles. Thus, the authors reversed their initial cynicism regarding the document's authenticity and concluded:

1) The original *Protocols of the Elders of Sion* text "was not a forgery. On the contrary, it was authentic. But it had nothing whatever to do with Judaism or an 'international Jewish conspiracy.' It issued, rather, from some Masonic organization or Masonically-oriented secret society that incorporated the word 'Sion.'"

2) The *Protocols* "included a program for gaining power, for infiltrating Freemasonry, for controlling social, political, and economic institutions. Such a program would have been perfectly in keeping with the secret societies of the Renaissance . . ."

3) Sergei Nilus initially brought the *Protocols* to the attention of the czar "with the intention of discrediting the esoteric enclave at the imperial court . . . who were members of the secret society in question."

4) The *Protocols* has become a "radically altered text." The remaining original "vestiges" though virtually "irrelevant to Judaism," are "extremely relevant to a secret society. . . . [T]hey were—and still are—of paramount importance to the Prieuré de Sion."[37]

The *Protocols*, discussed in greater detail in the next chapter as they relate to modern "Bible code" treatises, are believed to have originated centuries before even Rothschild is alleged to have come upon them. Their likeliest earliest origin being the secret Prieuré de Sion. Between 1773 and 1901 their whereabouts remain uncertain.[37]

## References

1. Knight C and Lomas R. *The Hiram Key: Pharaohs, Freemasons and the Discovery of the Secret Scrolls of Jesus.* Rockport, MA: Element Books, 1997, pp. 326-331.

2. Baigent M, Leigh R and Lincoln H. *Holy Blood Holy Grail.* New York: Dell, 1983, pp. 79-80; See also Icke D. *The Biggest Secret.* Scottsdale, Arizona, 1999, pp. 79, 160-67, 241-43, wherein the author noted that initiates of the esoteric knowledge could read the Bible differently than Christian and Jewish believers. Initiates could recognize the "symbolism, numerology, and the esoteric codes," while believers simply took the text literally and were thus manipulated, enslaved by doctrine, and ultimately ended up the victims of an organized "scam."

The word "SPECTRE" has esoteric connections as well. Made famous by Ian Flemming's James Bond "007" novels, *Webster's Dictionary* defines it as "a visible disembodied spirit," and cross references it to "spy" and the "spectrum" of electromagnetic energies or frequencies of sound waves. David Icke also noted that the European spy networks originated "under the influence of [Sir Francis] Bacon and other esoteric magicians like John Dee and Sir Francis Walsingham. . . . Dee signed his reports 007." Ian Flemming was apparently privy to this knowledge through his friend Aleister Crowley who practiced black magic, and whose writings heavily influenced Adolf Hitler.

3. David Icke presented extensive background research on King James's association with Francis Bacon, alias William Shakespeare, and their Rosicrucian-linked hidden obsession with the occult, numerology, Tarot, and astrology. According to Icke, "it was Bacon, with Robert Fludd, Grand Master of the Priory of Sion (see figure 3.2, p. 89), who oversaw the translation of the King James version of the Bible. . . ." See: Icke D. *Ibid.* pp.160-173; See also: van Helsing J. *Secret Societies and Their Power in the 20th Century.* Gran Canaria, Spain: Ewertverlag S.L., 1995, p. 34.

4. Baigent et al, *Op cit.,* p. 42 (for passage of ancient treasure eventually to the Cathars and/or the Templars. Otherwise pp. 73-77).

5. Gardner L. "Bloodlines of the Holy Grail." A lecture presentation recorded at Yale University in 1994. See: Gardner L. *Bloodline of the Holy Grail: The Hidden Lineage of Jesus Revealed.* Rockport, MA: Element Books, 1996.

Author David Icke likewise discerned Lawrence Gardner as a member of the "Babylonian Brotherhood" and purveyor of disinformation. Icke's thesis, however, denied Christ's existence entirely and argued the Christian myth, like every other religious myth, was secreted by alien-human crossbreeds who practiced "black magic." The skull and bones, for instance, Icke wrote, "is symbolic, in part, of the black magic rituals the Brotherhood have employed since their very earliest days and these same sickening rituals, often involving human sacrifice, are still going on today." As partial evidence Icke showed the skull and bones on "the Vatican or papal crest" in the "dome of St. Peter's Basilica and the crossed keys of Peter . . ." as well as on high ranking Nazi officers. "They're all in it together," he concluded. See: Icke D. *Op. cit.*, p. 135.

6. Baigent et al, *Op cit.*, pp. 106-152.

7. Loftus J and Aarons M. *The Secret War Against the Jews.* New York: St. Martin's Press, 1994, pp. 112-113, 142, 168-169; for MI6 information see p. 182.

8. Hunt L. *Secret Agenda: Nazi Scientists, The United States Government, and Project Paperclip*, 1945 to 1990. New York: St. Martin's Press, 1991, pp. 4;145-147 (for information on General Bolling); p. 186 (for Naval Medical Research Institute's employment of Paperclip Nazis for biological weapons testing); and p. 256 (for Dow Chemical employment of convicted Nazi Otto Ambros).

9. Horowitz LG. *Emerging Viruses: AIDS & Ebola—Nature, Accident or Intentional?* Rockport, MA: Tetrahedron, Inc. 1997, pp. 335-336; for William Colby's Congressional testimony see pp. 275-300.

10. Hervet F. Knights of darkness: The Sovereign Military Order of Malta. *Covert Action Information Bulletin* (Winter)1986;25:27-38.

11. van Helsing J. *Secret Societies and Their Power in the 20th Century.* Cran Canaria, Spain: Ewertverlag S.L., (ISBN 3-89478-654-X) 1995, pp. 32.

12. Stevenson W. *The Bormann Brotherhood*. New York: Harcourt, Brace, Jovanovich, 1973, pp. 82-85.

13. Scott PD. How Allen Dulles and the SS preserved each other. *Covert Action Information Bulletin* (Winter)1986;25:4-14.

14. Farago L. *Aftermath: Martin Bormann and the Fourth Reich*. New York: Avon, 1975, pp. 204-213 and pp. 370 (for Skorzeny);187 (Rudel); 305 (Rauff); 427 (Stangl); 289 (Eichmann); .

15. Bower T. *Klaus Barbie: The Butcher of Lyons*. London: Granada, 1984, p. 179.

16. Stevenson, *Op. cit.*, n. 11, p. 227.

17. Farago, *Op. cit.*, n. 13, p. 220.

18. Manning P. *Martin Bormann: Nazi in Exile*. Secaucas, NJ: Lyle Stuart Inc., 1981, pp. 29, 56, 64, 69, 113-118, and 134-135.

19. Covert NM. *Cutting Edge: A History of Fort Detrick, Maryland 1943-1993*. Fort Detrick, Maryland: U. S. Army Garrison Public Affairs Office (SHSD-PA; 301-619-2018), 1993, pp. 17, 20, and 39.

20. Manning, *Op. cit.*, p. 56.

21. Chaitkin A. Population control, Nazis, and the U.N.: Rockefeller and mass murder. Internet: Sumeria, 1996, http://www.livelinks.com/sumeria/politics/eugenics.html; see also: Kuhl S. *The Nazi Connection: Eugenics, American Racism, and German National Socialism*. Oxford: Oxford University Press, 1994.

22. Horowitz, *Op cit.* pp. 476. Based on personal communications with blood bank officials and Alfred P. Sloan Foundation reports from 1967-1969; For Rockefeller monopoly over American medicine see: Starr P. *The Social Transformation of American Medicine*. New York: Basic Books, 1982.

23. Baigent et al, *Op cit.*, pp. 122-123; 141; 150.

24. van Helsing, *Op cit.*, pp. 28-34; 39-40; for Bavarian Illuminati details see p.113; for Freemasonry in America see p. 120; for Clinton's life membership in the "Masonic Order of DeMolay" for boys see p.130; for Gary Allen's quote regarding Adam Weishaupt see p. 145; for Professor Quigley's quotes regarding Rhodes, The "Committee of 300," "The Round Table," and MI6 see pp. 145-147; for early "Brotherhood of the Snake" details see p. 374.

25. *Webster's Dictionary* defines "alchemy" as "a medieval chemical science and speculative philosophy aiming to achieve the transmutation of the base metals into gold, the discovery of a universal cure for disease, and the discovery of a means of indefinitely prolonging life."

26. Nodier C. *Contes*, p. 4ff. As cited in: Baigent *et al.*, *Op cit.*, pp. 150-152.

27. Rhodes C. Documents presented in the Rhodes House, Oxford, England. In: Aydelotte F. *The Vision of Cecil Rhodes: A Review of the First Forty Years of American Scholarships.* London: Geoffrey Cumberlege Oxford University Press, 1946, pp. 3-5.

28. Monteith S. *Is America Destined for Dictatorship?* A course manual published by Dr. Stanley Monteith, Radio Liberty-KKMC 880 AM, P.O. Box 13, Santa Cruz, CA 95063. (Copies may be ordered by calling: 888-2-4-LIBERTY.)

29. Quigley C. *The Anglo-American Establishment: From Rhodes to Cliveden.* In: *Ibid.*, p. 11.

30. Cuddy D. *President Clinton Will Continue the New World Order.* Oklahoma City: Southwest Radio Church, 1993, p. 5.

31. Quigley C. *Tragedy and Hope: A History of The World in Our Time.* New York: Macmillan Company, 1966, p. 952.

32. *Webster's Dictionary* defines "éminence grise" as the "gray eminence" and *"exercising unsuspected or unofficial power."* A related term is "grisaille" defined as a "decoration in tones of a single color and esp. gray designed to produce a three-dimensional effect."

33. McLamb J. *Operation Vampire Killer 2000.* Phoenix, AZ: Police Against the New World Order, 1996, p. 16.

34. Goldwater B. *With No Apologies: The Personal and Political Memoirs of United States Senator Barry M. Goldwater.* New York: William Morrow and Company, Inc., 1979, pp. 278-279.

35. The Publishers. *What's Behind the New World Order?* Jemison, AL: Inspiration Books East, Inc., 1991. Backcover.

36. Carr WG. *Pawns in the Game.* Clackamas, OR: Emissary Publications, 1994.

37. Baigent et al., *Op cit.*, pp. 190-195.

# Chapter 4.
## *The Bible Code, The Protocols* and Effectively Manipulating the Masses

A s evidenced in the two previous chapters, Masonic leaders have consistently encrypted intelligence, as well as disseminated counterintelligence, to achieve their goals in the continued acquisition of power and wealth. If Baigent *et al.* are accurate, and all indications suggest that they are, the Prieuré de Sion is still effectively operating "behind the scenes" to orchestrate the economic alignment of the superpowers and impact world history. For the New World Order, the secret society continues to influence the media and the public's assimilation of facts and fiction.

Could a flurry of books that claimed to have exposed secret Bible codes be part of this Masonic illusion? As this chapter reveals, such concerns are justified. *The Protocols of the Elders of Sion* [1] itself, having now been identified as originally Masonic, contained several passages that spoke to this likelihood and reliable methods of mass manipulation, and even mass destruction, through public delusion.

By way of background, consider the following "protocol:"

"Our States, marching along the path of peaceful conquest, has the right to *replace the horrors of war by less noticeable and more satisfactory sentences of death*, necessary to maintain the terror which tends to produce blind submission," asserted Masonic strategists. Emphasis here was added to accent the relationship of this recurring theme. Replacing the "horrors of war" in the New World Order with war substitutes will be substantially demonstrated and documented in the final chapters of this book.

Mention has already been made of the use of fear to successfully manipulate the masses. As detailed in Dr. Horowitz's previous publication,[3] biological weapons are the most effective implements of mass destruction for population control. In recent years they have also been used to render terror and fear in support of political agendas such as the antiterrorism bill of 1998 that was passed by the United States Congress.

"Protocol No. 2" states that "in the hands of the States of today there is a great force that creates the movement of thought in the people, and this is the press. The part played by the press is to keep pointing out requirements supposed to be indispensable; to give voice to the complaints of the people, and to express and to create discontent. It is in the press that the triumph of freedom of speech finds its incarnation. But the [manipulated] States have not known how to make use of this force; and it has fallen into our hands. Through the press we have gained the power to influence while remaining ourselves in the shade; thanks to the Press we have got the gold in our hands, notwithstanding that we have had to gather it out of oceans of blood and tears. . . (See Appendix figure 13 for CFR members in the media.)

"Moreover, [Protocol No. 5 states] the art of directing masses and individuals by means of cleverly manipulated theory and verbiage, by regulations of life in common, and all sorts of other quirks, in which the [manipulated] understand nothing, belongs likewise to the specialists of our administrative brain. Reared on analysis, observation, on delicacies of fine calculation, in this species of skill we have no rivals, any more than we have either in the drawing up of plans of political actions and solidarity. In this respect the Jesuits alone might have compared with us, but we have contrived to discredit them in the eyes of the unthinking mob as an overt organisation, while we ourselves all the while have kept our secret organization in the shade. However, it is probably all the same to the world who is its sovereign lord, whether the head of Catholicism or our despot of the blood of [S]ion! . . .

"For a time perhaps we might be successfully dealt with by a coalition of the [manipulated] of all the world: but from this danger we are secured by the discord existing among them whose roots are so deeply seated that they can never now be plucked up. . .

"The principle object of our directorate consists in this: to debilitate the public mind by criticism; to lead it away from serious reflections calculated to arouse resistance; to distract the forces of the mind towards a sham fight of empty eloquence. . . . [Our] orators will speak so much that they will exhaust the patience of their hearers and produce an abhorrence of oratory.

"In order to put public opinion into our hands we must bring it into a state of bewilderment by giving expression from all sides to so many contradictory opinions and for such a length of time as will suffice to make the [manipulated] lose their heads in the labyrinth and come to see that the best thing is to have no opinion of any kind in matters political . . . ."

As continued in Protocol No. 7, "We must compel the governments of the [manipulated] to take action in the direction favoured by our widely conceived plan, already approaching the desired consummation, by what we shall represent as public opinion, secretly prompted by us through the means of the so-called "Great Power"—the Press, which, with a few exceptions that may be disregarded, is already entirely in our hands. . . .

"In a word, to sum up our system of keeping the governments of the [manipulated] . . . in check, we shall show our strength to one of them by terrorist attempts and to all, if we allow the possibility of a general rising against us, we shall respond with the guns of America, or China, or Japan. . . ."

And to facilitate the New World Order, "Protocol No. 10," documented: "By such measures we shall obtain the power of destroying, little by little, step by step . . . the constitutions of States to prepare for the transition to an imperceptible abolition of every kind of constitution, and then the time is come to turn every form of government into our despotism.

"The recognition of our despot may also come before the destruction of the constitution; the moment for this recognition will come when the peoples, utterly wearied by the irregularities and incompetence—a matter which we shall arrange for—of their rulers, will clamor: 'Away with them and give us one king over all the earth who will unite us and annihilate the causes of discords—frontiers, nationalities, religions, state debts—who will give us peace and quiet, which we cannot find under our rulers and representatives.'

"But you yourselves perfectly well know that to produce the possibility of the expression of such wishes by all the nations it is indispensable to trouble, in all countries, the people's relations with their governments so as to utterly exhaust humanity with dissension, hatred, struggle, envy, and even by the use of torture, by starvation, *by the inoculation of diseases*, by want, so that the [manipulated] see no issue than to take refuge in our complete sovereignty in money and in all else." (The emphasis added on inoculated diseases refers to vaccine officials injecting mercury, aluminum, formaldehyde, and more. See Dr. Horowitz's earlier book, *Emerging Viruses: AIDS & Ebola—Nature, Accident or Intentional?*, as well as to chapters 8-12 herein.)

Finally, "Protocol No. 12" also deals extensively with the press and the shadow governors' capacity to direct it along with the population at large. It answers its own rhetorical question, "What is the part played by the press today? It serves to excite and inflame those passions which are needed for our purpose, or else it serves selfish ends of (other) parties. It is often vapid, unjust, mendacious, and the majority of the public have not the slightest idea what ends the press really serves. We shall saddle and bridle it with a tight curb: we shall do the same also with all productions of the printing press [book publishers], for where would be the sense of getting rid of the attacks of the press if we remain targets for pamphlets and books? The produce of publicity, which nowadays is a source of heavy expense owing to the necessity of censoring it, will be turned by us into a very lucrative source of income to our State: We shall lay on it a special stamp tax and require deposits of caution-money before permitting the establishment of any organ of the press or of printing offices; these will then have to guarantee our government against any kind of attack on the part of the press. For any attempt to attack us, if such still be possible, we shall inflict fines without mercy. . . . The pretext for stopping any publication will be the alleged plea that it is agitating the public mind without occasion or justification. I beg you to note that among those making attacks upon us will also be organs established by us, but they will attack exclusively points that we have predetermined to alter.

"Not a single announcement will reach the public without our control. Even now this is already being attained by us inasmuch as news items are received by a few agencies, in whose offices they are focused from all parts of the world. These agencies will then be already entirely ours and will give publicity only to what we dictate to them. . . .

"Literature and journalism are two of the most important educative forces and therefore our government will become proprietor of the majority of the journals. This will neutralize the injurious influence of the privately owned press and will put us in possession of a tremendous influence upon the public mind. . . If we give permits for ten journals, we shall ourselves found thirty, and so on in the same proportion. This, however, must in no ways be suspected by the public.

"For which reason all journals published by us will be of the most opposite, in appearance, tendencies, and opinions, thereby creating confidence in us and bringing over to us our quite unsuspicious opponents, who will thus fall into our trap and be rendered harmless.

"In the front rank will stand organ[ization]s of an official character. [Such as the American Medical and Dental Associations, the World Health Organization, the National Press Club, etc.] They will always stand guard over our interests, and therefore their influence will be comparatively insignificant.

"By discussing and controverting, but always superficially, without touching the essence of the matter, our organ[ization]s will carry on a sham fight . . . with the official newspapers (operating) solely for the purpose of giving occasion for us to express ourselves more fully . . . (superficially, self-generated) attacks upon us will also serve another purpose, namely, that our subjects will be convinced of the existence of full freedom of speech, and so give our agents an occasion to affirm that all organ[ization]s which oppose us are empty babblers, since they are incapable of finding any substantial objections to our orders.

"Methods of organization like these, imperceptible to the public eye, but absolutely sure, are best calculated to succeed in bringing the attention and the confidence of the public to the side of our government. Thanks to such methods, we shall be in a position as from time to time may be required, to excite or to tranquilize the public mind on political questions, to persuade or to confuse, printing now truth, now lies, facts or their contradictions, accordingly as they may be well or ill received, always very cautiously feeling our ground before stepping upon it. We shall have a sure triumph over our opponents since they will not have at their disposition organ[ization]s of the press in which they can give full and final expression to their views owing to the aforesaid methods of dealing with the press. We shall not even need to refute them except very superficially."[1]

## Applied Protocols and Deception in *The Bible Code*

A particularly relevant example of the protocol "to persuade or to confuse, printing now truth, now lies, facts or their contradictions, accordingly as they may be well or ill received . . . " is the book *The Bible Code*—the *New York Times* bestseller by Michael Drosnin.

Drosnin's past relationships with the *Washington Post*, as well as to National Security Agency "code-breaker" Harold Gans, makes his work suspect. He used his book, *The Bible Code,* to advance the thesis that computers are required to access God's codes. Drosnin's work is shown here to be a contemporary decoy to throw people off the track to discovering the true Bible codes.

Drosnin has described himself as "a reporter, formerly at the *Washington Post* and the *Wall Street Journal*"—two publications largely represented by CFR members as cited in appendix figure 13. The *New York Times* is widely suspected of disseminating both filtered news and Central Intelligence Agency (CIA) propaganda.

During the Nixon administration, for instance, J. Edgar Hoover ordered the FBI to break ties with *The Washington Post* due to its insidious connections with the CIA. In *Emerging Viruses: AIDS & Ebola*, Dr. Horowitz found *The Post*'s Bob Woodward held a military intelligence association with Alexander Haig. Haig, believed by most Watergate authorities to be the infamous "Deep Throat," was the man who most likely funneled intelligence to Woodward and Bernstein during their historic investigation that resulted in Nixon's resignation.[3]

Thus, regarding Drosnin's work, it was remotely suspicious that his second consecutive *New York Times* bestseller was *The Bible Code*. His first, in 1986, was called *Citizen Hughes*. It provided a biography of the politically influential aerospace industry leader Howard Hughes. Further information regarding Hughes-related organizations and projects will be discussed later.

Drosnin's work was said to be based on the work of Israeli mathematician Dr. Eliyahu Rips, "one of the world's leading experts in group theory, a field of mathematics that underlies quantum physics." Two other research assistants performed the analyses including Doron Witztum and Yoav Rosenberg. The Witztum et al. scientific publication appeared in the journal *Statistical Science*, as shown in figure 4.1. The journal's editor, Robert Kass, whose reviewers remained "baffled" by the study and its apparent statistical validity, excused the paper's publication as "a challenging puzzle."[6]

Following publication of *The Bible Code*, all three *Statistical Science* authors began to distance themselves from the book because of Drosnin's careless mixing of statistically significant "pairs of conceptually related words" with those believed to be insignificant, according to a CNN news story available on its website. Later, Witztum stated, "I was the first one to investigate the possibility of divining the future through these codes. Following logical and empirical tests, I found incontrovertible evidence proving it's impossible to predict the future with the hidden codes."[6]

Yet, as "prophesied" in the *Protocols*, Drosnin's deceptive effort began alleging he had *predicted* Israeli Prime Minister Yitzhak Rabin's assassination. He published excerpts from the warning he allegedly sent Rabin: "The reason I'm telling you about this is that the only time your full name—Yitzhak Rabin—is encoded in the Bible, the words, 'assassin that will assassinate' cross your name. . . . I think you are in real danger, but that the danger can be averted."[2]

How did Drosnin suddenly gain interest in investigating ancient Bible codes? Through his U.S. and Israeli intelligence agency connections, no less. *The Bible Code* stated that he allegedly went to Israel by invitation of "the chief of Israeli intelligence," to discuss "the future of warfare." (A topic of clear relevance to the later chapters of this book.) He made no mention on whose behalf he was laboring. As if to say the future of warfare in the Middle East had already been planned and Drosnin was privileged, by assignment, as a matter of fact, to cover the future apocalypse for the benefit of humanity?

Just "coincidentally," Drosnin's special interest in biblical encryption was hastened by "a senior code-breaker at the top secret National Security Agency, the clandestine U.S. government listening post near Washington," implicated in the failed attempt to assassinate Joey. According to Drosnin, Harold Gans, who "had spent his life *making* and breaking codes for American intelligence . . . decided to investigate" the codes independently of Drosnin and the American intelligence community.

"In evaluating the Bible code," Gans later admitted, "I was doing the same kind of work I did at the Department of Defense."

As Joey read *The Bible Code*, he recognized how similar Drosnin's writing style and even book's content was to Richard Preston's book *The Hot Zone* that had been critically examined and exposed by Dr. Horowitz as propaganda in *Emerging Viruses: AIDS & Ebola.*[3]

Like Preston's work, and the *Protocols* prescribed "terror which tends to produce blind submission . . . (and that will) finally distract their minds," Drosnin focused on horrific events: assassinations—including Kennedy's and Rabin's; wars—including the holocaust;

# Fig. 4.1. Equidistant Letter Sequences Report in *Statistical Science*

*Statistical Science*
1994, Vol. 9, No. 3, 429-438

# Equidistant Letter Sequences in the Book of Genesis

## Doron Witztum, Eliyahu Rips and Yoav Rosenberg

*Abstract.* It has been noted that when the Book of Genesis is written as two-dimensional arrays, equidistant letter sequences spelling words with related meanings often appear in close proximity. Quantitative tools for measuring this phenomenon are developed. Randomization analysis shows that the effect is significant at the level of 0.00002.

*Key words and phrases:* Genesis, equidistant letter sequences, cylindrical representations, statistical analysis.

## 1. INTRODUCTION

The phenomenon discussed in this paper was first discovered several decades ago by Rabbi Weissmandel [7]. He found some interesting patterns in the Hebrew Pentateuch (the Five Books of Moses), consisting of words or phrases expressed in the form of equidistant letter sequences (ELS's)—that is, by selecting sequences of equally spaced letters in the text.

As impressive as these seemed, there was no rigorous way of determining if these occurrences were not merely due to the enormous quantity of combinations of words and expressions that can be constructed by searching out arithmetic progressions in the text. The purpose of the research reported here is to study the phenomenon systematically. The goal is to clarify whether the phenomenon in question is a real one, that is, whether it can or cannot be explained purely on the basis of fortuitous combinations.

The approach we have taken in this research can be illustrated by the following example. Suppose we have a text written in a foreign language that we do not understand. We are asked whether the text is meaningful (in that foreign language) or meaningless. Of course, it is very difficult to decide between these possibilities, since we do not understand the language. Suppose now that we are equipped with a very partial dictionary, which enables us to recognise a small portion of the words in the text: "hammer" here and "chair" there, and maybe even "umbrella"

*Eliyahu Rips is Associate Professor of Mathematics, Hebrew University of Jerusalem, Givat Ram, Jerusalem 91904, Israel. Doron Witztum and Yoav Rosenberg did this research at Jerusalem College of Technology, 21 Havaad Haleumi St., P.O.B. 16031, Jerusalem 91160, Israel.*

elsewhere. Can we now decide between the two possibilities?

Not yet. But suppose now that, aided with the partial dictionary, we can recognise in the text a pair of conceptually related words, like "hammer" and "anvil." We check if there is a tendency of their appearances in the text to be in "close proximity." If the text is meaningless, we do not expect to see such a tendency, since there is no reason for it to occur. Next, we widen our check; we may identify some other pairs of conceptually related words: like "chair" and "table," or "rain" and "umbrella." Thus we have a sample of such pairs, and we check the tendency of each pair to appear in close proximity in the text. If the text is meaningless, there is no reason to expect such a tendency. However, a strong tendency of such pairs to appear in close proximity indicates that the text might be meaningful.

Note that even in an absolutely meaningful text we do not expect that, deterministically, every such pair will show such tendency. Note also, that we did not decode the foreign language of the text yet: we do not recognise its syntax and we cannot read the text.

This is our approach in the research described in the paper. To test whether the given text may contain "hidden information," we write the text in the form of two-dimensional arrays, and define the distance between ELS's according to the ordinary two-dimensional Euclidean metric. Then we check whether ELS's representing conceptually related words tend to appear in "close proximity."

Suppose we are given a text, such as Genesis (*G*). Define an equidistant letter sequence (ELS) as a sequence of letters in the text whose positions, not counting spaces, form an arithmetic progression; that is, the letters are found at the positions

$$n, n + d, n + 2d, \ldots, n + (k - 1)d.$$

133

plagues and earthquakes; terrorist attacks—especially the Oklahoma City bombing; depopulation, cosmic cataclysms, Armageddon, and finally, the apocalypse.

"It's interesting that God wouldn't have placed more pleasant events in the Bible as well," Joey considered.

Moreover, Drosnin's bias clearly surfaced during his discussion of Timothy McVeigh and the Oklahoma City bombing for which an Oklahoma Grand Jury determined the conspiracy extended far beyond this government patsy and Terry Nichols. Striking evidence that McVeigh and Nichols had not acted alone was blatantly censored.[7] Drosnin wrote: "Government investigators claimed that McVeigh wanted to avenge the Koresh cult, an Apocalyptic religious group . . . And there was a disturbing echo of that cult's insanity in the verse of the Bible where the Oklahoma tragedy was encoded: "the terror of God was upon the cities that were around them."[2]

In fact, as evidenced in the International Documentary Association 1997 Feature Award winning film *Waco: Rules of Engagement*, Drosnin's prose was seriously counterintelligent. This 1998 Academy Award nominee for "best documentary" detailed, in living color, an entirely different story than the one offered by Drosnin and government spin doctors.[8] The Waco tragedy had apparently been orchestrated by government agents and agencies well in advance of Waco becoming an inferno.

Despite its widespread popularity, one of *The Bible Code*'s critical reviewers, Ed Christian, reported on the Internet that Drosnin's effort was a complete "hoax." In this regard, here's what the obviously intelligent Hebrew scholar offered:

> How does the Bible Code work? It's a giant 'find the word' puzzle with a number of tricks which make it easier to find words. These tricks should be apparent to someone with even the most rudimentary knowledge of Hebrew, but in the book the Hebrew letters were shown in the code samples, but they were never analyzed.

Drosnin never mentioned whether the "word" he found was generally translated the way he translated it, or whether his way was an unusual alternative with many more likely translations. For example, the word he translated "assassin" in connection with Yitzak Rabin's assassination is generally translated "murder" or "murderer" in the Bible.

While some of the discoveries seemed unlikely, difficult to account for, here are some things to bear in mind when considering the validity of the code:

1. Bear in mind that in finding the code, the Torah was placed on the computer-equivalent of a cylinder which was expanded or contracted until a match was found. With every letter added to the horizontal length of the lines, a whole new set of words became possible vertically and diagonally (they remained the same horizontally). The reference to the ten commandments being computer-generated is found in a segment only ten letters wide, whereas some words have letters spaced chapters apart—which can be juxtaposed only by expanding the cylinder to a thousand letters or more in width.

2. The hardest part to find was a person's name, but given that the name could be read in any direction, with any number of equidistant spaces between the letters, and that the computer could adjust the line length, and that any possible variation of spelling was allowed, and that abbreviations, initials, and nicknames were allowed, the wonder would be if any name could not be found (See figure 4.2, page 28 of *The Bible Code*.) Drosnin generally found the names vertically by expanding or contracting the line length, then he looked for the words around it.

3. The Hebrew used is "unvocalized," it does not use vowel pointings, but Drosnin used the letters aleph, ain, vau, and jod as semi-vowels where convenient. These semi-vowels could be used to approximate a number of vowels (yod might represent IH, EE, EYE, EH, EI, for example). Thus, exact spelling was not essential—"sounds similar" was close enough. If none of these semi-vowels occurred, the word was simply read without vowels. (For example, President Clinton's name was spelled Q L Y N T W N. "President" is N S Y A which means "leader" or "ruler" and is in fact the Hebrew word for "president" today, though it could also be seen as "Nazi." "Hitler" was found as H Y T L R, and "Nazi" as N A D Z Y. "Shakespeare" occurs as Sh Q S P Y R, "Macbeth" as M Q B T, and "Hamlet" as H M L T. Note the cavalier attitude toward vowels.)

135

Fig. 4.2. Computer Generated Letter Matrix From *The Bible Code*

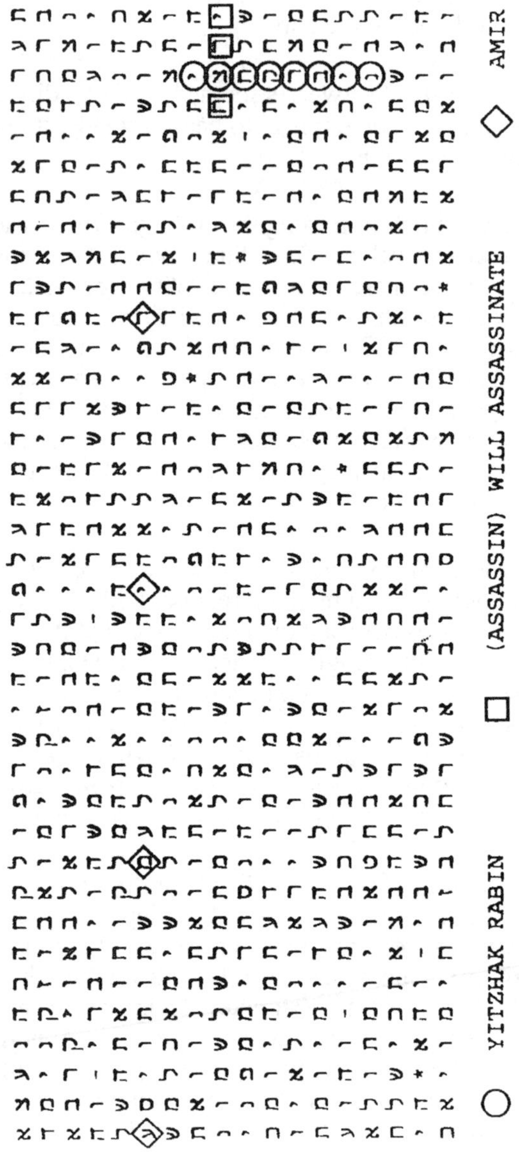

According to to Israeli mathemeticians and Michael Drosnin, author of *The Bible Code*, this figure shows a section of the Book of Genesis in which the name "YITZHAK RABIN" and the phrase "ASSASSIN WILL ASSASSINATE" are encoded. This work has been heavily criticized and largely refuted. It evidences how sophisticated counterintelligence propaganda is disseminated through the media. From: Drosnin M. *The Bible Code.* New York: Simon & Schuster, 1997, p. 28.

4. In giving the computer names to search for, every possible spelling was used whether or not the spelling had ever been used. This increased the likelihood of a match. Also, usually the words used were Hebrew, but sometimes they were English (names).

5. Without vowel points, a three letter Hebrew root may have many meanings, this possibly quintupled the likelihood of a match. For example, the Hebrew root 'Ayin–Lamed–He, "'LH," with one set of vowels, can mean to ascend, or break, or excel, or fall, or offer (and many more), or with different vowels it means "holocaust," or "burnt offering," or with yet other vowels it means a "branch," or "leaf," or with other vowels it means "occasion," or with other vowels, "iniquity." But Drosnin translated words in whatever way seemed convenient for the meaning he wanted to find.

6. Many modern Hebrew words were based on old words with ancient but related meanings. This made it easier to find 'modern' words in the ancient text, even though when written, the words did not have the modern meanings. For example, the word for "missile."

7. Hebrew has letters which represent different sounds but might be transliterated in English by the same letter. For example, "he" and "heth" might both be represented by an H, but the latter has a guttural CH sound. Kaph and Qoph might be written as K, Q, or C. Taw and teth might both be written as a T. Samech, sin, shin, and zayin all might be seen as S sounds. These are not used interchangeably in Hebrew, nor do scholars who transliterate Hebrew in books and articles use them interchangeably, but they are in *The Bible Code*, whenever convenient. This increased the chance of a match.

8. The letter field was not made up of random letters, but made up of Hebrew words without vowels. This increased the chance of a horizontal match in Hebrew, of course, even if one rearranged the letters. That is to say, on any page, whatever the line length, there will be many Hebrew words already there, read right to left. Read left to right, some of these words have other meanings. If one begins with the second letter in a word rather than the first letter, one may get yet more words.

9. [In Hebrew] Dates are based on a letter/number code in which each letter represents a number. As the Torah is all letters, this also makes a match more likely. Also, modern Hebrew dates often leave off the millennium number (1891 would be written, in Hebrew letters, 891). Thus, Drosnin's finding of dates such as "2013" could as well be 1013 or 3013. He never explained this to his readers, and finally,

10. Most "pages" have a thousand or more letters to choose from, nearly every three of which constitute a Hebrew word root, in any direction. The chance of finding something somewhat significant on a page with a name on it is quite high. If nothing is found, perhaps the computer might find the name elsewhere.

In a competing and more serious work that will be discussed in the next section of this book, Del Washburn, the author of *The Original Code in the Bible: Using Science & Mathematics to Reveal God's Fingerprints*,[6] additionally debunked *The Bible Code.* Among the entries was a signed statement issued by forty-five prominent scientists and mathematicians who testified:

There is a common belief in the general community to the effect that many mathematicians, statisticians, and other scientists consider the ["Equidistant Letter Sequences," or "ELS" also referred to as "Torah codes," and "the Bible code"] claims to be credible. This belief is incorrect. On the contrary, the almost unanimous opinion of those in the scientific world who have studied the question is that the theory is without foundation. The signatories to this letter have themselves examined the evidence and found it entirely unconvincing. (http://math.caltech.edu/code/petition.html).

To add insult to injury, Washburn relayed the analysis conducted by Brendan McKay of Australia National University." McKay, a career debunker of "egregious" claims, took a page from *Moby Dick*—"obviously not a Divine inspiration," wrote Washburn. He laid the text on an ELS grid following Drosnin's method and decoded the following words:

PRINCESS DIANA
ROYAL
DODI
HENRI PAUL
MORTAL IN THESE JAWS OF DEATH

All propaganda told, it is easy to understand why Drosnin's *Bible Code* became a *New York Times* bestseller. Its machinations had been described in the *Protocols of the Elders of Sion*. The book's purpose was described in the *Protocols* under the utility of the "press" to deceive. Relatedly, the fourteenth century English verb "press" is defined in *Webster's Dictionary* as to "beseech, entreat" or "try hard to persuade." *The Bible Code* went to great lengths to do just that. The question is why?

You will soon learn the answer as well as the extraordinary nature of at least one of the legitimate Bible codes that Drosnin's work helped obscure.

### *The Original Code in the Bible:*

Among more recent and serious contributions to Bible code devotees was Del Washburn's *The Original Code in the Bible*.[6] At first glance this work seemed refreshingly similar to the approach Jeshua had inspired Joey to advance. Even the Pythagorean skein appeared modestly represented among Washburn's more complex decoding methods. It was the complex nature of his methods that initially raised Joey's suspicions.

The *Protocols* had, after all, explained the utility of publishing books like *The Bible Code*, and then, "the most opposite, in appearance, tendencies, and opinions"—books that created "confidence" in the masses of manipulated "unsuspicious opponents, who will thus fall into our trap and be rendered harmless."[1] Following a thorough review of Washburn's "*Theomatics*" methods, Joey concluded that *The Origi-*

*nal Code in the Bible* served a similar hidden propagandist agenda as Drosnin's.

According to Washburn, *Theomatics*, first published in 1978, was purchased by almost ninety-thousand mainly Christian readers who learned of it through "the *700 Club* with Pat Robertson, *PTL Network*, [and] on Christian TV across Canada. . . ."

In 1994, he published *Theomatics II*, a 663-page treatise that needed to be "severely edited," prompting Washburn to write a "300-page scientific work called *Theomatics and the Scientific Method*." This work, he claimed, provided "serious and compelling evidence—a complete scientific testing and analysis by computer. It is available for review by mathematical scientists, scholars, and anyone out there who is skeptical," Washburn wrote.

More recently he was "contacted," then commissioned, by his "Washington, D.C." publisher to produce *The Original Code in the Bible*—a condensed "volume that was more practical and appealing to the general reader," a "fast-food society—sort of . . . 'McTheomatics' version that people could read while sitting on airplanes or in waiting rooms."[6]

Before Joey, and later Dr. Horowitz, entertained Washburn's method of decoding the Bible, it seemed prudent to review his biography and, according to Joey, his biography contains significant Masonic parallels.

For fifteen years Washburn worked in the field of church design and architecture. He even referred to "masons" when he discussed the "heavenly languages" of Hebrew and Greek." Born in Columbia, South America, "to evangelical Christian missionaries," Washburn related Bible encryption to "the following analogy . . . "

> Have you ever watched a large brick building under construction? Surrounding the building is a complete network of scaffolding, planks, tarps, masons, and bricklayers. The entire thing looks like a mess. However, after the job is complete and each brick has been neatly laid, the scaffolding is removed, the brick is cleaned, and a beautiful structure is the result.[6]

Joey looked up the term 'mason' in *Webster's Dictionary* and found it meant virtually the same as "bricklayer." "Why would Washburn and his editors, allegedly interested in condensing this version, allow for such repetition?" he questioned. He wondered whether it had been a simple editing oversight, a "Freudian slip," or a subtle tease.

Joey's fundamental question, however, if Washburn's thesis was correct, that "Every word in the Bible was designed by God, from eternity past, to be part of a very organized and systematic grammatical structure. . . ," then why had God, in all His grace and love for humanity, obscured important codes in the Bible. For instance, as you will soon learn, why had Numbers 7:12-83 provided completely nonsensical repeating verses such as: "One spoon of ten shekels of gold, full of incense."? Moreover, why would God, who loves even simple things and people, have required the masses to learn the complex "science" of "Theomatics" to gain a full appreciation of "His" hidden treasures—methods so complex that even mathematicians and statisticians found them demanding? If you were God, and you had the choice to make law easy or difficult, which would you choose? Jesus had that choice and simplified Mosaic law, God's instructions, even further.

According to Washburn, God created an extremely complex encryption that requires seven steps, some very tedious, to decypher the Bible. Apparently Joey was not the only one put off by this. John MacArthur, Jr. a well known Christian evangelist, wrote in *Charismatic Chaos*:

> The words of scripture are to be interpreted the same way words are understood in ordinary daily use. God has communicated his Word to us through human language, and there is every reason to assume he has done it in the most obvious and simple fashion possible. . . .[9]

Washburn did, however, agree in *Theomatics II*. Here he noted that "With just the simple written words in the Bible, and their simple literal interpretation, God has given us everything we need for both life and Godliness in this present age. Nothing else is essential." Then he

## Fig. 4.3. The "Gematria" Upon Which Theomatics Practice is Based

| HEBREW ALPHABET | | GREEK ALPHABET | |
|---|---|---|---|
| א | 1 | α | 1 |
| ב | 2 | β | 2 |
| ג | 3 | γ | 3 |
| ד | 4 | δ | 4 |
| ה | 5 | ε | 5 |
| ו | 6 | ς' | 6 ** |
| ז | 7 | ζ | 7 |
| ח | 8 | η | 8 |
| ט | 9 | θ | 9 |
| י | 10 | ι | 10 |
| כ — ך | 20 * | κ | 20 |
| ל | 30 | λ | 30 |
| מ — ם | 40 * | μ | 40 |
| נ — ן | 50 * | ν | 50 |
| ס | 60 | ξ | 60 |
| ע | 70 | ο | 70 |
| פ — ף | 80 * | π | 80 |
| צ — ץ | 90 * | ο | 90 ** |
| ק | 100 | ρ | 100 |
| ר | 200 | σ - ς | 200 * |
| ש | 300 | τ | 300 |
| ת | 400 | υ | 400 |
| | | φ | 500 |
| | | χ | 600 |
| | | ψ | 700 |
| | | ω | 800 |

\* These double letters are the same. The second letter is used in place of the first letter when it occurs as the last letter in a word.

\*\* Those who are familiar with New Testament Greek may be surprised to see the addition of the letters *vau* (number value = 6) and *koppa* (number value = 90). The letter *vau* appears in Revelation 13:18 as the numerical value of the number 6 in the number 666. In the early history of the Greek language both these letters existed, but later became extinct. They have always retained their numerical equivalency (see *Webster's Dictionary*).

Figure shows the number values of letters in the Hebrew and Greek alphabets, and words, according to an encrypted numerical system termed the "gematria" detailed in: Washburn D. *The Original Bible Code*. Washington, DC: Madison Books, 1998.

proceeded to outline his "numerical system or code of awesome proportions—that will ultimately unlock the deeper and symbolical meanings present."

The first step in *The Original Bible Code* recognized, as Joey had, that numerical values could be assigned to every letter in the Hebrew and Greek alphabets. Unlike Joey's thesis, however, Washburn's ruled out the use of the English language in deciphering the hidden Bible codes. Moreover, though Washburn's letter/number codes contained a similar repeating 1–9, 1-8 pattern, Washburn applied a "Denary System . . . based upon 10s, 100s, and 1000s as shown in figure 4.3.

In "Step 2: Every Word Has a Numeric Value" he added, like Joey had, the numeric values of each letter of virtually every word in the New Testament. To give credit where credit appears due, this took him "almost 800 hours!" He also explained that phrases added up to significant numbers.

In "Step 3: Multiples" the process became a bit more challenging, though still reasonable. Here Washburn stated that everything in theomatics operated "on the principle of multiples and multiple structures based upon prime numbers." Joey was earnestly intrigued when he read here, ". . . if you examine specific references to Jesus the Son of God, you will find that they all contain multiples of the same number [in the set of "1–9" possibilities]. The many different references to Satan are all structured around multiples of another number.

"Step 4: Clusters" got Joey more excited with the potential validity of Washburn's work. As seen in the example reprinted in figure 4.4, a "clustering of numbers around these multiples" was routinely observed. Washburn offered this reasonable explanation:

> These circles or clusters are rather like shooting a basketball through a hoop. . . . Everything in theomatics operates on this principle. One example in creation demonstrates the principle of clusters. In the universe, galaxies are all structured around clusters of stars. The largest concentration of stars exists toward the center of the galaxy. But farther out from the center, the stars become fewer and fewer.[6]

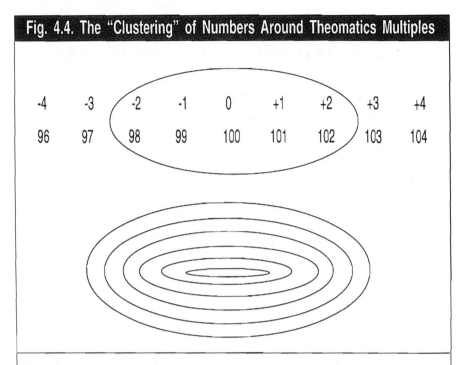

### Fig. 4.4. The "Clustering" of Numbers Around Theomatics Multiples

| -4 | -3 | -2 | -1 | 0 | +1 | +2 | +3 | +4 |
|----|----|----|----|----|----|----|----|----|
| 96 | 97 | 98 | 99 | 100 | 101 | 102 | 103 | 104 |

Figure shows circles, reminiscent of frequency vibrations, fundamental to theomatics and all of nature. These clusters were said to be found only in Hebrew and Greek Bibles. "Everything in theomatics operates on this principle," *The Original Bible Code* author argued. From: Washburn D. *The Original Bible Code*. Washington, DC: Madison Books, 1998, p. 31.

Joey immediately recognized the possible implications of this part of Washburn's thesis regarding resonant frequencies. Like the notes of the Solfeggio, or the expanding waves of water created when a pebble drops into a pond, these waves expand to infinity until they are somehow blocked by a counter force. This was consistent with Washburn's galaxy example.

Washburn began to lose Joey's attention in "Step 5: The Grammar of the Hebrew and Greek Languages." Joey had already shown how the Pythagorean skein might apply to the English as well as the Hebrew and Greek alphabets. Washburn stated, "in reality" there were only "two heavenly languages" that God spoke. Had God left the masses of illiterate Hebrew and Greek people in the lurch? It was in this section that Washburn advanced his "mason" analogy.

For "Step 6: Putting It All Together," Washburn put it together elsewhere, then left his readers to seek his "detailed explanation" in another text—*Theomatics II*. He alleged this would spare us from "extremely laborious reading," the mere four pages of which he might have graciously provided in his appendix section.

The final rule largely rehashed earlier steps, but summarized them in "the golden rule of theomatics." That is, "every single word or phrase that is used for a theomatic feature must come right out of the text in exactly the same manner as God put it there" in Greek or Hebrew. Otherwise, he insisted, this method was unreliable.[6]

Washburn then advanced the most controversial condition underlying his thesis, once again, reminiscent of the *Protocols*'s helter-skelter prescription for world domination. In this regard he wrote:

> All schools of prophecy, both futurist and preterits, follow the predisposed premise of *literalism*. As a rule, you interpret all prophetic passages in a grammatical-historical literal manner, as much as is reasonably possible. Everything is to be understood in a specific earth-time sequential manner. This principle is especially true for premillennial dispensationalism; it is the very cornerstone of the [religious] system[s]. Such a method of interpretation will send Christians away from the truth—in the exact opposite direction.

> Dispensationalism [as defined in *Webster's* as "a system of revealed commands and state or ordering of things," and "pertaining to a particular arrangement, or provision esp. of providence or nature,"] detests the idea that God might use numbers symbolically in the Bible. Most evangelical scholars won't touch the subject. It is an area of biblical interpretation that few dispensationalists (or futurists) know how to deal with, so it is basically ignored. Dispensationalists would much prefer to debate other issues. Their standard position is that since everything is to be taken literally, numbers are no exception. According to them, "We have no reason to believe that there is any significance to the numbers mentioned in the Bible, other than their quantitative value."

> *To admit that God may have imparted a symbolic principle to numbers in the Bible would in effect destroy their system. The very fact that theomatics exists—the very fact that God has put a*

> *hidden and symbolical system of this nature in the Bible—is going to knock the pilings out from underneath the entire grammatical-historical-literal premise.* [Emphasis not added.][6]

Joey felt these conclusions seriously undermined Washburn's effort. It seemed a direct contradiction of purpose, a thesis/antithesis dialectic that left the masses more confused and divided. On the one hand the numerical codes throughout the Bible were "the fingerprints of God." On the other, Washburn declared all literal interpretations of the numbers and Bible, every chapter and verse, was potentially a deception. It just didn't add up without taking the related *Protocols* into account.

In the same vein that Washburn followed (divide the "sheeple" to conquer the flock), Lawrence Gardner addressed the limitations of literal Bible interpretations, and at the same time acknowledged the "encrypted" Bible codes. His Yale lecture included the following observations:

> There is an allegory within the Gospels—a use of words that we don't understand today. We now know [for example] that baptismal priests were called "fishes." We know that those who aided them by hauling the baptismal candidates into the boats in large nets were called "fishermen." And we know that the baptismal candidates themselves were [also] called "fishes." The apostles James and John were both ordained "fishes." The brothers Peter and John were lay "fishermen," and Jesus promised Peter and Andrew priesthood within the new ministry saying, "I will make you to become fishers of men." We now know that there was a particular jargon of the Gospel era. A jargon that would have been readily understood by anyone reading the Gospels in the first century and beyond.
>
> These jargonistic words have been lost to later interpretation. Today, for example, we call our top entertainers "stars." But what would a reader in some far distant culture, 2,000 years further off in time, make of, "He went to Hollywood to talk to the stars?"

The Gospels are full of these jargonistic words. The "poor," the "lepers," the "multitude," the "blind," none of these were what we presume them to mean today. Definitions of such words as "cloud," "sheep," "fishes," "loaves," and a variety of others were all related, just like "stars," to people.

When the Gospels were written in the first century they were issued into a Roman controlled environment. Their content had to be disguised against Roman scrutiny. The information was often political [and thus,] it was coded. It was veiled. And where important sections appeared, they were often heralded by the words "This is for those with ears to hear." [In other words] for those who understood the code.

It was no different from the coded information passed between members of oppressed groups throughout history. [For instance, t]here was a code in documentation found passed between the Jews in Germany in the late 1930s and 1940s, jargons, cryptic wording.

By use of knowledge of this Bible cryptology we can now determine dates and locations with very great accuracy. We can uncover many of the hidden meanings in the Gospels, down to the extent that the miracles themselves take on a whole new context. In doing this, this does not in any way decry the fact that a man like Jesus, and, in fact, specifically Jesus, was obviously a very, very special person with enormously special powers.

Sadly, Washburn and Gardener's conclusions fulfill protocols fourteen through seventeen:

We have long past taken care to credit the priesthood of the [manipulated], and thereby to ruin their mission on earth which in these days might still be a great hindrance to us. Day by day its influence on the peoples of the world is falling lower. Freedom of conscience has been declared everywhere, so that now only years divide us from the moment of the complete wrecking of that Christian religion. . . .

The King of the Jews will be the real Pope of the Universe, the patriarch of an international Church. But, in the meantime, while we are reeducating youth in new traditional religions and afterwards in ours, we shall not overtly lay a finger on existing churches, but we shall fight against them by criticism calculated to produce schisms. . . .

Our philosophers will discuss all the shortcomings of the various beliefs of the [manipulated]. But no one will ever bring under discussion our faith from its true point of view since this will be fully learned by none save ours who will never dare to betray its secrets.

In countries known as progressive and enlightened we have created a senseless, filthy, abominable literature. . . . In order that the masses themselves may not guess what they are about we further distract them with amusements, games, pastimes, passions, people's palaces [etc.] . . .

. . . [T]he weapons in our hands are limitless ambitions, burning greediness, merciless vengeance, hatreds and malice.

It is from us that the all-engulfing terror proceeds. We have in our service persons of all opinions, of all doctrines, . . . monarchists, demagogues, socialists, communists, and utopian dreamers of every kind. We have harnessed them all to the task: each one of them on his own account is boring away at the last remnants of authority, is striving to overthrow all established form of order. By these acts all States are in torture; they exhort to tranquility, are ready to sacrifice everything for peace: but we will not give them peace until they openly acknowledge our international Super-Government, and with submissiveness.[1]

## Conclusions on Washburn, Gardner and the *Protocols*

Counterintelligence propaganda commonly presents many truths, but when combined they paint only a partial picture. By selectively avoiding certain important aspects of the entire reality, propagandists facilitate misinterpretations and mass deceptions. By so doing, people can be easily divided, conquered, or manipulated to kill or be killed.

Whole truths, on the other hand, resonate absolute certainty on all levels—physical, mental, emotional, social, intuitive and/or spiritual. At this time when God's secrets, his hidden codes, and those of the ruling elite are being unveiled, increasingly it seems that people are developing an acute "sixth sense"—like Willi Apel's "secret ear"—to "feel" the resonate frequencies of whole truths and distinguish them from the "energy vibrations" that partial truths and outright lies provide—vibes that mislead, separate, and destroy humanity.

In this chapter the techniques by which such mass manipulation, separation, and destruction, largely through the media, were revealed in the Masonic document called the *Protocols of the Elders of Sion*. This document explained how selected truths or partial truths are used in the press of old, and the contemporary media, to effect political agendas for an "illumined" few. (An additional example involving healing herbs and *TIME* magazine is included in the appendix.) In this context the works by Drosnin, Washburn and Gardner, though grossly different in content, are very similar in effect.

Gardner, for instance, presented an in-depth historic reinterpretation of the Gospels and the genealogy of royal bloodlines including Christ's. He based his oration and written works on new truths provided, as he said, by thirty-three (33) royal families and the Celtic church. He alleged that the Knights Templar evolved to protect and promote the Nazarene theology—Christ's most holy loving teachings.

Yet, despite his factual precision, as in Washburn's case, Gardner's offering left Joey in doubt. Why, for instance, if Jesus was merely a unique "person," could periodic miracles be happening for so many people who invoke his name, or pray, like Joey, for his intervention? In other words, if Jesus wasn't the messiah, then all those praying to him, all the angels responding to these calls, and all the miracles created as a result, would be, according to Gardner and Washburn, part of a cosmic tragedy, if not a deception. How might we explain Jeshua's revelations to Joey? If Jesus was merely an "illumined" and powerful mortal then this book would not exist.

Moreover, had the Templars been so sincerely moved to share the truth about Christ's love and teachings with mankind, as Gardner alleged, then why, after all these years, did they not reveal the codes that

King James et al. kept hidden? The highest levels of Freemasonry, as you will see in Chapter 5, knew how critical and powerful the arcana that Jeshua was about to reveal to Joey truly is. If the Templars cared so much about Nasorean Christianity, why would they help to keep the power and the glory of the truth from the people?

Similarly, for Washburn's work there are paradoxes to be reconciled. On the one hand he evidenced the omnipotence of God, and claimed "simple" public access to God's infinite wisdom. On the other hand his methods and prose fostered sectarianism, and intellectual and cultural elitism.

By understanding the authenticity of the *Protocols*, the motives of those who wrote them, and the ways in which they are being actualized today, such perceived paradoxes in popular literature, in the media at large and, as a result in the public's mind, can be more easily reconciled.

## References

1. van Helsing J. *Secret Societies and Their Power in the 20th Century.* Gran Canaria, Spain: Ewertverlag S.L., 1995, pp. 41-95.

2. Drosnin M. *The Bible Code.* New York: Simon & Schuster, Inc., 1997, pp. 12, 18, and 23.

3. Horowitz L. *Emerging Viruses: AIDS & Ebola—Nature, Accident or Intentional?* Sandpoint, ID: Tetrahedron Publishing Group, 1998, pp. 228, 549; for evidence of Richard Preston's work on behalf of U.S. counterintelligence see "Marburg, Ebola and Chilling Propaganda in *The Hot Zone, Ibid.* pp. 385-400 and 475-479.

4. Horowitz L. *Deadly Innocence: The Kimberly Bergalis Florida Dental AIDS Tragedy.* Rockport, MA: Tetrahedron Publishing Group, 1993.

5. NCI staff. *The Special Virus Cancer Program: Progress Report #8.* Office of the Associate Scientific Director for Viral Oncology (OASDVO). J. B. Moloney, Ed., Washington, D. C.: U.S. Government Printing Office, 1971. Note: This publication is a very hard to locate.

Few libraries carry it including the NCI Library at Fort Detrick, Maryland. It is available through the Davis Library, The University of North Carolina, Chapel Hill, Government Documents Department Depository, Reference # HE 20.3152:V81. The incriminating contracts are contained in "Bionetics Research Laboratories, Inc., A Division of Litton Industries. Progress report on investigation of carcinogenesis with selected virus preparations in the newborn monkey." *Ibid..*, pp. 273-278; See also: NCI staff. *The Special Virus Cancer Program: Progress Report #9* Office of the Associate Scientific Director for Viral Oncology (OASDVO). J. B. Moloney, Ed., Washington, D. C.: U.S. Government Printing Office, 1972.

6. Washburn D. *The Original Code in the Bible: Using Science & Mathematics to Reveal God's Fingerprints.* Lanham, Maryland: Madison Books, 1998, pp. 231-235.

7. Personal communication with retired Col. Ben Partin, Oklahoma City bombing expert, following his presentation at the "American Heratage Festival," Precious Moments Conference Center, Carthage, Missouri, Sunday, July 19, 1998.

8. *"Waco: The Rules of Engagement,"* the 136-minute documentary—winner of the 1997 IDA Feature Award, and Academy Award nominee, by Sam Ford Entertainment and Film Estate Productions, Mike McNulty, producer, is available from The Free American Group, U.S. Highway 380—Box 2943, Bingham, New Mexico 87832; 505-423-3250; e-mail:-freeamerican@etscl.net.

9. MacArthur J. *Charismatic Chaos.* Grand Rapids, Michigan: Zondervan Press. 1990, pp. 88-92.

# Chapter 5.
# Exposing Deception
# and Decoding Truth

J oey was still missing knowledge about the ancient Solfeggio. What was the spiritual significance of its notes? What meaning(s) did they convey? Were they really hidden to disempower the masses? What about the important hymn to John the Baptist? Where might that be found, and what meaning(s) did it hold? These and other questions tormented him.

"Nobody wants to talk to me about this stuff," Joey complained to John the bookstore owner one afternoon.

"Maybe if you go to the Vatican, you can find out what you need to know," John replied half joking.

Another friend overheard their conversation. "Maybe you'd be better off dropping this whole investigation," he suggested. "You're uncovering some arcana that nobody wants out. They've burned castles, killed kings, murdered the Cathars, destroyed the Templars, and everywhere you go people are telling you to get off the subject. Maybe you'd better listen to them."

"How can a seeker of truth just stop?" Joey returned. "I'm being spiritually led! Therefore, I needn't be afraid."

## The Answers Revealed

Later that snowy afternoon Joey pondered his predicament. Peering out his picture window at the wind swept crystal flakes that melted then ran down the glass, there were only two things he needed. First were the definitions of the mysterious sacred tones—the ancient Solfeggio. That knowledge, he suspected, would likely provide users with divine powers that might be used to create and heal. Second, there were the missing books of the Bible contained in the Protestant Apocrypha. These were also likely to contribute to his knowledge about the elusive hymn to John the Baptist. So he prayed to Jeshua for help in this quest.

Within seconds Jesus appeared before Joey in the window. He smiled broadly.

"You have the Apocrypha," Jeshua advised.

"Where is it?"

"Close your eyes," Jeshua commanded.

Joey complied. Then suddenly an image came to him—a box full of Bibles. "That's my box!" he declared.

The Bible box had been given to him about a year earlier by the minister of a church in Sandpoint. The minister explained that their church's recently deceased caretaker, whom Joey had befriended, had willed it to Joey.

Joey ran to the storage closet where he kept the gift. He opened the box, rifled through the top layers of Bibles and, lo and behold, there it was—an old Greek Apocrypha.[1]

Now, I'm missing only the Latin tone information he thought. So he returned to the window to consult Jeshua. "Thanks for the Apocrypha," Joey said, "Now can you help me find the missing Solfeggio?"

Jeshua smiled and repeated: "Webster. Webster."

"Are you kidding? *Webster's Dictionary*?" Joey asked incredulously.

Jeshua laughed and said, "Yes."

Joey ran to his library, grabbed his *Random House Webster's College Dictionary* from the shelf, and opened it as though magnetically guided to the sample page viii. His eyes immediately caught the phrases: "hidden entry" and "cross reference to a hidden entry." Joyously he cried, "Oh my glorious God!" (See figure 5.1.)

## The Apocrypha and Webster

As it turned out, Joey later learned, Noah Webster, if not a Freemason, was heavily influenced by Masons including several delegates to the U. S. Constitutional Convention. Like King James, he was enam-

## Fig. 5.1. Reference to "Hidden Entry" and "Cross Reference to a Hidden Entry" Found in *Webster's*

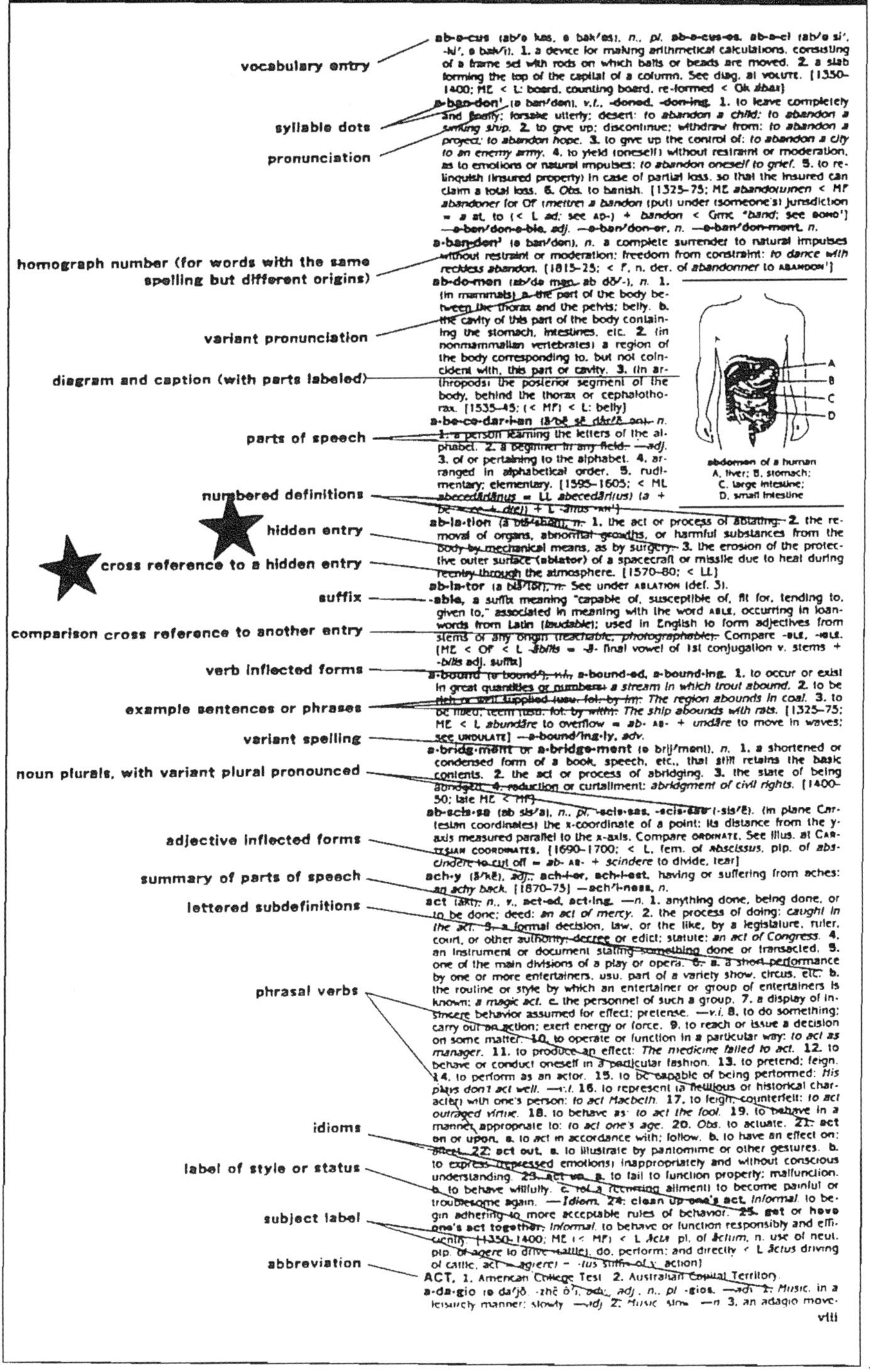

**Labels (left column):**

- vocabulary entry
- syllable dots
- pronunciation
- homograph number (for words with the same spelling but different origins)
- variant pronunciation
- diagram and caption (with parts labeled)
- parts of speech
- numbered definitions
- hidden entry
- cross reference to a hidden entry
- suffix
- comparison cross reference to another entry
- verb inflected forms
- example sentences or phrases
- variant spelling
- noun plurals, with variant plural pronounced
- adjective inflected forms
- summary of parts of speech
- lettered subdefinitions
- phrasal verbs
- idioms
- label of style or status
- subject label
- abbreviation

**Dictionary text (right column):**

ab-a-cus (ab'ə kəs, ə bak'əs), n., pl. ab-a-cus-es, ab-a-ci (ab'ə si', -ki', ə bak'i). 1. a device for making arithmetical calculations, consisting of a frame set with rods on which balls or beads are moved. 2. a slab forming the top of the capital of a column. See diag. at VOLUTE. [1350–1400; ME < L: board, counting board, re-formed < Gk ábax]

a-ban-don¹ (ə ban'dən), v.t., -doned, -don-ing. 1. to leave completely and finally; forsake utterly; desert: to abandon a child; to abandon a sinking ship. 2. to give up; discontinue; withdraw from: to abandon a project; to abandon hope. 3. to give up the control of; to abandon a city to an enemy army. 4. to yield (oneself) without restraint or moderation, as to emotions or natural impulses: to abandon oneself to grief. 5. to relinquish (insured property) in case of partial loss, so that the insured can claim a total loss. 6. Obs. to banish. [1325–75; ME abandounen < MF abandoner for OF (mettre) a bandon (put) under (someone's) jurisdiction = a at, to (< L ad; see AD-) + bandon < Gmc *band; see BOND¹] —a-ban'don-a-ble, adj. —a-ban'don-er, n. —a-ban'don-ment, n.

a-ban-don² (ə ban'dən), n. a complete surrender to natural impulses without restraint or moderation; freedom from constraint: to dance with reckless abandon. [1815–25; < F, n. der. of abandonner to ABANDON¹]

ab-do-men (ab'də mən, ab dō'-), n. 1. (in mammals) a. the part of the body between the thorax and the pelvis; belly. b. the cavity of this part of the body containing the stomach, intestines, etc. 2. (in nonmammalian vertebrates) a region of the body corresponding to, but not coincident with, this part or cavity. 3. (in arthropods) the posterior segment of the body, behind the thorax or cephalothorax. [1535–45; (< MF) < L: belly]

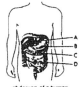

abdomen of a human
A, liver; B, stomach;
C, large intestine;
D, small intestine

a-be-ce-dar-i-an (ā'bē sē dâr'ē ən), n. 1. a person learning the letters of the alphabet. 2. a beginner in any field. —adj. 3. of or pertaining to the alphabet. 4. arranged in alphabetical order. 5. rudimentary; elementary. [1595–1605; < ML abecedāriānus (a + bē + cē + dē + -ARIUS) + -AN; see ABC]

ab-la-tion (a blā'shən), n. 1. the act or process of ablating. 2. the removal of organs, abnormal growths, or harmful substances from the body by mechanical means, as by surgery. 3. the erosion of the protective outer surface (ablator) of a spacecraft or missile due to heat during reentry through the atmosphere. [1570–80; < LL]

ab-la-tor (a blā'tər), n. See under ABLATION (def. 3).

-able, a suffix meaning "capable of, susceptible of, fit for, tending to, given to," associated in meaning with the word ABLE, occurring in loanwords from Latin (laudable); used in English to form adjectives from stems of any origin (teachable, photographable). Compare -IBLE, -ABLE. [ME < OF < L -ābilis = -3- final vowel of 1st conjugation v. stems + -bilis adj. suffix]

a-bound (ə bound'), v.i. 1. to occur or exist in great quantities or numbers: a stream in which trout abound. 2. to be rich or well supplied (usu. fol. by in): The region abounds in coal. 3. to be filled, teem (usu. fol. by with): The ship abounds with rats. [1325–75; ME < L abundāre to overflow = ab- AB- + undāre to move in waves; see UNDULATE] —a-bound'ing-ly, adv.

a-bridg-ment or a-bridge-ment (ə brij'mənt), n. 1. a shortened or condensed form of a book, speech, etc., that still retains the basic contents. 2. the act or process of abridging. 3. the state of being abridged. 4. reduction or curtailment: abridgment of civil rights. [1400–50; late ME < MF]

ab-scis-sa (ab sis'ə), n., pl. ab-scis-sas, -scis-sae (-sis'ē). (in plane Cartesian coordinates) the x-coordinate of a point: its distance from the y-axis measured parallel to the x-axis. Compare ORDINATE. See illus. at CARTESIAN COORDINATES. [1690–1700; < L, fem. of abscissus, plp. of abscindere to cut off = ab- AB- + scindere to divide, tear]

ach-y (āk'ē), adj., ach-i-er, ach-i-est. having or suffering from aches: an achy back. [1870–75] —ach'i-ness, n.

act (akt), n., v., act-ed, act-ing. —n. 1. anything done, being done, or to be done; deed: an act of mercy. 2. the process of doing: caught in the act. 3. a formal decision, law, or the like, by a legislature, ruler, court, or other authority; decree or edict; statute: an act of Congress. 4. an instrument or document stating something done or transacted. 5. one of the main divisions of a play or opera. 6. a. a short performance by one or more entertainers, usu. part of a variety show, circus, etc. b. the routine or style by which an entertainer or group of entertainers is known: a magic act. c. the personnel of such a group. 7. a display of insincere behavior assumed for effect; pretense. —v.i. 8. to do something; carry out an action; exert energy or force. 9. to reach or issue a decision on some matter. 10. to operate or function in a particular way: to act as manager. 11. to produce an effect: The medicine failed to act. 12. to behave or conduct oneself in a particular fashion. 13. to pretend; feign. 14. to perform as an actor. 15. to be capable of being performed: His plays don't act well. —v.t. 16. to represent (a fictitious or historical character) with one's person: to act Macbeth. 17. to feign; counterfeit: to act outraged virtue. 18. to behave as: to act the fool. 19. to behave in a manner appropriate to: to act one's age. 20. Obs. to actuate. 21. act on or upon, a. to act in accordance with; follow. b. to have an effect on; affect. 22. act out, a. to illustrate by pantomime or other gestures. b. to express (repressed emotions) inappropriately and without conscious understanding. 23. act up, a. to fail to function properly; malfunction. b. to behave willfully. c. (of a recurring ailment) to become painful or troublesome again. —Idiom. 24. clean up one's act, Informal. to begin adhering to more acceptable rules of behavior. 25. get or have one's act together, Informal. to behave or function responsibly and efficiently. [1350–1400; ME < MF < L āctus pl. of āctum, n. use of neut. pip. of agere to drive (cattle), do, perform; and directly < L āctus driving of cattle, act < agere] —tus suffix —L act/on]

ACT, 1. American College Test. 2. Australian Capital Territory.

a-da-gio (ə dä'jō, -zhē ō), adj., n., pl. -gios. —adj. 1. Music. in a leisurely manner; slowly. —adj. 2. Music. slow. —n. 3. an adagio movement

viii

ored with the Bible and, according to historians, used the Bible as the foundation for his definitions. "In other words," Joey explained, "He too included encryptions. If you had a Bible, and an encrypted *Webster's Dictionary*, that's all you needed. You could go anywhere in the world and be a secret agent for the Illuminati.

"Nikola Tesla, the great grandfather of electromagnetic technologies, also worked his miracles by referencing the Bible codes," Joey continued. "Tesla knew how to read the codes to get the magnificence. He and Keely said in many of their works: 'If you only knew the magnificence of the 3s, 6s and 9s you'd have a key to the universe.'

"Besides knowing the codes," Joey speculated, "Webster likely knew of the Illuminati's covenant. That everything had to be presented up front. That was God's covenant. The Templars knew it. The evil demiurges knew it too.

"So right in *Webster's Dictionary* what do you find?" Joey continued by opening his dictionary to the word "Bible." Under 'BOOKS OF THE OLD TESTAMENT,' between 'JEWISH SCRIPTURE' and 'BOOKS OF THE NEW TESTAMENT,' was 'PROTESTANT APOCRYPHA.' (See figure 5.2.)

"Everybody's Bible just has the Old and New Testaments. But why does Webster say the 'books of the Bible'? He doesn't say the 'real' books, or the 'non-real' books. He includes the Apocrypha.

"Now the Catholic Church says the Apocrypha is not worth including," Joey continued, "But Webster, quoted in law books, puts it right there in black and white as a book of the Bible.

Then, Joey asked rhetorically, "Where are they? The only good one was done by Goodspeed in a 1939 edition, and it had nothing to do with the Council of Bishops or the clergy. Goodspeed, his brother, and a bunch of scholars sought to study the *Greek Septuagint,* and its direct translation in the Apocrypha that was originally found."

Goodspeed described the history of these important writings this way:

# BOOKS OF THE OLD TESTAMENT

| ROMAN CATHOLIC CANON | PROTESTANT CANON | ROMAN CATHOLIC CANON | PROTESTANT CANON |
|---|---|---|---|
| Genesis | Genesis | Wisdom | |
| Exodus | Exodus | Sirach | |
| Leviticus | Leviticus | Isaiah | Isaiah |
| Numbers | Numbers | Jeremiah | Jeremiah |
| Deuteronomy | Deuteronomy | Lamentations | Lamentations |
| Joshua | Joshua | Baruch | |
| Judges | Judges | Ezekiel | Ezekiel |
| Ruth | Ruth | Daniel | Daniel |
| 1 & 2 Samuel | 1 & 2 Samuel | Hosea | Hosea |
| 1 & 2 Kings | 1 & 2 Kings | Joel | Joel |
| 1 & 2 Chronicles | 1 & 2 Chronicles | Amos | Amos |
| Ezra | Ezra | Obadiah | Obadiah |
| Nehemiah | Nehemiah | Jonah | Jonah |
| Tobit | | Micah | Micah |
| Judith | | Nahum | Nahum |
| Esther | Esther | Habakkuk | Habakkuk |
| Job | Job | Zephaniah | Zephaniah |
| Psalms | Psalms | Haggai | Haggai |
| Proverbs | Proverbs | Zechariah | Zechariah |
| Ecclesiastes | Ecclesiastes | Malachi | Malachi |
| Song of Songs | Song of Solomon | 1 & 2 Maccabees | |

## JEWISH SCRIPTURE

| | | | |
|---|---|---|---|
| *Law* | 1 & 2 Kings | Nahum | Song of Songs |
| Genesis | Isaiah | Habakkuk | Ruth |
| Exodus | Jeremiah | Zephaniah | Lamentations |
| Leviticus | Ezekiel | Haggai | Ecclesiastes |
| Numbers | Hosea | Zechariah | Esther |
| Deuteronomy | Joel | Malachi | Daniel |
| *Prophets* | Amos | *Hagiographa* | Ezra |
| Joshua | Obadiah | Psalms | Nehemiah |
| Judges | Jonah | Proverbs | 1 & 2 Chronicles |
| 1 & 2 Samuel | Micah | Job | |

## PROTESTANT APOCRYPHA

| | | | |
|---|---|---|---|
| 1 & 2 Esdras | Ecclesiasticus | Prayer of Azariah | Bel and the |
| Tobit | or the Wisdom | and the Song of | Dragon |
| Judith | of Jesus Son | the Three Holy | The Prayer of |
| Additions to Esther | of Sirach | Children | Manasses |
| Wisdom of Solomon | Baruch | Susanna | 1 & 2 Maccabees |

# BOOKS OF THE NEW TESTAMENT

| | | | |
|---|---|---|---|
| Matthew | Romans | 1 & 2 Thessalo- | James |
| Mark | 1 & 2 Corinthians | nians | 1 & 2 Peter |
| Luke | Galatians | 1 & 2 Timothy | 1, 2, 3 John |
| John | Ephesians | Titus | Jude |
| Acts of the Apostles | Philippians | Philemon | Revelation |
| | Colossians | Hebrews | *or* Apocalypse |

The Apocrypha formed an integral part of the King James version of 1611, as they had all of the preceding English versions from their beginning at 1382. But they are seldom printed as part of it any longer, still more seldom as part of the English Revised Version, and were not included in the American Revision. This is partly because the Puritans disapproved of them; they had already begun to drop them from the printings of their Geneva Bible by 1600, and began to demand copies of the King James version omitting them, as early as 1629. And it is partly because we moderns discredit them because they did not form part of the Hebrew Bible, and most of them have never been found in any Hebrew forms at all.

But they were part of the Bible of the early church, for it is used in the Greek version of the Jewish Bible, which we shall call the *Septuagint*, and these books were all in that version. They passed from it into Latin and the great Latin Bible edited by St. Jerome about A.D. 400, the Vulgate [the Hebrew Bible], which became the Authorized Bible of western Europe and England, and remained so for a thousand years. But Jerome found that they were not in the Hebrew Bible, and so he called them the Apocrypha, the hidden or secret books.

. . . They are scattered here and there through the Vulgate, much as they are through the Greek Bible. They are also scattered through the versions made from the Vulgate—the Wyclif-Purvey English translations and the old German Bible, both products of the fourteenth century. It remained for Martin Luther to take the hint Jerome had dropped eleven hundred years before, and to separate them in his German Bible of 1534 from the rest of the Old Testament, and put them after it. This course was followed the next year by Coverdale, in the first printed English Bible, of 1535; and the English Authorized Bibles, the Great Bible; the Bishops' and the King James, all followed the same course. The Catholic English Old Testament of 1610, however, followed the Vulgate arrangement and left them scattered among the books which we include in our Old Testament. It still contains them. But on the Protestant side, both British and American Bible societies, more than a hundred years ago (1827), took a definite stand against their publication, and they have since almost disappeared.

Great values reside in the Apocrypha . . . The strong contrast they present in sheer moral values to the New Testament is most instructive. And they form an indispensable part of the historic

Christian Bible, as it was known in the ancient Greek and Latin churches, in the Reformation and the Renaissance, and in all Authorized English Bibles, Catholic and Protestant.

It has been said that no one can have the complete Bible, as a source book for the cultural study of art, literature, history, and religion, without the Apocrypha. From the earliest Christian times down to the age of the King James Version, they belonged to the Bible; and, while modern critical judgments and religious attitudes deny them a position of equality with the Old and New Testament scriptures, historically and culturally they are still an integral part of the Bible. . . .[2]

In fact, the Apocrypha contained much of the missing numbering system that Joey needed to complete the Pythagorean skein, the Mediaeval hymn to John the Baptist, and other key insights he required to augment this work.

## Evolution of The Dark Ages

A brief review of religious history best explains how and why books like the Apocrypha, 152 spiritual hymns held by the Catholic Church, and much more, as you will soon see, disappeared or were markedly changed. Historic revelations also explain how the rift occurred between Christians and Jews, Catholics and Protestants, as well as the initial evolution of religious sectarianism.

Pastor Norm Franz, Director of the Institute of Prophetic Study, and one of America's foremost prophetic ministers explained it this way during a series of lectures entitled "Prophets and Prophetic Ministry:"[3]

"There was a time when the First Century [Christian] Church turned the religious world upside down. Then it died out. What happened? This is [a brief the history] of the church.

"From 33 A.D. to about 70 A.D. the Apostolic Church [based on the apostles and their direct teachings of Christ] grew. . . . It was spontaneous, powerful, and bold in the Lord because it had a proper foundation. It functioned according to . . . [the holy] men, the original twelve apostles [—the direct students of Christ].

"The Bible truths that were in the church at this time were [*as paraphrased*]: 1) 'salvation by grace' through the grace of God, 2) full immersion water Baptism, 3) Baptism by the Holy Spirit with the evidence of speaking in tongues, 4) all the gifts of the Holy Spirit—divined praise and worship, the laying on of hands [for healing], miracles, healings, deliverances, resurrection from the dead . . . and, 5) a five fold ministry of apostle, prophet, evangelist, pastor, and teacher. This movement was a Jesus movement. It was Messianic Judaism that was heresy to the Jews until they met the Messiah. Then it was the fulfillment of what they had been looking for.

"The denomination in those days was called: 'The Church of the Lord Jesus Christ,' 'The Body of Christ,' 'The Army of God,' 'The Temple of God,' 'The Temple of the Holy Spirit,' [or] 'The Way.' [In essence] there wasn't a denomination. It was all Jesus—the Body of Christ.

"The first time they tried to split up [the Body of Christ was when] . . . Paul said, 'Some of you say that I'm a Paul; some say I'm a Barnabus [false prophet], or an Apollos,' [and] Paul just rebuked them. Christ never divided, . . .

"Now you will begin to understand why we have all the denominations, and why all the mainline denominations are as messed up as they are.

"From 70 A.D. until about 313 A.D. [the Body of Christ became] the persecuted church. In 70 A.D. Titus and the Roman legions came into Jerusalem and destroyed the city and temple. The Jew [at that time] was the most hated and persecuted person on the face of the earth. Gentiles who now believed in the Jewish God, Jesus Christ, were not considered good Christians. They were considered 'good Jews.'"

Yet, people turned to Christ and followed the Bible despite the persecution. The term "Christians" started at Antioch, and was the term used to describe gentiles who now believed in the Jewish Messiah—Jesus Christ.

Likewise, at that time, Jews continued to love Christ and his teachings. According to the work of religious scholar Dr. Russ Weinstein, the vast majority of intelligent religious Jews who met Christ or knew of his deeds firmly believed he was the Messiah.[4]

So Christians and Jews alike were hated. They were persecuted. And the type of Christian Church at that time was one whose leaders were killed. "They were thrown in the lions' den," Pastor Franz continued. "They were sawed in two. They were hung, burned alive, and crucified. . . . [But] during this time, [despite the persecution] the church was still moving in dynamic power because it was pure before the Lord. The men that were involved included Justin who was beheaded in 160 A.D. because he refused to bow down to the Caesars."[3]

"Others were persecuted on July 17, 180 A.D., when Spiritus, Sidonus, Donetta, Secunda, Vestia, and others went before the Pro Council Saturnanus. He . . . [warned them that if they did not] stop being Christians, and start to worship the state religion, which was the Caesars—men proclaiming themselves as Gods—they would be executed. [They refused to cower so they were] killed by the sword.

"What were the Bible truths at that time?" Pastor Franz asked. "The same as always. The movement was called 'The Jesus Movement.' So the persecution continued."[3]

In 313 A.D., the Imperial Church, or the Constantine Church, began. It was born from Constantine's vision of a cross on a hill. He heard a voice say, "Under this sign you shall conquer." That's why the Crusaders began wearing the cross on their armor and uniforms. When Constantine had this vision he decided to become a "Christian." He had been a Pagan. Suddenly he was a "Christian" who hadn't been taught the ways of God. Instead of persecuting the church, he then started funding it. Pagan entities suddenly fell out of favor and were being abandoned. Then a Pagan form of "Christianity" suddenly became the order for the empire when the priests of the Pagan religions resigned to follow the money and politics. They quickly converted so that they could be priests in the new "Christian" church.[3]

Many of their Pagan idols and worship came with them. New doctrines began and the Bible began to include Pagan religions and customs. They called them "Christian rituals," but they were not. They put a Christian flavor on Pagan observances to assimilate Paganism into the state religion which made it more politically correct. One such inclusion was the worship of the sun god's birthday—December 25—today known as Christmas. They changed the first day of the week and called it Sunday in honor of their sun god. Monday was a tribute to their moon god. Tuesday was for the god Tunas. Thursday was named for Thor—the god of wind, and so on until all days were named after Pagan gods.[3]

"In the Bible, God never called them this, he called them 'the first day,' 'the second day,' and so on," Franz continued.

"The veneration of Mary was another addition of their 'Christianity.' Mary was deified and made a god. This dated back to ancient mother and child worship in Babylon with Nimrod and his mother—Cimeramous—named the 'mother of God' and 'Queen of Heaven.'" This evolved from the Egyptian goddess of fertility, Isis, called the 'great virgin.' She was also called the 'mother of God' and got into Egyptian religious ceremonies at that time."[3]

Soon the Roman Catholic Church began to partition the deceased saints—the Apostles Paul and Peter. This caused strife among the Christian ranks.

The state Pagan church began to place the names of gods and servants of gods over temple doorways and named their temples after them. Church buildings were built with Constantine's money which wasn't the case until his supposed "conversion." Prior to this, religious meetings were conducted in the home church or in the synagogue.

Pastor Franz discussed the advent of "an Apostate five-fold ministry that came into being. Instead of the apostle, prophet, evangelist, pastor and teacher, there was the pope, the cardinal, the archbishop, the bishop, and the priest. They began to call the leaders—the priests—

'father.' The Bible said to call no man 'father.' And the head priest was called the 'Holy Father.'"[3]

Instead of repenting, "penance" was done. Basically you paid your way through works so that God would forgive you. The only way you could be saved was through membership in the state church.

There were no miracles. Because, after all, the miracles had passed away with the First Century Church and the apostles and the prophets. In fact, as you will soon learn, the knowledge and electromagnetic technology for producing "mira gestorum"—that is, miracles—were then hidden from the masses.

"This movement was man-made, dead religion. It was apostasy and controlled by the state," Pastor Norm said. "Though this may seem to be a heavy indictment, if you study history at all, this is exactly what happened."[3]

The Dark Ages ran from 478 A.D. to 1500 A.D. The type of Pagan church that was around at that time destroyed the power of the church. "The life of God—the Holy Spirit of God—that brought life and light was refused," Pastor Norm reported. "They did not allow it to work. For all intensive purposes, God's power and God's light on the earth was censured and not allowed to be revealed or practiced." That was why the entire earth moved into the Dark Ages. "This was a time of spooky spiritual mysticism" that was designed around the Roman Catholic Church and the Orthodox Greek Church. Bibles containing God's word were taken away. Interpretation and reading of old doctrine could only be performed by clergymen. They had Holy Saints Days and ritual beads. They came out with many new signs and insignias including many new crosses—what may be seen as "graven images" in contrast to the pure word of God and the second commandment. This was the period of the Imperial Churches. They were state churches; they were not churches of God.

In the 1500s, many believe that God began to restore what the church had lost during the Dark Ages. Martin Luther, a Catholic monk, had read the Bible as only the clergy could during that period. As he did, the story goes, God's spirit inspired him to speak his heart.

Ephesians Chapter 2, verses 8 and 9 (the numbers for "God" and completion) told him, "For by grace are ye saved through faith; and that not of yourselves: *it* is the gift of God: Not of works, lest any man should boast." This moved Luther to avidly search the scriptures. As he did, God showed him that the doctrine of the Catholic Church was wrong because it kept people in bondage. It made people have to work their way into heaven rather than be saved by "grace" and through "faith."[3]

So Martin Luther, the Rosicrucian who bore his personal red rose and cross insignia, went to the Whittenburg Church and nailed his thesis to its door. The Catholics screamed heretic and persecuted him. But in the process, he restored major truths including salvation, justification by grace through faith, prayer by the people for the people, walking in peace and joy, and more. This movement was called the Protestant movement. Protestants, at that time, were considered, according to Pastor Norm, "radical protestors who dared to depart from the norm and come away from the establishment church of the world and say 'You're wrong, we're following God.'"[3]

The Lutheran Church, it is believed with a few incriminating exceptions,[3] evolved out of this spirit. With his ties to the Rosicrucians and the Prieuré de Sion, Luther developed his Bible.[3] The Protestants then developed their Bible with the addition of the Apocrypha. It was at this time that King James of Scotland and England, who was also a Freemason, allegedly embattled with the Roman Catholic Church, also developed his version of the Bible.

## Matrices in the Recovered Knowledge

The Roman Catholic Church, like King James, as you are about to learn, in distancing the masses from the truth, suppressed the matrices of thought required for divinity to be experienced and expressed by the masses. The personal relationships between God and man were sacrificed to everyone's detriment except for the ruling elite.

Matrices play intimate roles in every aspect of life. Matrices are found in computers, corporations, and institutions. They underlie thought, sound, healing, and light. In the Bible the word is found *thrice* in Exodus (13:12–15; and 34:19). Moses bade "sacrifice to the Lord all that openeth the matrix." This was done so the Hebrews could be freed. The word is repeated in Numbers (3:12 and 18:15) wherein God said, "Every thing that openeth the matrix in all flesh . . . shall be thine."

Webster defined the word "matrix" as:

> 1. something within or from which something else originates, develops, or takes form. . . . 4 a: the intercellular substance in which tissue cells (as of connective tissue) are embedded. . . . 5 a: a rectangular array of numbers, algebraic symbols, or mathematical functions [such as a clock or calendar] (as the coefficients of simultaneous linear equations) that can be combined to form sums and products with similar arrays having an appropriate number of rows and columns [or that can be added or multiplied following certain rules]. . . . b: a similar rectangle consisting of rows and columns of numbers and symbols [like a calendar] used in displaying statistical variables, linguistic features, or others [including music sheets, languages based on mathematics, tide tables, and solar and lunar cycles.] c: an array of circuit elements (as diodes and transistors) for performing a specific function. 6: a main clause that contains a subordinate clause. [For example] a *matrix sentence*—a sentence in which another sentence is imbedded in it. [Much like Webster's "hidden entry" clause.]

In essence, as you will soon see, directions for accessing the matrix of all creation, including spiritual development, human evolution, accurate dates and time, and natural healing was hidden and recovered by Joey through Jeshua when the former learned the secrets that the Protestant Apocrypha and *Webster's Dictionary* revealed.

As seen in figure 5.3 the ancient Solfeggio contained six tones with hidden meanings. They piqued Joey's curiosity and demanded his attention. Instructed by Jeshua to search *Webster's Dictionary* for their definitions, including the "hidden entries" behind their meanings, Joey compiled the information shown in figure 5.3.

## Exposing Deceptions

In the *King James Bible*, the word "Selah," a musical term that means to "sprout"—give rise to life—can be found seventy-one times. Only once the term "Higgaion" is used. The two are virtually interchageable as seen in Psalm 9:16. The term Higgaion means "a

## UT–quent laxis

1. a syllable used for the first note in the diatonic scale in an early solminzation system and later replaced by do. 2. the syllable sung to this note in a mediaeval hymn to St. John the Baptist. <Gk. -Gamut- 1. the entire scale or range; *the Gamut of dramatic emotion from grief to joy.* 2. *the whole series of recognized musical notes* [1425-75]; late ME (Middle English)> <ML (Mediaeval Latin)–contraction, of *Gamma*, used to represent the first lowest tone of (G) in the Medieval Scale Ut, Re, Mi Fa, So, La, Si. <Gk -Gamma- 1. the *third* letter of the Greek alphabet. 2. the *third* in a series of items. 3. a star that is usually the third brightest of a constellation. 4. a unit of weight equal to one microgram. 5. **a unit of magnetic field strength equal to $10^5$ power gauss.** (quent: needing), (laxis: loose; axis—an affiliation of two or more nations. Also Axis Powers.)

## RE–sonare fibris (Res-o-nance)

1 a: the state of quality of being resonant. b (1) *a vibration of large amplitude in a mechanical or electrical system caused by a relatively small periodic stimulus of the same or nearly the same period as the natural vibration period of the system* 2. the prolongation of sound by reflection; reverberation. 3a. Amplification of a source of speech sounds, esp. of phonation, by sympathic vibration of the air, esp. in the cavaties of the mouth, nose and pharynx. b. a characteristic quality of a particular voice speech sound imparted by the distribution of amplitudes among the cavities of the head, chest, and throat. 4a. *a larger than normal vibration produced in response to a stimulus whose frequency is close to the natural frequency of the vibrating system, as an electrical circuit, in which a value much larger than average is maintained for a given frequency.* 5a. a quality of *enriched significance, profundity, or allusiveness; a poem has a resonance beyond its surface meaning.* 6. the chemical phenomenon in which the arrangements of the valance electrons of a molecule changes back and forth between two or more states. (in percussing for diagnostic purposes) a sound produced when air is present [1485-95]; <MF (Middle French), <L Resonantia, Echo = Reson (are) to resound + Antia-ance.(Re–a prefix, occuring orig. in loan words from Latin, use to form verbs denoting action in a backward direction , *Action in answer to or intended to undo a situation*, or that *performance of the new action brings back an earlier state of affairs.* (fibris: fibre string, vocal cord.)

## MI–ra gestorum (Miracle)

1. *an extraordinary occurance that surpasses all known human powers or natural forces and is ascribed to a divine or supernatural cause esp. to God.* 2. a superb or surpassing example of something; wonder, marvel [1125-75]; ME <L Miraculum=Mira(Ri) to wonder at. *fr* (French): sighting, aiming to hold against the light. (gestorum: gesture; movements to express thought, emotion; any action, *communication*, etc. intended for effect.)

# FA–muli tuorum (Famulus,)

. . . plural Famuli, 1a. *servant/s, or attendant/s, esp. of a scholar or a magician* [1830-40 <L (Latin), servant, of family. (Tourum - quorum - 1. *the number of members of a group required to be present to transact business or carry out an activity legally. usu. a majority.* 2. *a particularly chosen group.* [1425-75; <L quorum of whom; from a use of the word in commissions written in Latin specifying a quorum.)

# SO-lve polluti (So-lve')

1. to find the answer or explanation for; clear-up; explain; to *solve a mystery* or puzzle, to work out the *answer or solution to (a mathematical problem.*) [1400-50; Late ME <L Solvere to loosen, release dissolve = so-var, after velarl, of se-set-luere to wash; (see Ablution.) Ablution n. 1. a cleansing with water or other liquid, esp. as a religious ritual. [1350-1400]. (Pollutii–pollute-luted, 1. to make foul or unclean,)

# LA–bii reatum (Labi-al)

1. of pertaining to or resembling a Labium. 2. of pertaining to the lips, 3. (of a speech sound) *articulated using one or both lips.* 4. of or designating the surface of a tooth facing the lips. 5. the labial speech sound, esp. consonant, [1585-95]; ML lingual. (Reatum - reaction - 1. *a reverse movement or tendency; an action in a reverse direction or manner.* 2. *a movement toward extreme political conservatism;* 3. *a desire to return to an earlier system or order.* 3. action in response to some influence, event, etc.; 4. a psysiological response to an action or condition. b. a physiological change indicating sensitivity to a foreign matter.) 6. mech. the *instantaneous response of a system to an applied force,* manifested as the exertion of a force equal in magnitude, but opposite in direction, to the applied force [1635-45].

# SI (Sancte Johannes)

1. a person of exceptional holiness, formally recognized by the Christian Church esp. by *Canonization.* 2. a person of great virtue or benevolence. 3. a founder or patron, as of a movement. 4. a member of any various Christian groups. 5. to acknowledge as a Saint. Canonize. [1150-1200]; ME Seinte. Canon: 1. an ecclesiastical rule or law enacted by a council or other competent authority and, in the Roman Catholic Church, approved by the Pope. 3. a body of rules, principles, or standards accepted as *axiomatic* and universally binding, esp. in a field of study of art.. 6. any officially recognized set of sacred books. 10. the part of the mass between Sanctus and the *communion.* 11. *consistent, note-for-note imitation of one melodic line by another, in which the second line starts after the first.* (axiomatic: 1. pertaining to or of t*he nature of an axiom; self-evident. 2. a universally accepted principle or rule. 3. a proposition in logic or mathematics that is assumed without proof for the sake of studying consequences that follow from it.*

**[Emphasis added in each definition denotes special relevance to text.]**

deep sound." This is important for those who sing hymns or chants. The perfect notes have an inspirational affect, and give rise to spiritual life which transforms physical nature through electromagnetic vibrations.

The Apocrypha contained the knowledge that these two items—Selah, arising into life or genesis, and Higgaion, a deep sound—should be added.

Oxygen or breath is required for both Selah and Higgaion. God is, of course, required for both as well. Again, the term God or "Yah Vah" in Hebrew means "to breathe is to exist." Moreover, in review, God's covenant involves the importance of oxygen-carrying blood.

Thus, a significant number of seventy-two (72) occurs when seventy-one (71) Selahs plus one (1) Higgaion yield seventy-two (72). Not only did this number represent completion whereby 7+2=9, but every 72 years one degree of astrological declination occurs. This changes the magnetic fields on earth and the cosmos, changes the rates of resonance, and alters the consciousness of the humans as well. These changes were of great significance in keeping people from developing the unseen ears and eyes that could hear and see into the spiritual realms.

The hymn to Saint John the Baptist, also found in the Apocrypha, that followed the tones of the Solfeggio, referred to this process of enlightening the masses to their optimal spiritual potential by washing away their "guilt" ( much of which had been laid upon them by the Church). As sung in Mediaeval Latin:

So that your servants
Can sing together
With the loose strings [the vocal cords]
The wonders of their deeds [potential miracles]
Oh Saint John
Wash away the guilt
of their polluted lips.

In other words, so people could live together in peace and communicate in harmony about the miracles in their lives, and how God blessed them to produce this "magic," people's true unpolluted spiritual natures required revelation. Such baptism could be best accomplished by washing away people's guilt, false judgements, and divisive dialects, that they had assumed due to deceptive manipulations perpetrated by those in control of the spiritual knowledge. Thus, to be "saved by grace" alone, this cleansing and illumination could be best achieved by singing or listening to hymns that used the Solfeggio notes.

Moreover, this hidden knowledge, and related vocal actions taken by "144,000" spiritually enlightened people, would bring about the social transformation of planet earth—that is, as described in figure 5.3 under "LA-bii reatum," the "reverse movement" back from mankind to "Godkind." Humanity could go from shackled to sovereign, hateful to trusting, fearful to empowered, all the while being protected by God's ever flowing love.

According to Revelation 7:4, the magical number of 144,000, is promised to be composed of "all the tribes of the children of Israel." This "FA-muli tuorum," or "family of scholarly magical servants,"(*Webster's* says) are "the people chosen by God." They will call forth the original concept of Israel—a place where "the lion lies down with the lamb;" where absolute peace would be enjoyed by the masses for 1,000 years. Revelation predicted that the 144,000 would be composed of 12,000 from each of twelve tribes. The Pythagorean skein numbers provided here are: nine (9) for 144,000, that is completion; three (3) each for 12,000 tribal representatives from each of twelve (12) tribes—that is, $3\times12=36=9$, or $3+3=6$, or $3\times3=9$, all numerologically powerful, if not magical. Remember what Tesla and Keely said, "If you only knew the power of the 3s, 6s and 9s!"

Those 144,000 "servants of God," according to Revelation 7:3, "were sealed" with "the seal of the living God." The term "seal," according to *Webster's Dictionary* derives from the old high German word *Selah*. Remember that the word *Selah* was used interchangeably in Psalms from the *King James Bible* with the word "Higgaion," musically meaning, "a deep sound," as is used "in meditation." The word Higgaion was referenced three times in James's "Biblical Cyclopedic Index," (Ps. 9:16; Ps. 19:14; and Ps. 92:3) but was only used once in Psalm 9:16. It is missing from Psalm 19:14—"Let the words of my mouth, and the meditation of my heart, be acceptable in thy sight, O Lord, my strength (Hebrew rock), and my redeemer (cross referenced to Isaiah 44:6)."

The term "rock" (or "strength") derives from "back and forth in, or as if in, a cradle," according to *Webster's Dictionary*, like the movement of vibrational frequencies of sound, or "to cause to shake violently" as is done to activate homeopathic medicines. Besides this, the term denotes "popular music usu. played on electronically amplified instruments," and "a large mass of stone . . . " such as a "rock crystal" as will be discussed later.

The term "redeemer," cross referenced to Isaiah 44:6, relates to *God's* "redeemer, the Lord of hosts," that is, "the Lord King of Israel." Isaiah said that God depended on the "Lord of hosts" for redemption. The term "host," in *Webster's* is defined first as "an army" of "a very large number" that might assemble "usu. for a hostile purpose," that is to do battle with an enemy. In this case a spiritual enemy. Moreover, *Webster's* cross references the term "host" with "guest"—"a stranger, enemy" who shares "the dwelling of another."

These passages relate to the great spiritual battle that will be shortly discussed as described in Revelation 7:4 and Psalm 91 when the army of 144,000 servants of God take "refuge" in His "fortress" (Psalm 91:2-3). Then all faithful will be delivered "from the snare of the fowler, and from the noisome pestilence." At the same time, they "will deliver him, and honour him." (See Psalm 91:14-15.)

In essence, deliverance of God by the chosen masses for the greatest "paradigm shift" in history simply depends on the sound frequencies sung by a "critical mass" of faithful and trusting servants.

Recall that in Psalms, Chapters 120–132, the seven "song of degrees" was a deception. The critical number was six. Similarly the use of seventy-one (71) "Selahs" and one (1) "Higgaion" produced nine (9), or completion of the spiritual work accomplished by the masses singing in unison the six degrees of tonal frequencies.

Thus, 144,000 people representing a *critical mass* singing in unison the notes of the Solfeggio, will likely produce what the previously hidden knowledge prescribed singing: 1) "UT"—the "whole series of . . . musical notes" to transmit a "magnetic field strength equal to 144,000 times $10^5$ power (100,000) gauss; 2) "RE"—to resonate a "relatively small periodic stimulus to a natural vibration" to produce "a vibration of large amplitude . . . of enriched significance, profundity, and allusiveness," to act and "undo" the estrangement of man from God and bring back the "earlier state of affairs;" 3) "MI"—"to produce an extraordinary occurrence that surpasses all known human powers or natural forces and is ascribed to a divine or supernational cause esp. to God. . . . "Sighting" this possibility, and "aiming to hold [it] against the light," while communicating for an "intended . . . effect; miracles will happen;" 4) "FA"—the 144,000 servants of God with this knowledge—that of "a scholar or a magician—to be present to transact [this] business or carry out . . . [the extraordinary] activity" as described in "SO" and "LA" below. That is, in Christian terms, "FA" implies "Jesus' bride," "the body of Christ," or for the Hebrews, God's "chosen people." 5) "SO"—Solving the "mystery or puzzle," and working out "the answer or solution to [the] mathematical problem" behind the spiritual "pollution" requiring an "ablution" or a "cleansing religious ritual;" and 6) "LA"—articulating using the lips the sound required to "reverse direction" and move "toward extreme political conservatism . . . to return to an earlier system or order"—world peace.

Finally, as seen in figure 5.3, by referencing the "hidden entries" in *Webster's Dictionary*, Joey learned that these definitions of the original six notes of the Solfeggio compared closely to the meanings of the words and overall message in the recovered hymn to John the Baptist.

"All I need to do is get this information into the hands and hearts of 144,000 enlightened people to bring about the transformation of this planet!" Joey realized most excitedly. "To reverse the spiritual movement of the planet using voice, communication, and electromagnetic frequencies to return mankind to "Godkind." I need to get this information out! I need someone like Dr. Horowitz. Jeshua, please send me someone like Dr. Horowitz to help me get your message to people."

## UnGodly Roman Time

Joey also discovered in the Apocrypha that the Roman time clock, that virtually everyone accepted without question, is completely reversed! As with the alpha numeric translation of Hebrew to English, this similar perversion is illustrated in figure 5.4. According to Genesis 1:5, and John 11:9, a new day always began in the evening. What we now refer to as 6 p.m. Likewise, in *Gregorian Chant*, Professor Apel, who taught at a Jesuit college and meticulously researched the early French literature, stated that during the early days of the Roman Catho-

---

## Fig. 5.4. Roman Versus Mosaic Time Clocks

### BACKWARDS ROMAN CLOCK

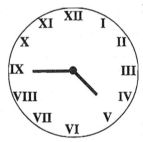

Venetians and Germans, both under Roman influence, developed the modern clock. According to authorities, and Roman Catholic Church archives, the first hour of the day began at what we now call 6 o'clock in the evening—directly opposite to the original time clock as described in the Bible. This was likely done to spiritually disorient and disempower people.

### STANDARD MOSAIC TIME CLOCK

For many thousands of years people began their days in the evening according to Genesis 1:5 and John 11:9. Theoretically, by reverting back to God's way of keeping time, left and right brain function will improve as will people's spiritual receptivity. This thesis was additionally supported by the number codes discovered in the Bible.

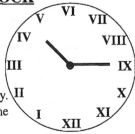

---

lic Church the first hour of the day *was* 6 p.m. Their church masses and spiritual hymns were all originally conducted in Hebrew and began at that time.

Further reflecting on Babylon, and consistent with the use of altered language for mass spiritual deception and strife, Latin followed Hebrew and further confused "communications"—the root of which is the French term *communis* and the Mediaeval Latin term communia, meaning "to receive Communion" or union with God, or "to open into each other." Thus, language that was originally developed to secure unity among people and with God. Once modified, however, it helped to obscure the inherently open door to divinity and peace on earth.

The Romans, with the Vatican's blessing, took Hebrew, a perfectly Godly language that provided the tones for "atonement," or oneness with God, and substituted Latin with little chance for the masses to recover their divine link.

Likewise, they took a perfectly functional clock and inverted it. In the process, they literally "dumb downed" the masses. The change supported dysfunction of the "right/left brain," and blocked spiritual integration, and hampered the Godly evolution of humanity.

Figure 5.5 provides further evidence of a conspiracy to deceive. Shown is a copy of the "Hieroglyphic Plan, by Hermes, of the Ancient Zodiac." This was published by Manly P. Hall in his book *An Encyclopedic outline of Masonic, Hermetic, Kabbalistic and Rosicrucian Symbolical Philosophy: Being an Interpretation of the Secret Teachings Concealed Within the Rituals, Allegories and Mysteries of All Ages.* This hieroglyphic adorned the roof of Hermes Temple in ancient Egypt where Jesus sojourned to study Greek and Egyptian theology. Viewed from space, that is, from the perspective of heavenly beings, the sixth house of Gemini lines up perfectly with the 6th hour on Moses's clock believed to have come from God. This provides additional evidence that the Mosaic clock was astronomically accurate, while the Roman clock is grossly inaccurate, that is, backwards.[5]

Another problem arose from the modification of the twelve-month leap year calendar originally in the Bible. The "leap year" occurred

## Fig. 5.5. Hermes Temple Hieroglyphic of the Ancient Zodiac as Superimposed on the Mosiac Clock

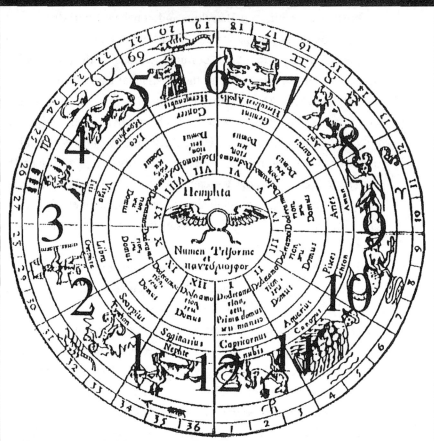

This hieroglyphic adorned the roof of Hermes Temple in ancient Egypt where Jesus sojourned to study Greek and Egyptian theology. Viewed from space, that is, from the perspective of heavenly beings, the sixth house of Gemini lines up perfectly with the 6th hour on Moses's clock believed to have come from God. This provides additional evidence that the Mosaic clock was astronomically accurate, while the Roman clock is grossly inaccurate. Adapted from: Hall MP. *An Encyclopedic outline of Masonic, Hermetic, Kabbalistic and Rosicrucian Symbolical Philosophy: Being an Interpretation of the Secret Teachings Concealed Within the Rituals, Allegories and Mysteries of All Ages.* Los Angeles: The Philosophical Research Society, Inc., (3910 Los Feliz Boulevard, Los Angeles, CA 90027), 1989, pp. LVI; CLXXVII.

every three years wherein the twelfth month was repeated as a thirteenth month. Joey discovered a similar pattern in the Apocrypha. This change clearly confused the high holy days, such as Passover, the true Hebrew New Year, and Yom Kippur—the "day of *Atonement*"—when the shofar, the ram's horn, was precisely and repeatedly blown to reinstate the masses' communion with God.

These changes also assured that the masses would never know the true dates of Christ's birth, his crucifixion, and his resurrection. Not to mention the correct astronomical and astrological knowledge that could be used for living a more spiritual life. (See appendix section for additional evidence and discussion.)

When the master Roman clock set the world standard, insidiously working was the force of *entrainment*. This word is also defined in *Webster's Dictionary*. The definition includes the power "to determine or modify the phase or period of circadian rhythms." Webster even included the example: "Entrained by a light cycle." Meaning? The world's most dominant clocks set the time through vibrations, sound, and even light. This effect was partly explained in figure 5.3 under the definition of "RE–sonare fibris"—"a vibration of large amplitude in a mechanical or electrical system caused by a relatively small periodic stimulus . . . "

"You're out of time," Jeshua told Joey, considering the inverted Roman clock. "You're going 'tock tick' instead of 'tick tock.'" Again, this helped assure that people's intuition, an electromagnetic, that is, spiritual function, would be kept to a minimum.

Why the Apocrypha was removed from the early Bibles, and why Guttenberg's Bible was likely destroyed and his presses burned, was because of this conspiracy to demote "Godkind" to mankind. The demiurges—the first churches and the Holy Roman Empire—withheld this vital knowledge from the masses who, because of their ignorance, could be most easily manipulated. Fear, hate and war replaced trust, faith and love as humanity's modus operandi.

The good news, Joey realized, is that God wants this sacred knowledge returned to the masses of spiritual people who long for it. By returning to God's clock, calendar, musical notes, and color scheme,[6] humanity will return to the matrices of thought that enable spirit to inspire natural "communion." That is, people who sing the notes of the Solfeggio, and practice the precepts therein, will be blessed with peace, health, harmonious social relationships, and oneness with God.

"Much like the concept of entrainment," Joey thought "when 144,000 people, aligned in the spirit, sing the notes of God in harmony with the Father, they will ring in world peace. What everyone really longs for—the messianic age—a millennium of bliss and love."

## Moses's Fourth Book of Numbers Decoded

From his new found knowledge in the Apocrypha, Joey was also able to glean *the vibrational frequencies used for creation and destruction.*

Excited by the meaning of the Solfeggio notes, including *Webster's* definition of "RE"—*"a vibration of large amplitude . . . caused by a relatively small periodic stimulus"* that could replicate a *"natural vibration"* to affect the matrices of spirit and matter, Joey prayed to Jeshua for his next step. He had thought about the **six-tone musical scale** for days. Jeshua quickly returned to guide Joey back to the **six-verse repeating code** he had found in **Numbers Chapter 7**. Just as the seven tone musical scale was a deception, you will soon see that *Numbers 7:12-83 offers a set of confusing repeating verses that camouflage the most vital six tone frequencies of the Solfeggio.*

Joey began again on "the first day"—verse 12—recalling from Professor Bullinger and Psalm 119 that the addition of "one degree" was often significant. Thus, he read verse 13 trying to decipher a numerical code. It read: "And his offering was one silver charger, the weight thereof was an hundred and thirty shekels, one silver bowl of seventy shekels, after the shekel of the sanctuary; both of them were full of fine flour mingled with oil for a meat offering:"

"This doesn't make any sense," Joey thought. Then after reading six verses further. "Bingo!" The verse was repeated. "Why would God repeat something so inane? Here's the code!"

Indeed, he discovered that Numbers 7:13 was repeated eleven more times, every six verses, including: 19, 25, 31, 37, 43, 49, 55, 61, 67, 73, and 79, for a total of twelve.

He found the same thing occurred for the next "one degree higher" verse 14, as well as verses 15, 16, 17, and 18.

That is, beginning with Numbers 7:12, between each increasing day, he noted twelve *consecutive repeating verses that revealed the frequency codes for all six Solfeggio notes!*

To determine these for yourself, recall that the first numerical code, or hidden pattern, demonstrated in figure 2.4 was "3, 9, 6." or "396." Turn back to pages 54 through 57 (Numbers, Chapter 7) and identify the subsequent codes for verses 13–17 as you did for verse 12. Use the Pythagorean skein to decipher each verse number down to a single digit. Then examine the patterns. You will discover all six of the hidden codes that are mathematically and harmonically related, and ultimately form the pattern 936 using the Pythagorean skein as seen in figure 5.6.

*These previously secret sound frequencies, or electromagnetic vibrations, are likely the primary ones associated with the matrix of creation and destruction. That is, they were likely the frequencies used by God to form the cosmos in six days, as well as the tones required to*

## Fig. 5.6. The Secret Solfeggio Frequencies: Sound Vibration Rates for Creation and Destruction

| | |
|---|---|
| 1. Ut = 396 = 9 | 4. Fa = 639 = 9 |
| 2. Re = 417 = 3 | 5. Sol = 741 = 3 |
| 3. Mi = 528 = 6 | 6. La = 852 = 6 |

Table shows the increasing frequencies encoded in modern Torahs and Bibles in NUMBERS, Chapter 7, verses 12–83. Initially encrypted by Levi priests who translated the original Torah into the Greek *Septuagint*, these six frequencies, apparently possess extraordinary spiritual power. Besides their link to the hymn to St. John the Baptist, and their likely association with creative and destructive events as detailed in the Bible, the third note—"MI" for "Miracles" or "528"—is the exact frequency used by genetic engineers throughout the world to repair DNA.[7]

*shatter Jericho's great wall in six days.* Additional evidence for this assertion comes from the fact that the third note—"Mi" for "Miracles," or "528"—is the exact frequency used by genetic engineers throughout the world to repair the blueprint of life, DNA, which is structurally supported by *six-sided hexagonal clustered water molecules.*[7]

This is the first time this information, held exclusively by the highest degree Freemasons and religious authorities, has been revealed to the public in at least 3,000 years, or possibly ever!

Additional revelations Joey received while studying the Apocrypha helped him better understand the generic meaning of the tones or what "a-'tone'-meant" in the days of old. (See appendix section for discussion on "atonement.")

Like any scientific technology these frequencies may be used for better or worse, for good or evil. Those who have hid this knowledge from the masses for their own selfish reasons, the few who, as you will soon learn, virtually control the world, will suddenly find themselves at a disadvantage as masses of loving Godly people awaken to this knowledge and use its inherent power to bring about the great healing.

## References:

1. Goodspeed EJ. and Powis-Smith, J.M. et al. *The Complete Bible: An American Translation. Fifth Edition*, Chicago, IL: Univ. of Chicago Press, Oct., 1942.

2. *Ibid.*, pp. iv-v.

3. Franz N. *Prophets and Apostles in the New Testament. In: Prophets and Prophetic Ministry, Course #1*. Institute of Prophetic Study, School of Prophetic Ministry (2100 W. Drake Road #115, Ft. Collins, CO 80526, 970-490-1543), Audiotape #7, 1996. The information provided here is either quoted or paraphrased from Pastor Franz's lecture.

Alternatively, author David Icke presented a more disturbing review of religious history including the "contribution" of Martin Luther. Icke linked the manufacture of all religious doctrines to the Illuminati—the Prieuré de Sion or the "Babylonian Brotherhood." Luther, he argued, was "one of their frontmen . . . a product of German secret societies and a Rosicrucian . . . [who] hated freethinking and open minded research." According to Icke and Arthur Findlay in *The Curse of Ignorance, A History of Mankind* (Vols. I and II, Headquarters Publishing Company, London, 1947), Luther wrote: "Damned be love into the abyss of hell, if it is maintained to the damage of faith. . . . It is better that tyrants should sin a hundred times against the people than the people should sin once against the tyrants. . . . the ass wants to be thrashed, the mob to be governed by force."

Icke wrote that the Rosicrucian Manifestos of 1614 and 1616, as well as the seal that Martin Luther carried, issued from the practices first advanced by the Royal Court of the Dragon in ancient Egypt, and in Martin Luther's time by the German esotericist, and Prieuré de Sion Grand Master, Johann Valentin Andrea following Robert Fludd's reign over this secret society. See: Icke D. *The Biggest Secret*. Scottsdale, Arizona: Bridge of Love Publications, 1999, pp. 160-61.

4. Weinstein R and Horowitz L. *Why It's Time Jews and Christians Unite*. Rockport, MA: Tetrahedron Publishing Group. 1998. (The audiotaped thesis and interview is available by calling 1-888-508-4787, or by writing the company at: P. O. Box 2033, Sandpoint, ID 83864.)

5. Hall MP. *An Encyclopedic outline of Masonic, Hermetic, Kabbalistic and Rosicrucian Symbolical Philosophy: Being an Interpretation of the Secret Teachings Concealed Within the Rituals, Allegories and Mysteries of All Ages*. Los Angeles: The Philosophical Research Society, Inc., (3910 Los Feliz Boulevard, Los Angeles, CA 90027), 1989, pp. LVI; CLXXVII.

According to Hall, "There were persistent rumors that Jesus visited and studied in both Greece and India, and that a coin struck in His honor in India during the first century has been discovered. Early Christian records are known to exist in Tibet, and the monks of a Buddhist monastery in Ceylon still preserve a record which indicates that Jesus sojourned with them and became conversant with their philosophy."

6. God's original color scheme, apparently, has also been modified. For more information see Chapter 4 and: Ghadiali, Dinshah P. *Spectralchromety Encyclopedia, Third Edition*. Malagut, NJ: Dinshah Health Society (100 Dinshah Drive, Malagut, NJ 08328) April, 1992, pp. 35; 51-52.

7. Personal communication from Dr. Lee Lorenzen, Ph.D., Vice Chairman, Japanese American Research Society, and world renowned nutritional biochemist, April 18, 1999. Dr. Lorenzen is the inventor of clustered water—considered by many health scientists and professionals to be the most promising discovery of the twentieth century.

Intimately related to this discussion of the six Solfeggio frequencies is the fact "528," the specific frequency used by genetic biochemists to repair DNA, the hereditary code for life, was impregnated into clustered water by Dr. Lorenzen. He and other investigators discovered that *six*-sided, *crystal*-shaped, hexagonal clustered, water molecules form the supportive *matrix* of healthy DNA. During aging and intoxication, these structurally supportive water clusters are depleted, thus, compromising the electrical potential and integrity of cellular DNA. This primary process underlying aging negatively affects virtually every physiological function.

According to biochemist and author Steve Chemiske, these six-sided crystal-clear water clusters that support the DNA double helix structure, "vibrate at specific resonant frequencies and these frequencies can help restore homeostasis to cell structures in the body through signal transduction . . . the process by which one form of energy is converted to another.

"When clustered water is consumed, high frequency information is transmitted to proteins . . . [and] this wave of information is carried throughout the body like a "wake-up call" to restore normal function."

Dr. Franco Bistolfi, a bioelectronics expert, theorized that intercellular communications, instantaneously affecting cells throughout the body, occurs "by means of piezoelectric interactions and photon/phonon transduction of electromagnetic signals of both endogenous and exogenous origin." In other words, tiny imperceptible electromagnetic signals, both man-made and natural, profoundly influence health status and the pathogenic processes involved in virtually every disease.

For scientific evidence regarding clustered water see: Liu K, Cruzan JD, and Saykally RJ. Water clusters. *Science,* February 16, 1996;271:929-931. See also: Chemiske, S. Clustered water: A summary of the work of Dr. Lee Lorenzen. Available from PacTech Life Systems, 15550-D Rockfield Blvd., Irvine, CA 92618, 949-855-3355; clustered water can be purchased by calling toll free 1-888-508-4787.

# Chapter 6.
# The Healing Codes

The ancient knowledge of how to summon the power to create or destroy matter was now in Joey's hands.

After learning how to decode the Bible using the Pythagorean skein, the Protestant Apocrypha, and *Webster's Dictionary*; and knowing the certain *"relatively small periodic"* tones that produced *"large amplitude vibrations"* could affect the matrices of spirit, matter, and energy, Joey realized how God had verbally commanded the universe into existence. He also realized how other biblical miracles could have been affected. Like the literal shattering of Jericho's great wall.

With regard to the miracle at Jericho, Joey realized that the secret Solfeggio scale of *six* tones, whose frequencies were defined in Numbers 7:12-83, also reflected the *six* chapter hidden code in Psalms 120 through 134.[1] (See reference for further explanation.) In Joshua, Chapter 6, God's advice enabled him to conquer the city of Jericho by marshalling "seven priests [with] seven trumpets" along with the ark of the covenant. The Ark was well known for its power and energy. It was therefore likely used to amplify the notes the priests blew *with their lips* for *six* consecutive days. Each advancing day added one degree of higher resonance, according to the Mosaic calendar, just as accomplished by the Solfeggio—six notes that increased the frequency of sound, each by one degree.

Most likely the major damage was done to Jericho's wall during the first six days when the masses were instructed to stay away. On day seven, the people were invited to participate by clapping and cheering. Then the wall crumbled. The citizenry falsely assumed they had caused the damage.

Moreover, in Joshua, Chapter 2, the two spies sent to Jericho, who took refuge in Rahab's house, warned her to protect herself and her family from what would soon befall other Jericho inhabitants. Her house shared a common wall with the great wall that would soon crumble. In verse 18 she was urged to "bind this line of scarlet thread in the window which thou didst let us down by," and no harm would come to that part of the wall, her house, and her family. The "scarlet thread" apparently acted like a "heat sink"—defined in *Webster's Dictionary* as "a device that collects or dissipates energy (as [electromagnetic sound] radiation)."

Universal creation was likewise a miraculous manifestation of mathematics and sound as described in the first three chapters of Genesis. When carefully studied with an eye for the mathematics, the "days of creation are exact descriptions of manifested intervals of which there are six, " wrote Dale Pond, an avid student of the late nineteenth century genius inventor John Keely.[2]

## Notes on Keely

During the late 1800s a syndicate of the world's wealthiest mining capitalists bought many of the abandoned gold mines across America. Following what amounts to a planned industry takeover, these mining magnates commissioned Mr. John Keely, a Philadelphia inventor, to demonstrate his new device that he claimed could easily and inexpensively "disintegrate quartz." Days later, in the Catskill mountains, Keely tunneled a four and a half feet wide groove through eighteen feet of quartz mountainside to demonstrate his "vibration" machine. The businessmen secured the technology, bound themselves to secrecy, and proceeded to make vast fortunes in gold mining. Keely went on to write volumes of detailed information on a wide array of inventions that employed his knowledge of how matter and energy could be manipulated through sound and light. Later, in response to a letter that asked Keely to define the "force" that expressed itself in "illuminated" people's desire to associate "in universal brotherhood," Keely replied: "I hold that ONE SUPREME FORCE, which we may term the incomprehensible, holds within itself all these sublime qualities, as an octave embraces its many tones. This force expressed in the human organisms, has what may be termed CONCORDANT CHORDSETTINGS . . . "

## Words From Tesla

Nikola Tesla, the genius inventor and great grandfather of modern day elecromagnetic technology, wrote in his essay on "Man's Greatest Achievement:"

> There manifests itself in the fully developed being –MAN – a desire mysterious, inscrutable and irresistible: to imitate nature, to create, to work himself the wonders he perceives. Inspired to this task he searches, discovers and invents, designs and constructs . . .

> What has the future in store for this strange being, born of a breath, of perishable tissue, yet immortal, with his powers fearful and divine? What magic will be wrought by him in the end? What is to be his greatest deed, his crowning achievement?

> Long ago he recognized that all perceptible matter comes from a primary substance . . . filling all space . . . luminiferous ether, which is acted upon by the lifegiving Prana or creative force, calling into existence, in never ending cycles, all things and phenomena. The primary substance, thrown into infinitesimal whirls of prodigious velocity, becomes gross matter; the force subsiding, the motion eases and matter disappears, reverting to the primary substance.

> Can man control this grandest, most awe-inspiring of all processes in nature?

> If he could do this, he would have powers almost unlimited and supernatural. . . . He could originate and develop life in all its infinite forms.

> To create and to annihilate material substance, cause it to aggregate in forms according to his desire, would be the supreme manifestation of the power of Man's mind, his most complete triumph over the physical world, his crowning achievement, which would place him beside his Creator, make him fulfill his ultimate destiny.[2]

## Healing Colors

Keely wrote, "When one realizes that the human body is composed of molecular, atomic and subatomic particles and that energies are

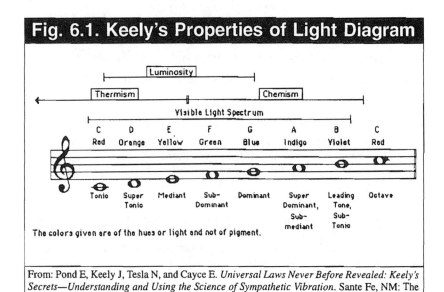

## Fig. 6.1. Keely's Properties of Light Diagram

The colors given are of the hues or light and not of pigment.

From: Pond E, Keely J, Tesla N, and Cayce E. *Universal Laws Never Before Revealed: Keely's Secrets—Understanding and Using the Science of Sympathetic Vibration*. Sante Fe, NM: The Message Company, p. 210.

manifested in these particles, one can then begin to see that to evoke a harmonious condition (health) in the bodily functions these particles must not be left out of the prognosis."[3]

In his essay the "Scale of the Forces in Octaves," Keely provided a technical explanation to the relationship between the octaves of healing tones and light.[4] Figure 6.1 graphs this relationship while figure 6.2 relays the "spectro-chrome color" and "sound equivalent frequency" of each color and musical note as recorded by Dinshah.[5]

Based partly on Keely's and Tesla's century old work, modern healers from various disciplines have used color and music therapy on patients with mixed results.

Much inefficacy in color therapy may stem from the fact that God's original color scheme was, like the Mosaic clock, Solfeggio, and apparently even the Bible, modified for mass consumption and deception.

Dinshah Ghadiali, for example, among the leaders in this field, refined Keely's research on octaves. He further theorized the relationship between sound, light, and healing by writing:

| Fig. 6.2. Dinshah's Sound/Color Equivalent Chart | | | |
|---|---|---|---|
| Color | Frequency | Musical Note | Note Frequency |
| Red | 397.3 | G | 392 |
| Orange | 430.8 | A | 440 |
| Yellow | 464.4 | A# | 466 |
| Lemon | 497.9 | B | 494 |
| Green | 531.5 | C | 523 |
| Turquoise | 565.0 | C# | 554 |
| Blue | 598.6 | D | 587 |
| Indigo | 632,1 | D# | 622 |
| Violet | 665.7 | E | 659 |
| Purple | 565.0* | A# and E | 562* |
| Magenta | 531.5* | G and E | 525* |
| Scarlet | 497.9* | G# and D | 501* |

* denotes reverse polarity.

From: Dinshah GP. *Spectralchrometry Encyclopedia*, Third Edition. Malagut, NJ: Dinshah Health Society (100 Dinshah Drive, Malagut, NJ 08328) April 1992, p. 112.

In the Bible in Genesis, the First Book of Moses, Chapter 1, verse 3, is written, "And God said, Let there be light: and there was light." . . . God spoke to make light. The sound preceded light. On the oscillatory frequency principle this is very correct because sound is an energy acting on a lower scale. The fact of light appearing on a forty-ninth octave explains its divine origin and relation. . . . The number forty-nine is made by seven times seven, and stands for each circle having been traversed seven times in cosmogenesis. Before light came into being was seven spectral colors. The beauteous energy was preceded by sound with its seven musical notes in a number seven keeping pace with the scales of evolution.[5]

If this complex concept of repeating sevens to generate the cosmos befuddles you, simply refer again to the manner in which Jericho's wall was made to fall. Joshua was told by God to employ "seven priests" blowing "seven trumpets of rams' horns" to circle the city for "seven days" and on the seventh day "compassed the city . . . seven times." Then the "wall fell down flat." (See: Joshua, Chapter 6.)

Regarding the falsification of the color scheme for mass consumption, Dinshah wrote:

The triad of primary colors exemplified by Bruster, adopted by Babbott, as red, yellow and blue, follows evolutionary rules in the same manner. The difference is that red, yellow and blue *are not the fundamentals of light.* Hence after years of thought, experienced research analysis, synthesis in the study of geometrical, mathematical, and chromatic, chemical, physical, physiological, spectroscopic, radiant, metaphysical, pathological and clinical phenomena involved, I scrapped all the theories enmasse, and established the finality on the basis of precision; which all the points ring true and actually produce the long sought resultant in the instances without guesswork. *The true triad of primary colors is red, green and violet. The true triad of secondary colors are yellow, blue and magenta. . . .*"[5] (Emphasis added.)

Dinshah went on to report a study in which the primary colors red, green and violet were projected onto a screen to produce white light. The same method using Babbott's "primary colors" red, yellow and blue, that had been promoted by the Catholic Church and commonly set in their stained glass, produced muddy brown.

## The Healing Codes

Now that Joey had the Bible codes, the frequencies related to creation and destruction, and knowledge of their relationship to sound and light, it was time for him to fulfill his covenant with Jeshua—to use this knowledge to inspire mass healing.

After learning how to crack the codes of the Bible and use the dictionary to recover the numerical values that match sound, light, and color, Joey took a pathology book from his shelf. From it he compiled a list of diseases and their associated numbers. Beginning with the first disease under letter A, abscesses, through the letter Z, each illness was given a number based on the Pythagorean skein. This list is presented in figure 6.3.

"There were really only nine numbers," Joey explained. "Jeshua told me this too."

So with both Hebrew and English alphabets decoded (numbers that ran from one through nine, one through nine, and one through eight) Joey simply took each disease, and added their letter values reduced to the Pythagorean single digit.

In other words, Joey believed that God chose to make things easy rather than hard. As today, the same went for mechanical functions— simple was preferable.

For instance, regarding the first disease listed— "abscess"—Joey simply added A=1 + B=2 + S=1 + C=3+ E=5 + S=1 + S=1, or 1+2+3+5+1+1, which totaled 14. Reduced to the Pythagorean skein single digit, the number became 5.

Being a practicing herbalist, having *faith* and *trust* in the numerous biblical references to God's healing herbs and botanicals,[6] Joey began to compile a list of remedies for the diseases listed in figure 6.3. To develop "combination remedies," he referenced works by virtually all the leading bioelectric researchers including Tesla,[7] Rife,[8] Dinshah,[9] Goldman,[10] Ott,[11] Gerber,[12] and herbalists Tierra,[13] Rector-Page,[14] Mindell,[15] Mowrey,[16] Reid,[17] Theiss,[18] and Buchman.[19]

"I took all the codes, and these people's research, to find out what was behind the mathematical sequences, and the work of the great healers who were curing people using herbal medicine and bioelectric technologies," Joey explained. "Including people whose efforts were largely, or entirely, suppressed or destroyed.

"If I had, for example, a number five disease, I went to all the number five herbs. By looking each herb up in my reference books to determine their systemic effects, I combined herbs that I believed would have a primary or even secondary affect on the physical structures or systems requiring support. I used secondary herbs to help 'orchestrate' healing.

"Anyone can do this for any disease, or any symptom, by simply taking the alphabet and associated "number equivalents" from the Pythagorean skein, and deciphering the single digit number equivalent for the disease or treatment."

For example, if someone was suffering with a "skin problem," Joey looked up the number equivalent for skin (in figure 6.3) and saw it was an eight (8). Next he looked up all of the number 8 herbs listed in figure 6.4. He chose only those that his reference books indicated

## Fig. 6.3. Pythagorean Skein Number Equivalents for Diseases

| Disease/ Condition | # | Disease/ Condition | # |
|---|---|---|---|

| **A** | | **B** (cont.) | |
|---|---|---|---|
| Abscess | 5 | Bed=2 Wetting=8 | 1 |
| Acidosis | 7 | Bee=3 Sting=6 | 9 |
| Acne | 5 | Beriberi | 5 |
| Addiction | 7 | Bite | 7 |
| Addisons | 4 | Bitots=4 Spots=8 | 3 |
| Addisons=4 Disease=3 | 7 | Bladder | 1 |
| Adrenal | 1 | Bladder=1 Cancer=8 | 9 |
| Adrenal=1 Disorders=3 | 4 | Bladder=1 Infection=5 | 6 |
| Age | 4 | Body | 1 |
| Age=4 Spots=8 | 3 | Boil | 2 |
| Aging | 2 | Bone | 9 |
| Aging=2 Body=1 | 3 | Bone Spur | 2 |
| AIDS | 6 | Bone=9 Fractures=3 | 3 |
| Alcoholism | 8 | Breast | 2 |
| Alkalosis | 9 | Breast=2 Cancer=8 | 1 |
| Allergies | 7 | Breast=2 Infection=5 | 7 |
| Alopecia | 8 | Brights=2 Disease=8 | 1 |
| Aluminum Toxicity | 1 | Bronchitis | 9 |
| Alzheimers | 8 | Bruising | 9 |
| Alzheimers=8 Disease=8 | 7 | Bruxism | 7 |
| Anemia | 7 | Bulemia | 4 |
| Anorexia | 6 | Burns | 2 |
| Anorexia=6 Nervosa=4 | 1 | Bursitis | 9 |
| Appetite | 2 | Cadmium Toxicity | 9 |
| Appetite=2 Poor=1 | 3 | Cancer | 8 |
| Apthous Ulcers | 7 | Candidiasis | 2 |
| Arsenic | 6 | Canker | 7 |
| Arsenic=6 Poisoning=1 | 7 | Canker=7 Sores=4 | 2 |
| Arterioschlerosis | 7 | Cardiovascular | 3 |
| Arthritis | 5 | Cardiovascular=3 Disease=8 | 3 |
| Asthma | 8 | Cataracts | 5 |
| Athersclerosis | 6 | Celiac | 6 |
| Athletes=9 Foot=2 | 2 | Celiac=6 Disease=8 | 2 |
| Autism | 2 | Cervical | 1 |
| | | Cervical=1 Cancer=8 | 9 |
| **B** | | Chemical | 9 |
| Backache | 7 | Chemical=9 Allergies=7 | 9 |
| Baldness | 4 | Chemical=9 Poinsoning=1 | 1 |
| Barr | 3 | Chicken=8 Pox=1 | 9 |
| Bed=2 Sores=4 | 6 | Cholesterol=6 Problems=1 | 9 |

## Fig. 6.3. (Cont.) Pythagorean Number Equivalents for Diseases

| Disease/ Condition | # |
|---|---|
| **C** (cont.) | |
| Chronic=7 Fatigue=6.................4 | |
| Chronic=7 Fatigue=6 Syndrome=5...9 | |
| Circulatory=1 Problems=1.......2 | |
| Cirrhosis...............................1 | |
| Cold....................................7 | |
| Cold=7 Sores=4.....................2 | |
| Colitis.................................6 | |
| Colon=5 Cancer=8.................4 | |
| Common=1 Cold=7..............8 | |
| Constipation.......................2 | |
| Copper=1 Toxicity=8............9 | |
| Cramps...............................7 | |
| Crohns=5 Disese=8............4 | |
| Croup.................................1 | |
| Cyst....................................4 | |
| Cystic=7 Fibrosis=7.............5 | |
| Cystitis..............................7 | |
| **D** | |
| Dandruff.............................2 | |
| DDT=1 Poisoning=1............2 | |
| Depression.........................7 | |
| Dermatitis...........................1 | |
| Diabetes.............................1 | |
| Diabetes=1 Insipidus=3........4 | |
| Diabetes=1 Mellitus=3........4 | |
| Diarrhea.............................1 | |
| Disease..............................8 | |
| Disorders...........................3 | |
| Diverticulitis.............9 | |
| Dog=8 Bite=9.....................8 | |
| Drug..................................5 | |
| Drug=5 Reaction=4...........9 | |
| Drug=5 Addiction=7...........3 | |
| Dyspepsia..........................6 | |
| **E** | |
| Ear......................................6 | |
| Ear=6 Infection=5.............2 | |

| Disease/ Condition | # |
|---|---|
| **E** (cont.) | |
| Eating=2 Disorders=3............5 | |
| Eczema..............................8 | |
| Edema................................1 | |
| Emphysema.........................6 | |
| Endometriosis......................3 | |
| Endometrium=2 Cancer=8.......1 | |
| Environmental.................4 | |
| Environmental=4 Toxicity=8....3 | |
| Epilepsy.............................8 | |
| Epstein=5 Barr=3 Virus=8........7 | |
| Eye....................................8 | |
| Eye=8 Problems=1...............9 | |
| **F** | |
| Fatigue..............................6 | |
| Fever.................................2 | |
| Fibrocystic=3 Breast=2 Disease=8...4 | |
| Fibrosis....................7 | |
| Flu.....................................3 | |
| Food=4 Poisoning=1............5 | |
| Food=4 Allergies=7...........2 | |
| Foot...................................2 | |
| Fractures.....................3 | |
| Frigidity.....................8 | |
| Fungus.........................7 | |
| **G** | |
| Gallbladder=6 Disorders=3.....9 | |
| Gangrene............................8 | |
| Glands...............................3 | |
| Glaucoma............................9 | |
| Gout..................................9 | |
| Growth Problems.................8 | |
| Gum Disease......................4 | |
| **H** | |
| Hair Loss...........................2 | |
| Halitosis...................4 | |
| Hayfever.....................9 | |
| Headache....................8 | |

## Fig. 6.3. (Cont.) Pythagorean Number Equivalents for Diseases

| Disease/ Condition | # | Disease/ Condition | # |
|---|---|---|---|
| **H** (cont.) | | **L** (cont.) | |
| Heart Problems | 8 | Legionnaires Disease | 9 |
| Heel Spur | 2 | Leukemia | 4 |
| Hemophilia | 6 | Leukorrhea | 6 |
| Hemorrhoids | 6 | Liver=3 Cancer=8 | 2 |
| Hernia, Hiatal | 7 | Lung | 9 |
| Herpes | 8 | Lung=9 Cancer=8 | 8 |
| Herpes=8 Simplex=8 | 7 | Lupus | 8 |
| High Cholesterol | 4 | Lyme Disease | 9 |
| Hyperactivity | 1 | | |
| Hypertension | 6 | **M** | |
| Hyperthyroid | 9 | Malabsorption | 2 |
| Hypoglycemia | 4 | Manic Depressive | 9 |
| Hypothyroid | 1 | Mastitis | 2 |
| Hysterectomy | 5 | Measles | 2 |
| | | Memory Loss | 1 |
| **I** | | Menieres Syndrome | 3 |
| Impotence | 1 | Meningitis | 2 |
| Indigestion | 8 | Menopause | 1 |
| Infection | 5 | Menstrual Cramps | 4 |
| Infertility | 7 | Mercury Toxicity | 3 |
| Inflammation | 1 | Migraine | 4 |
| Influenza | 9 | Mold=8 Allergies=7 | 6 |
| Insect Allergy | 6 | Mononucleosis | 3 |
| Insect Bite | 7 | Motion Sickness | 5 |
| Insomnia | 3 | Mouth=5 Cancer=8 | 4 |
| Irritable Bowel | 7 | Multiple Sclerosis | 2 |
| | | Mumps | 1 |
| **J** | | Muscle=1 Cramps=7 | 8 |
| Jaundice | 4 | Myocardial Infarction | 3 |
| | | Melanoma | 2 |
| **K** | | | |
| Kidney=5 Problems=1 | 6 | **N** | |
| Kidney Stones | 7 | Nephritis | 1 |
| Kidney Cancer | 4 | Nervousness | 9 |
| | | Neurosis | 3 |
| **L** | | Nickel Toxicity | 8 |
| Larynx | 4 | Nose Bleeds | 1 |
| Larynx Cancer | 3 | | |
| Lead Poisoning | 5 | | |
| Leg Ulcers | 3 | | |

## Fig.6.3. (Cont.) Pythagorean Number Equivalents for Diseases

| Disease/ Condition | # | Disease/ Condition | # |
|---|---|---|---|
| **O** | | **S** (cont.) | |
| Obesity | 5 | Stomach=7 Cancer=8 | 6 |
| Osteoporosis | 5 | Strains | 1 |
| Ovarian=8 Cancer=8 | 7 | Stress | 1 |
| Ovarian=8 Cyst=3 | 2 | Sulfite=2 Allergies=7 | 9 |
| | | Sunburn | 5 |
| **P** | | Syndrome | 5 |
| Pancreatitis | 9 | | |
| Parkinsons Disease | 2 | **T** | |
| Pneumonia | 9 | Temporomandibular Joint Pain | |
| Poison Ivy | 9 | Syndrome | 4 |
| Poisoning | 1 | Testicular=2 Cancer=8 | 1 |
| Polyps | 4 | Throat=1 Cancer=8 | 9 |
| Premenstrual Syndrome | 5 | Thrush | 4 |
| Prostatitis | 4 | Tonsillitis | 5 |
| Prostate Cancer | 5 | Toxicity | 8 |
| Psoriasis | 8 | Tuberculosis | 2 |
| | | Tumors | 7 |
| **R** | | | |
| Radiation Poisoning | 2 | **U** | |
| Raynauds Disease | 3 | Ulcers | 6 |
| Reyes Syndrome | 5 | Underweight | 8 |
| Rheumatic Fever | 1 | Urinary Tract Infection | 3 |
| Rheumatoid Arthritis | 2 | Uterine=2 Cancer=8 | 1 |
| Rickets | 4 | | |
| | | **V** | |
| **S** | | Vaginitis | 2 |
| Schizophrenia | 7 | Varicose Veins | 8 |
| Seborrhea | 1 | Venereal Disease | 9 |
| Senility | 5 | Vertigo | 6 |
| Shingles | 3 | Viral Infections | 5 |
| Sinusitis | 4 | Vitiligo | 4 |
| Skin=8 Disorders=3 | 2 | | |
| Skin Cancer | 7 | **W** | |
| Snake Bite | 5 | Warts | 9 |
| Sore Throat | 4 | Weakened Immune System | 1 |
| Sores | 4 | Weight Problems | 1 |
| Spider Bite | 8 | Worms | 7 |
| Sprains | 6 | | |
| Spur | 2 | **Y** | |
| Sting | 6 | Yeast Infection | 3 |

191

## Fig. 6.4. Pythagorean Skein Number Equivalents for Herbs

| Herb Name and Number | Herb Name and Number |
|---|---|
| **1** | **2** |
| American Arnica | Arame |
| Balmony | Astragalus |
| Barley=9 Grass=1 | Bayberry=6 Bark=5 |
| Bay | Bears Foot |
| Beet=5 Root=5 | Birds Nest |
| Bilberry | Bittersweet |
| Buchu | Black |
| Calendula | Burdock |
| Cherry=5 Bark=5 | Butternut=6 Bark=5 |
| Chia Seeds | Celery=5 Seed=6 |
| Cleavers Herb | Chaga |
| Dill Ephedra | Chestnut |
| Frostwort | Cinnamon |
| Grass | Corn=5 Silk=5 |
| Hounds Tongue | Cotton Root |
| Huckleberries | Cramp=6 Bark=5 |
| Iceland Moss | Devils=8 Claw=3 |
| Leaves | Dogwood |
| Life Root | Fennel |
| Maidenhair | Fenugreek |
| Milkweed | Foot |
| Mistletoe | Frank Incense |
| Myrrh | Grape |
| Oats | Helleborne American |
| Passion=3 Flower=7 | Hydrangea |
| Penny=4 Corns=6 | Leverwood |
| Pipsissewa | Licorice |
| Prickly Ash=5 Bark=5 | Lions Root |
| Psyllium | Lobelia |
| Reishi Mushroom | Maple |
| Rose Hips | Mint |
| Sawpalmetto | Motherwort |
| Shepherd Spurse | Sage=5 Leaf=6 |
| St. Johns Wort | Slippery elm=6 Bark=5 |
| Tongue | Strawberry Leaf |
| Valerian | Tea Tree Oil |
| Vera | Trailing |
| Walnut | White=2 Willow=4 Bark=5 |
| Weed | Wild Yam Root |

## Fig. 6.4. Pythagorean Skein Number Equivalents for Herbs

| Herb Name and Number | Herb Name and Number |
|---|---|
| **3** | **4** |
| Agrimony | Alder |
| Alpalfa | American=1 Ginsing=3 |
| Anise | Ash Tree |
| Arbutus | Asparagus |
| Black=2 Walnut=1 | Barberry=8 Root=5 |
| Bladder Wrack | Bean |
| Blue Flag | Bearberry |
| Borage | Beech Drop |
| Bugleweed | Berries |
| Calamus=7 Root=5 | Bethroot |
| Carrot | Birch |
| Chives | Blackberry=7 Leaf=6 |
| Claw | Buckthorn |
| Clover | Calico Bush |
| Elm | Canabis |
| Eryngo | Capsicum |
| Feverweed | Castor Oil |
| Fireweed | Cayenne |
| Five Finger Grass | Celandine |
| Ginseng | Cloves |
| Gotu Kola | Comfrey |
| Horse Radish Root | Echinacea |
| Hyssop | Female Fern |
| Irish=9 Moss=3 | Fiber |
| Ivy American | Flax=7 Seed=6 |
| Juniper | Goldenrod |
| Ladys Slipper | Goldenseal |
| Liver | Goldthread |
| Milk=9 Thistle=3 | Hawthorne |
| Oak Tree | Henbane |
| Propolis | Hops |
| Red=9 Clover=3 | Horse=2 Chestnut=2 |
| Spikenard Root | Indigo |
| Thistle | Ironweed |
| Tree | Linden |
| Urvaursi | Lungwort |
| Wood Betony | Mallow |
| | Mandrake |
| | Nettle |
| | Oat=9 Fiber=4 |

Fig. 6.4. Pythagorean Skein Number Equivalents for Herbs

| Herb Name and Number | Herb Name and Number |
|:---:|:---:|
| **4** (cont.) | **5** |
| Onion | Almond |
| Oregon Grape | Apple |
| Pepper | Arbutus=3 Trailing=2 |
| Pleurisy=8 Root=5 | Balsom Fir |
| Sassafras | Bark |
| Schizandra | Bee=3 Pollen=2 |
| Wild Cherry Bark | Beech |
| Willow | Beet |
| Yellowdock Root | Berry |
| Yucca Root | Black Indian Hemp |
| | Blue=4 Cohosh=5 Root=5 |
| | Celery |
| | Cherry |
| | Corn |
| | Cranberry |
| | Cranes Bill |
| | Dragon Root |
| | Foti |
| | Garden Nightshade |
| | Garlic |
| | Gelsemium |
| | Ginkgo=9 Biloba=5 |
| | Gum Plant |
| | Haircap Moss |
| | High |
| | Kidney=5 Liver=3 Leaf=6 |
| | Marigold=7 Flower=7 |
| | Mullein |
| | Mushroom |
| | Periwinkle |
| | Pricklyash |
| | Primrose |
| | Raspberry |
| | Red Raspberry |
| | Red Root |
| | Sage |
| | Skullcap |
| | Squawvine |
| | Strawberry |
| | Suma Root |

## Fig. 6.4. Pythagorean Skein Number Equivalents for Herbs

| Herb Name and Number | Herb Name and Number |
|---|---|
| **6** | **7** |
| Alaria | Adders=6 Tongue=1 |
| Aloe | Aloe=6 Vera=1 |
| Arsesmart | Alum=2 Root=5 |
| Blessed=3 Thistle=3 | Angelica |
| Butchers=6 Broom=9 | Basil |
| Butternut | Bitter Root |
| Cardamon Pods | Black Root |
| Chaparral | Black=2 Cohosh=5 |
| Crawley | Blackberry |
| Cypress | Blackhaw |
| Dandelion | Blue=4 Vervain=3 |
| Fir | Burdock=2 Root=5 |
| Gillenia | Calamus |
| Ginger | Cascarasagrada |
| Herb Leaf | Chamomile |
| Papaya | Cowslip |
| Parsley | Cramp=6 Bark=5 High=5 |
| Pepper=4 Mint=2 | Crow Foot |
| Plantain | Dongquai |
| Raspberry=5 Leaves=1 | Dulse |
| Rosemary | Flax |
| Seed | Gentian |
| Shitake=1 Mushroom=5 | Gravel Root |
| Soapwort Root | Horse Radish |
| Valerian=1 Root=5 | Juniper=3 Berries=4 |
| Wild Yam | Kava Kava |
| | Labrador Tea |
| | Licorice=2 Root=5 |
| | Marigold |
| | Paudarco |
| | Quassia Chips |
| | Sarsaparilla |
| | Seneca Root |
| | White=2 Oak=9 Bark=5 |
| | Wild=3 Indigo=4 |
| | Witch Hazel |

| Fig. 6.4. Pythagorean Skein Number Equivalents for Herbs | |
|---|---|
| **Herb Name and Number** | **Herb Name and Number** |
| **8** | **9** |
| Alenhoof | Artichoke |
| Amaranthus | Barley |
| Arnica=1 Flower=7 | Birch=4 Bark=5 |
| Barberry | Blue=4 Cohosh=5 |
| Beech Tree | Broom |
| Blood Root | Buckthorn=4 Bark=5 |
| Boneset | Caraway |
| Bupleurum Root | Catnip |
| Calendula=1 Flower=7 | Chicory |
| Camomile | Comfrey=4 Root=5 |
| Castor Bean | Evening=4 Primrose=5 |
| Centaury | Eyebright |
| Chickweed | Feverfew |
| Colts=6 Foot=2 | Horehound |
| Couch Grass | Ladys=7 Mantle=2 |
| Elder | Lippa |
| Elecampane Root | Magnolia |
| Eucalyptus | Marshmallow |
| Fringe Tree | Mugwort |
| Hawthorne=4 Berries=4 | Oak |
| Horsetail | Oat |
| Jasmine | Oil |
| Kelp | Olive |
| Larkspur | Red |
| Lavender Flowers | Simson Weed |
| Siberian=5 Ginsing=3 | Suma |
| Tea | Yerbamate |
| Thyme | |
| Turmeric | |
| Wild Cherry | |
| Yarrow | |
| Yarrow Flowers | |
| Yellow Dock | |
| Yucca | |

would be beneficial for treating skin problems. If he desired to expand the treatment, or orchestrate additional support, he sought additional number equivalents by expanding the definition of the illness. In the case of "skin" he added "skin *disorders*." This gave him another number from which to work in selecting additional herbs. In this case he researched number 2 herbs, as well as number 8 herbs, for their beneficial effects on the skin or related ailments.

In time, virtually anyone who practices herbal healing using this technique can become a master herbalist. (Until then, it is imperative that you consult with reputable health professionals for more accurate, potentially life-saving, diagnoses and treatments.)

Moreover, this work will stand the test of time because it is based on God's simple and powerful laws and promise. As Revelation 22:1-3 and 22:14 predicted "a pure river of water of life, clear as crystal, proceeding out of the throne of God" will once again flow.[20] On "either side of the river" will grow trees whose "leaves were for the healing of the nations." People in tune with the melody of God are "they that do his commandments." They will "have right to the tree of life, and may enter in through the gates into the [Holy] city."[20]

### References:

1. When Psalms 120 through 134 are carefully examined, these fifteen chapters, mostly titled "A Song of degrees," are each one degree higher than the chapter before it relating to the frequency codes provided in Numbers, Chapter 7. The two stanzas containing seven chapters each, in Psalms 120 through 134, are broken or separated by Psalm 127 entitled "A Song of degrees for Solomon." Thus, seven is the deception. *The critical power number is six.* The reduction from seven chapters to *six* here is accomplished by repeating "A Song of degrees of David" in Psalms 122, 124, 131, and 132. Similar to the use of "Selah," 71 times and its synonym "Higgaion" that is used once. The second "Song of degrees of David," that is Chapters 124 and 132, concealed the key number of six.

2. Harte R. Disintegration of stone. In: Pond D, Keely J, Tesla N. and Cayce E. et al. *Universal Laws Never Before Revealed: Keely's Secrets—Understanding and Using the Science of Sympathetic Vibration.* Sante Fe, NM: The Message Company (RR2 Box 307 MM, Sante Fe, NM 87505; 505-474-0998), 1996, pp. 9-15.

Also, the February 1990 issue of *Nature* cited the findings of two teams of astronomers, one British and the other American. "We may be living among [a] huge honeycomb [that is, hexagonal shaped, a] . . . galaxy [of] clusters," concluded David Koo of the University of California at Santa Cruz. Contrary to the "Big Bang Theory" of random universal creation and arrangement, this new evidence proved "the regularity of galactic structures" were, like the molecularly clustered healing waters of the world, arranged in six-sided groupings.

3. Tesla N. Man's greatest achievement. In: Pond D, Keely J, Tesla N. and Cayce E. et al. *Universal Laws Never Before Revealed: Keely's Secrets—Understanding and Using the Science of Sympathetic Vibration.* Ibid. p. 187.

4. Keely J. The role of atomic forces in healing. In: Pond D, Keely J, Tesla N. and Cayce E. et al. *Universal Laws Never Before Revealed: Keely's Secrets—Understanding and Using the Science of Sympathetic Vibration.* Ibid. p. 118.

5. Ghadiali, Dinshah P. *Spectralchrometry Encyclopedia,* Third Edition. Malagut, NJ: Dinshah Health Society (100 Dinshah Drive, Malagut, NJ 08328) April 1992, p. 35; 51-52.

6. Staff writers. Bible cures revealed. *Sun.* August 4, 1998 pp. 20-21. (See appendix section for herbs cited in the Bible.)

7. Tesla N. Coil for Electro-Magnetics. U.S. Patent Office, Serial Number 479,804, July 7, 1893 Bifilar coils as opposed to standard mono-filament coils.

8. Davidson A. *The Royal R. Rife Report.* Bayside, CA: Borderland Sciences, 1988.

9. Ghadiali, Dinshah P. Op cit.

10. Goldman J. *Healing Sounds: The Power of Harmonics.* Rockport, MA: Element Books, Inc., 1992.

11. Ott J. *Health and Light: The effects of natural and artificial light on man and other living things*. New York: Pocket Books, 1976. See also: *Light, Radiation and You: How to Stay Healthy*. Marco Island, FL: Dewin Adiar Pub, 1985.

12. Gerber R. *Vibrational Medicine: New Choices for Healing Ourselves*. Sante Fe, NM: Bear & Company, 1988.

13. Tierra L. *The Herbs of Life: Health & Healing Using Western & Chinese Techniques*. Unpublished manuscript, 1992.

14. Rector-Page LG. *How to be Your Own Herbal Pharmacist*. Sonora, CA: Healthy Healing Publications, 1994.

15. Mindell E. *Earl Mindell's Herb Bible*. New York: Simon & Schuster/Fireside, 1992.

16. Mowrey DB. *The Scientific Validation of Herbal Medicine*. Dunvegan, ON, Canada: Cormorant Books, 1986.

17. Reid DP. *Chinese Herbal Medicine*. Boston: Shambhala Publications, Inc. 1992.

18. Theiss B and Theiss P. *The Family Herbal Guide*. Rochester, VT: Healing Arts Press, 1993.

19. Buchman DD. *Herbal Medicine: The Natural Way to Get Well and Stay Well*. New York: Gramercy Publishing Company, 1980.

20. It seems extraordinary that Revelation predicted that the Messianic Age would be accompanied by "crystal clear water" flowing through the rivers and streams, that the book revealed are "the people," in light of Dr. Lee Lorenzen's research in clustered water. It is remarkable that the structure upholding the "tree of life"—DNA—as seen in figure 3.5 (page 106), is not a snake, but in reality snowflake-shaped, hexagonal (six-sided), water clusters. In its healthy state, the crystal cluster supported double helix acts as an electromagnetic energy receiver and transmitter. Many scientists believe this is the primary function of DNA.

Moreover, the structure of more than 4,000 enzymes that regulate virtually every body function largely depends on these same hexagonal-shaped crystal water clusters.

See reference 7 in Chapter 5 for further discussion and citation.

*Healing Codes for the Biological Apocalypse*

# Chapter 7.
# Mad Cows and Madder Men

Not long after Joey completed his herbal directory he prayed again to Jeshua for help. "Can you please help me get this information out to your people?" Realizing that his speaking and writing skills were unpolished, he prayed, "Jeshua, please send me someone like Dr. Horowitz who can help deliver these important teachings to the world."

The next day, Errol Owen, a friend of Joey's, who routinely listened to the Art Bell show — America's most listened to late night radio program — brought Joey a tape.

"Joey, you've got to listen to this," Errol said. "This is Art Bell's interview of Dr. Leonard Horowitz. Dr. Horowitz is the author of the book *Emerging Viruses: AIDS & Ebola — Nature, Accident or Intentional?*

"I know of Dr. Horowitz's work," Joey replied. "I've even been praying to meet him. I'd love to listen to the tape. I read Dr. Horowitz's book, and watched his video, and just yesterday I asked Jeshua for someone like him to help me get my information out to the people."

So Joey listened to the tape. Afterwards he prayed again, "Jeshua, you've got to help me meet this guy."

## Another "Eagle" Landing

About a year earlier Dr. Horowitz had been a featured speaker at the "Conscious Living Conference" in Spokane, WA. With a day off he decided to rent a car and travel with his agent to "check out the mountains north of Coeur D'Alene.

"Jackie and I are looking for a place to move with the two girls," he told Kathy. "I don't think the northern tip of Metropolis is a very healthy place to raise our kids anymore."

Since the time he graduated from Tufts School of Dental Medicine in 1977, Harvard School of Public Health in 1981, and Interface Foundation's training program in holistic health studies in 1982, the public health educator program in holistic health studies in 1982, the public health educator had called Rockport, Massachusetts, his home. Suddenly it seemed time to leave. "We see the 'End Times' prophecies quickly coming true," he explained.

"Revelation talks about the last days in which the kings and wealthiest men of all the nations were deceived by men who practiced 'sorcery.' The earliest word for sorcery, from *Strong's Concordance*, is the Greek root word 'pharmacopeia' or pharmacy. I interpret that to mean the Rockefeller directed pharmaceutical industrialists have deceived international leaders. The Rothschilds, Rockefellers and their friends also largely control the International Monetary Fund (IMF). Their 'sorcery' is not only associated in the Bible with the great plagues, it's linked to the onslaught of 'beasts' as well. The beasts are predicted to kill billions more. The *Strong's Concordance* root word for 'beasts' is the Hebrew word [#2416] 'chay' meaning 'alive; having an appetite for raw flesh,' like the flesh eating bacteria. And in the Greek Lexicon, the original word [#2342] for 'beasts' is 'therion' meaning 'a little beast or little animal.' That sounds like little bacteria and viruses to me.

"The Rockefeller Foundation and the Merck Fund, that is, Merck, Sharp and Dohme—the world's leading vaccine maker—are among the leading funding sources for world depopulation. The earth's greatest depopulation event is prophesied to be associated with little beasts and the great plagues. The bacteria, viruses, and pieces thereof—infectious agents most insidiously spread precisely and extensively in vaccines and contaminated blood—are bringing about the plagues that were predicted to kill half of the world's population. Isn't it interesting that the Rockefellers largely control the pharmaceutical, blood, sterilization, and population control industries?

"'God's wrath,' in Revelation, is predicted to be poured out largely because of these people and the masses who worship them. People who worship Babylon's idols above God get killed.

My mother, for example, died in 1992 of cancer and a disease commonly linked to flu vaccines—Guillain Barré. My mother believed that M.D.s were medical deities. She routinely followed her doctors' recommendations and got her flu vaccines. For this reason, I believe she was ultimately killed. Given the Nazi links to the Rockefellers,[1] I believe the Nazis my mother escaped from, after scrubbing the streets of Vienna at gunpoint in 1939, killed her in 1992.

"Today, as modern medical science is idolized, and continues to dramatically alter the gene pools of plants, animals, bacteria, viruses, foods, and humans, the people who made vast fortunes during World War II continue to wreak havoc, play God, devastate populations, and make vast fortunes along the way.

"Revelation predicted how those who 'fornicated' with the devil, and stole the blood of 'prophets and saints,' would surely succumb to God's wrath. It was Laurance Rockefeller who organized the New York City Blood Council—the council of doctors that established the New York City Blood Bank. They became the international blood 'banksters.' They allowed the 10,000 hemophiliacs in the United States, and countless others throughout the world to get AIDS. They knew the blood was contaminated between 1980 and 1986 but did little to clean it up. They also knew the blood was filled with hepatitis B and hepatitis C viruses that are now spreading cancer throughout the world.

"Revelation also predicted that, during Babylon's fall, deadly red 'wine' will flow full of impurities into the rivers and streams of people, infecting millions at a time of the great plagues. That's what's happening!"

Later that afternoon, Len drove into downtown Sandpoint, Idaho. "Let me run into this real estate office to pick up a listing sheet," he said to Kathy. A few minutes later he returned with some literature. "I got a magnetic business card from a really nice realtor named Lou," he said. "She promised to send us more listings as they come available."

Once home, Len gave the business card to his wife Jackie who stuck it on their refrigerator door where it remained for weeks.

Months later, after their Massachusetts house sold, it was time for the doctor, his wife, and their two young girls to move. The business card had been long discarded and forgotten when the Horowitz family packed their belongings into a thirty-four foot motorhome and headed west in search of a new "homestead."

During the next eight weeks, they drove through Colorado, Utah, Wyoming, Montana, Oregon and Washington State looking for possible places to settle. Nothing felt quite right. Northern Idaho was their next stop.

But Len had run out of time. A booking at the American College of Advanced Medicine (ACAM) in Florida required him to fly to Ft. Lauderdale from Spokane leaving Jackie and the kids to search on their own. The next day Jackie was to have driven south to check out the "constitutional community" being established by Jack McLamb a couple hours south of Spokane. But intuition stopped her.

"After Len left," Jackie explained, "I woke up the next morning, and looked at a map. Len said that Coeur D' Alene was very pretty, and I thought I'd check it out. But when we got there and saw how suburbanized it was, I thought I would drive north towards Canada where my family lives."

Sandpoint was on the way, and when Jackie got to town, without knowing it, she saw the same real estate office in which Len had met Lou. Jackie walked in and there she was.

Later that night, after a few hours of touring Lou's listings, Jackie called Len in Florida and said. "We're definitely moving to Sandpoint."

"Are you kidding? How do you know that?"

"I can just feel it. This is the right place. It's beautiful. It reminds me of the ferry ride from Vancouver to Victoria. Wait till you see it. . . ."

Len couldn't believe that their long search might be over. After all, they hadn't checked out a number of other places on their possibility list.

Unassured Len replied, "Well, we'll see."

The next morning, at the ACAM meeting, Jackie's choice was quickly confirmed. Within twenty minutes, two doctors walked up to Len, and like messengers from God, he recalled, introduced themselves. "The first one said to me, 'D'ya know? I have someone you need to meet. You're really interested in these new viruses and their effect on people's immune systems. I have a friend who produces some of the world's best nutritional supplements for boosting immunity."

"Is that right?," Len asked, "Where's his company?"

"Sandpoint, Idaho," the man said.

"You've got to be kidding. My wife just phoned me from there last night and told me, in no uncertain terms, that's where we're moving."

Fifteen minutes later, another doctor walked up to Len and said, "You're really into the current and coming plagues, and how they fulfill Bible prophecy. I have someone for you to meet."

"Who?"

"Well it's a guy and his buddy who had a lot of money. More than $10 million. They're Christians. About ten years ago they read Revelation. They felt the plagues were pretty much assured, and would cause so much illness that they decided to put all of their wealth into developing advanced bioelectric technologies to help people heal."

"Is that right? Where do they live?"

"Well, they just moved from Phoenix, Arizona. They sold their factory there because they wanted to be far away from urban areas. They think the 'End Times' prophecies are about to happen. They just moved to *Sandpoint, Idaho*."

"What! Are you serious? I can't believe this!" Len exclaimed. Then he looked up, raised his arms to heaven, and said, "Thank you God."

He then explained to the doctor what Jackie had said the night before, and what the other doctor had mentioned only minutes earlier—*Sandpoint*. "It's clearly a sign," Len said. The Christian doctor agreed.

## "Eagle" Gatherings

Months later, on the 4th of July, after Len and Jackie had relocated to Sandpoint, Len approached a lemonade vendor at a street stand.

"Can I have one large lemonade please?"

The tall earthy-looking blonde woman behind the counter looked up from her register. After a double-take of Len she declared, "You're Dr. Len Horowitz!"

"That's right. Hello, and who are you?"

"I'm Ingri Cassel. I'm a big fan of yours. I heard you lecture in Spokane last year. I rounded up all my friends and drove them down to see you. You were great! I've been praying for you to come here! "

Ingri explained, "I'm really into what you talk about. My mother is Walene James. You've probably heard of her. She wrote the book *Immunization:The Reality Behind the Myth.* We talk about you all the time. We need a lot of help in this area waking people up to the dangers of vaccinations, and really, I kid you not, I've been praying for you to come."

"Well, it's nice to meet you," Len replied. "Let me introduce you to my wife Jackie, and our girls—Alena and Aria."

And so it was that Len met Ingri, who later introduced him to Errol Owen, who arranged a dinner meeting between Len and Joey.

"I prayed to meet you," Joey told Len that night after dinner, "but I never expected Jeshua to deliver you personally to my home."

Joey relayed his story to Len and when finished asked, "Can you help me write a book and get this information out?"

"Well, my schedule is insane. But I'll try. Maybe Errol and Ingri can help with some of the writing and editing."

As he drove home from Joey's house that night, Len reflected back to a workshop he attended in 1982 as part of his holistic education master's program. During a meditation and guided imagery session designed to elicit an image associated with Len's spiritual identity, a vision of a giant eagle appeared in his mind's eye. The eagle swooped down from behind a great golden pyramid. It grabbed Len by the back of his neck and lifted him off the ground and whisked him away. It carried him to a place high in the clouds where everything was alight with a golden glow of peace. When the session ended, Len was asked to paint a picture of his experience. Today, the painting hangs in his office on the wall behind his desk. "The 'gathering of eagles,'" Len thought. "Isn't that interesting."

A few nights later, Len met with Joey again. This time, Joey relayed information and his suspicion that mad-cow disease might be a madman creation. Based on evidence he had gathered, the small protein, called a "prion," associated with transmissible spongiform encephalopathies, or TSEs, including "mad cow disease" in cattle, "scrapie" in sheep, and "Creutzfeldt-Jakob disease," or CJD, in humans, was likely a man-made biological weapon suitable for population control.

Joey had seen the U.S. Government contracts reprinted in Len's book, *Emerging Viruses: AIDS & Ebola—Nature, Accident or Intentional?*, that showed how numerous AIDS-like and Ebola-like viruses had been engineered by Litton Bionetics, a leading Army biological weapons contractor administering a largely funded mostly secret "Special Virus Cancer Program." The clandestine operation began on February 12, 1962, and ran to the mid 1970s.[2] Len also discovered and reprinted the contracts under which Dr. Maurice Hilleman, the world's leading vaccine developer for the Merck pharmaceutical company, developed the vaccines that most likely delivered AIDS to the world. Hilleman himself testified bringing the AIDS virus into North America in contaminated monkeys destined for vaccine research and development at Merck.[3] The suspected vaccine was given to gay men in New York City and Blacks in Central Africa beginning in 1974.

Len learned that, much like his investigation, Joey was being spiritually directed to discover the truth about mad cow disease.

"We need to get together again," Joey explained. "I need to bring you up to date on my most recent findings."

"How about next week," Len replied. "I'm scheduled to travel to Salt Lake City this weekend. A group of Mormons are bringing me in to speak at BYU on the subject of vaccine-related injuries and deaths."

"Fine," Joey said. "Call me next week when you get back and we'll schedule a get-together."

## Mad Cows and Poisoned Milk

That weekend Len presented his research following sessions by authors Howard Lyman and Robert Cohen. Lyman, the cattleman who learned of the deadly "mad cow" prion disease, became famous for alerting America about contaminated beef on the Opra Winfrey Show. The telecast caused such sagging beef sales that a Texas cattle association decided to sue Winfrey and Lyman for "food disparagement." They lost the highly publicized case. Robert Cohen, the second presenter, wrote *Milk: the Deadly Poison.* He relayed his concerns about Monsanto's genetically engineered bacteria that delivered a toxic growth hormone to dairy cows, and subsequently to humans through dairy products.[4]

Following their presentations and a vegetarian dinner, Robert and Len had the opportunity to compare notes.

"'Mad cow disease' has been around for at least a couple hundred years," Robert advanced matter-of-factly.

"Wait a minute," Len replied. "How do you know that?"

"Because that's what everyone has reported."

"Who's everyone?"

"Well Richard Rhodes in *Deadly Feasts* for one,"[5] Robert defended.

"Are you kidding? Richard Rhodes! You believe him? He's most probably a counterintelligence agent just like Richard Preston, the author of *The Hot Zone* undoubtedly is. I exposed Preston in *Emerging Viruses.*"[6]

"Well, [Carlton] Gajdusek said the same thing," Robert justified, "I spoke to him personally."

"Well of course he did!" Len admonished. "Let me give you some background about who's pulling the strings before we discuss Rhodes and Gajdusek."

## Socio-Economic and Political Background

Len explained why he first became suspicious of Carlton Gajdusek's early "mad cow disease" studies. In the 1960s, when the "Special Virus Cancer Program" began, the disease was still called "kuru" and Gajdusek was studying it in the Fore people of New Guinea.[7] Of all the diseases that he could have studied, and the World Health Organization (WHO) desired to fund, why they chose kuru seemed suspicious to Len. Kuru, after all, was a disease that only struck a few cannibals a year. They became paralyzed, demented, and then laughed themselves to death. Later he learned that you could heat the prion to a thousand degrees and not destroy it. You could drench it with acid, formaldehyde, and formalin and still not shatter it. It obviously held the potential to be an interesting biological weapon or population destroyer.

That the WHO was heavily funded and influenced by the Rockefeller family, along with the United Nations and World Bank, added to Len's curiosity. Further fueling his suspicions was the fact that John D. Rockefeller's business managers and lawyers, John Foster and Allen Dulles, had created the partnership between the world's largest oil conglomerate and I. G. Farben—Germany's leading industrial organization prior to World War II. Farben, Len explained to Robert, for all practical purposes became the Third Reich. Farben's top executives were Hitler's highest ranking SS officers.[8]

Near the war's end, Hitler's economic director, Martin Bormann, along with the top Nazis and Third Reich partners—Rockefeller and Farben—absconded with their loot. Virtually the entire Nazi war chest, all the gold, confiscated valuables, and the Nazis themselves, escaped through the "rat lines." These underground railroads and secret escape routes were mainly organized by the Dulles brothers in service to the Rockefeller family as well as the *Vatican*. The normal Rockefeller-controlled American and International Red Crosses issued false identifications to help many of Hitler's finest escape. One major "Ratline" ran underground from Germany directly to Rome, and the Vatican played a major role along with the Freemason and Prieuré de Sion-linked Sovereign Military Order of Malta (SMOM).[9-11]

## Kissinger's Roles

Len continued to relay to Robert what he had learned about the Rockefellers and Nelson Rockefeller's protégé Henry Kissinger. Kissinger had: 1) been a chief administrator in Germany facilitating "Project: Paperclip"—the Nazi escape program, 2) had virtually ordered the development of immune system ravaging microorganisms for germ warfare as alternatives to nuclear weapons in 1969 as National Security Advisor (NSA) under Richard Nixon, 3) had gotten to this highest level position in American intelligence by serving Rockefeller family members and advancing their political and economic interests, 4) ordered the deployment of nuclear weapons in Europe, and, at home, 5) ordered CIA Director William Colby to be prepared to deploy biological weapons illegally in the "grey areas" of operation that included Central Africa in the early-to-mid 1970s, 6) written National Security Memorandum 200 that called for massive Third World depopulation, 7) served Nixon along side Litton Bionetics's President—Roy Ash—Nixon's alternate for the NSC advisor post he gave Kissinger, and after all this, was knighted by Queen Elizabeth at Windsor Castle! To this day, he has remained a principal advisor to the Board of Directors of the Merck pharmaceutical company where the vaccine that most likely delivered AIDS to the world was made.

Within a year of Kissinger's assignment to the NSA post, Roy Ash's medical subsidiary—Litton Bionetics—received: 1) the contract to develop numerous immune system destroying and carcinogenic agents for "cancer research" and germ warfare (See figure 7.2), 2) the contract to supply all the monkeys and monkey viruses to America's biological weapons contractors, as well as the world's leading cancer researchers and vaccine developers, 3) the contract to administer all of the grants and programs ongoing at America's premier biological weapons testing center—Fort Detrick, Maryland, and 4) $2 million annually in funding during the late 1960s and early 1970s, delivered under the guise of "cancer research," to develop and test viruses that were descriptively and functionally identical to today's AIDS and Ebola viruses; and according to the *Congressional Record* in 1969 (See figure 7.1.), $180,000 in additional biological weapons contracts. Earlier that year, Kissinger had apparently selected the option to develop immune system destroying agents for germ warfare. Secretary of Defense Melvin Laird had investigated this for him in 1969. Litton Bionetics had been developing and testing these types of population reducers at that exact time.[12]

## Serving Up *Deadly Feasts*

"So when I saw kuru on the list of infectious agents being studied by Litton Bionetics," Len told Robert, "red flags waved. I suspected Rhodes as soon as I cracked his book. He immediately acknowledged funding from the Alfred P. Sloan Foundation. They funded Richard Preston's book *The Hot Zone*, and also Laurie Garrett's book, *The Coming Plague*."

A section of *Emerging Viruses* is called "The Sloan/Hot Zone/ Plague Connection" in which Dr. Horowitz exposed the fact that both the Sloan and Rockefeller Foundations maintained similar cancer virus and population control investments and agendas. Sloan had plenty of incentive to fund these misleading books. Their propaganda effectively confused the public and scientific community regarding AIDS, Ebola and other immune system destroying viruses that were created in many of the labs the Sloan and Rockefeller Foundations collectively funded.

"Laurance Rockefeller was, in fact, chairman of the board of the Memorial Sloan-Kettering Cancer Center, and a trustee for the Sloan Foundation, at the time their researchers supplied Robert Gallo [the alleged 1984 AIDS virus (HIV) discoverer] with the reagents he needed to develop [by 1972] viruses that were descriptively and functionally identical to HIV.[13] Both the Sloan Foundation and the Rockefellers were heavily connected with, and major shareholders of, the Merck pharmaceutical company.[14] The science indicated they spread the virus

211

# Fig. 7.1. 1970 DOD Appropriations Request for AIDS-like Virus

# DEPARTMENT OF DEFENSE APPROPRIATIONS FOR 1970

UNITED STATES SENATE LIBRARY

# HEARINGS

BEFORE A

## SUBCOMMITTEE OF THE COMMITTEE ON APPROPRIATIONS HOUSE OF REPRESENTATIVES

NINETY-FIRST CONGRESS

FIRST SESSION

SUBCOMMITTEE ON DEPARTMENT OF DEFENSE

GEORGE H. MAHON, Texas, *Chairman*

ROBERT L. F. SIKES, Florida
JAMIE Ơ. WHITTEN, Mississippi
GEORGE W. ANDREWS, Alabama
DANIEL J. FLOOD, Pennsylvania
JOHN M. SLACK, West Virginia
JOSEPH P. ADDABBO, New York
FRANK E. EVANS, Colorado [1]

GLENARD P. LIPSCOMB, California
WILLIAM E. MINSHALL, Ohio
JOHN J. RHODES, Arizona
GLENN R. DAVIS, Wisconsin

R. L. MICHAEL, Ralph Preston, John Garrity, Peter Murphy, Robert Nicholson, ROBERT FONTER, *Staff Assistants*

[1] Temporarily assigned

*H.B. 15090*

## PART 5

RESEARCH, DEVELOPMENT, TEST, AND EVALUATION

Department of the Army
Statement of Director, Advanced Research Project Agency
Statement of Director, Defense Research and Engineering

Printed for the use of the Committee on Appropriations

U.S. GOVERNMENT PRINTING OFFICE
WASHINGTON : 1969

36-334

# DEPARTMENT OF DEFENSE APPROPRIATIONS FOR 1970

## SYNTHETIC BIOLOGICAL AGENTS

There are two things about the biological agent field I would like to mention. One is the possibility of technological surprise. Molecular biology is a field that is advancing very rapidly and eminent biologists believe that within a period of 5 to 10 years it would be possible to produce a synthetic biological agent, an agent that does not naturally exist and for which no natural immunity could have been acquired.

Mr. SIKES. Are we doing any work in that field?

Dr. MACARTHUR. We are not.

Mr. SIKES. Why not? Lack of money or lack of interest?

Dr. MACARTHUR. Certainly not lack of interest.

.Mr. SIKES. Would you provide for our records information on what would be required, what the advantages of such a program would be, the time and the cost involved?

Dr. MACARTHUR. We will be very happy to.

(The information follows:)

The dramatic progress being made in the field of molecular biology led us to investigate the relevance of this field of science to biological warfare. A small group of experts considered this matter and provided the following observations:

1. All biological agents up to the present time are representatives of naturally occurring disease, and are thus known by scientists throughout the world. They are easily available to qualified scientists for research, either for offensive or defensive purposes.

* 2. Within the next 5 to 10 years, it would probably be possible to make a new infective microorganism which could differ in certain important aspects from any known disease-causing organisms. Most important of these is that it might be refractory to the immunological and therapeutic processes upon which we depend to maintain our relative freedom from infectious disease.

* 3. A research program to explore the feasibility of this could be completed in approximately 5 years at a total cost of $10 million.

4. It would be very difficult to establish such a program. Molecular biology is a relatively new science. There are not many highly competent scientists in the field, almost all are in university laboratories, and they are generally adequately supported from sources other than DOD. However, it was considered possible to initiate an adequate program through the National Academy of Sciences-National Research Council (NAS-NRC).

The matter was discussed with the NAS-NRC, and tentative plans were made to initiate the program. However, decreasing funds in CB, growing criticism of the CB program, and our reluctance to involve the NAS NRC in such a controversial endeavor have led us to postpone it for the past 2 years.

* It is a highly controversial issue and there are many who believe such research should not be undertaken lest it lead to yet another method of massive killing of large populations. On the other hand, without the sure scientific knowledge that such a weapon is possible, and an understanding of the ways it could be done, there is little that can be done to devise defensive measures. Should an enemy develop it there is little doubt that this is an important area of potential military technological inferiority in which there is no adequate research program.

Source: Department of Defense Appropriations for 1970. Hearings Before a Subcommittee of the Committee on Appropriations House of Representatives, Ninety-First Congress, Tuesday, July 1, 1969, Page 129. Washington: U.S. Government Printing Office, 1969.

through contaminated vaccines given to New York gays and Central African Blacks in 1974 and likely later as well."

The Rockefellers initiated the cancer and eugenics industries in the 1920s. Their eugenics program called for the mass sterilization and elimination of minority populations in America, and largely supported Hitler's racial hygiene program. Sloan and the Rockefellers benefitted most from Preston's *The Hot Zone*, Garrett's *The Coming Plague*, and Rhodes's *Deadly Feasts*—works that present eighty percent truth, but censor the material that is most incriminating.

For example, Rhodes described chief kuru investigator Carleton Gajdusek's history, personality, and Nobel Prize winning "genius" in great detail. He portrayed Gajdusek to be a humanitarian and pediatric devotee. He neglected to mention, however, that Gajdusek was a convicted pedophile.

In fact, to show how contemporary propaganda distorts the *whole* truth, regarding Gajdusek's pedophilia, Rhodes wrote:

"In 1963 Carlton Gajdusek had begun adopting children from New Guinea and Micronesia. He wanted a family and he wanted to help the premodern tribal groups that had welcomed him into their lives by educating some of their children. The first child he brought home with him was a twelve-year-old Anga boy named Mbaginta'o who had worked with him for years assisting with kuru examinations and autopsies. . . . Mbaginta'o was the first of thirty-eight children Gajdusek would impoverish himself to import into the U.S. across the next thirty years, seven or eight at a time, and sponsor through high school and college. When Gajdusek established a branch of his NIH laboratory in a Level Four containment facility the U.S. Army made available at Fort Detrick, in Frederick, Maryland, northwest of Baltimore, a wealthy friend loaned the maverick pediatrician an elegant eighteenth-century manor house sited on a hilltop estate outside town. The house . . . filled up with children and "came to look like an ethnographic museum, chockablock with hundreds of artifacts Carleton had brought home, along with the kids, from his Pacific bailiwick: pots, spears, shields, masks and canoes (hanging from the ceiling)."[15]

"What Rhodes failed to write," Len told Robert, "is that Gajdusek was convicted of sexually abusing at least some of these children.

"Now let me show you this." Len pulled out a copy of *Emerging Viruses: AIDS & Ebola*, and turned to the pages shown in figure 7.3. "This is an official U.S. Government document reprinted.[16] It is Litton's report to the National Cancer Institute in 1971. It lists the menu of mutant viruses and infectious agents that Litton Bionetics—the Army's sixth top biological weapons contractor—held in their labs at the time they shipped contaminated chimpanzees and monkeys from Africa to Dr. Hilleman in New York—animals used to develop the experimental hepatitis B vaccine in 1974 that most plausibly initiated the international AIDS pandemic.

"Count eleven agents down on the right hand column, and what do you see?" Len handed the book to Robert.

"Kuru!"

"Right."

"And when was this published?" Robert asked.

"1971," Len answered. "But they likely isolated the kuru agent, the prion, before that."

"That's incredible! I thought Stanley Prusiner only discovered the infectious agent in 1982. He won the Nobel Prize in Medicine for it in 1997."[17]

"Obviously," Len replied, "they had an infectious agent or material that initiated kuru more than a decade before that. Again, Prusiner's prize and mention seems like distractive propaganda to me."

"I'm going to call Richard Rhodes and Gadjusek when I get home and ask them about this."

"You do that," Len encouraged.

## Tuskegee in New Guinea?

Days later Robert called to report the results of his further investigation. "Len, I think you're on to something," he said.

Fig. 7.2. Bionetics Contract to Investigate AIDS-like Viruses

BIONETICS RESEARCH LABORATORIES, INC. (NIH-71-2025)

Title: Investigations of Viral Carcinogenesis in Primates

Contractor's Project Directors:  Dr. John Landon
Dr. David Valerio
Dr. Robert Ting

Project Officers (NCI):  Dr. Roy Kinard
Dr. Jack Gruber
Dr. Robert Gallo

Objectives: (1) Evaluation of long-term oncogenic effects of human and animal viral inocula in primates of various species, especially newborn macaques; (2) maintenance of monkey breeding colonies and laboratories necessary for inoculation, care and monitoring of monkeys; and (3) biochemical studies of transfer RNA under conditions of neoplastic transformation and studies on the significance of RNA-dependent DNA polymerase in human leukemic tissues.

Major Findings: This contractor continues to produce over 300 excellent newborn monkeys per year. This is made possible by diligent attention to reproductive physiological states of female and male breeders. Semen evaluation, artifical insemination, vaginal cytology and ovulatory drugs are used or tried as needed.

Inoculated and control infants are hand-fed and kept in modified germ-free isolators. They are removed from isolators at about 8 weeks of age and placed in filtered air cages for months or years of observation. The holding area now contains approximately 1200 animals up to 5 years old. Approximately 300 are culled every year at a rate of about 25 per month. This is necessary to make room for young animals inoculated with new or improved virus preparations.

During the past year macaques were inoculated at birth or in utero with the Mason-Pfizer monkey mammary virus, Epstein-Barr virus, Herpesvirus saimiri, and Marek's disease virus. EB virus was given with immunostimulation and immunosuppression (ALS, prednisone, imuran). Australia antigen was given to newborn African green monkeys.

The breeding and holding colonies were surveyed for antibody to EBV. All breeders were positive and their offspring contain maternal antibody for several months. Colony-born offspring that have lost maternal antibody and are sero-negative will be surveyed periodically for conversion to the EB positive state.

An RNA-dependent DNA polymerase similar to that associated with RNA tumor viruses was detected in human leukemic cells but not in normal cells stimulat by phytohemagglutinin. The enzyme was isolated, purified and concentrated 200-fold, making possible its further characterization and study in relation to the leukemic process in man.

Significance to Biomedical Research and to the Program of the Institute: Inasmuch as tests for the biological activity of candidate human viruses will not be tested in the human species, it is imperative that another system be developed for these determinations and, subsequently for the evaluation of vaccines or other measures of control. The close phylogenetic relationship of the lower primates to man justifies utilization of these animals for these purposes. Further study of altered transfer RNA and polymerase enzymes would determine their significance in neoplastic change and provide a basis for selection of therapeutic agents.

Proposed Course: Continuation with increased emphasis on monitoring and intensive care of inoculated animals to determine if active infection occurs, effects of infection, and degree of immunosuppression when used. Further studies of human neoplasms at a molecular level will continue.

Date Contract Initiated: February 12, 1962.

BIONETICS RESEARCH LABORATORIES, INC. (NIH 71-2025)

Title:  Investigations of Viral Carcinogenesis in Primates

Contractor's Project Director:  Dr. Harvey Rabin

Project Officers (NCI):  Dr. Roy Kinard
                         Dr. Jack Gruber
                         Dr. Gary Pearson

Objectives:  (1) Evaluation of long-term oncogenic effects of
human and animal viral inocula in primates of various species,
especially newborn macaques; (2) maintenance of monkey breeding
colonies and laboratories necessary for inoculation, care and
monitoring of monkeys; and (3) biochemical studies of transfer
RNA under conditions of neoplastic transformation and studies
on the significance of RNA-dependent DNA polymerase in human
leukemic tissues.

Major Findings:  This contractor continues to produce over
300 excellent newborn monkeys per year.  This is made possible
by diligent attention to reproductive physiological states of
female and male breeders.  Semen evaluation, artifical
insemination, vaginal cytology and ovulatory drugs are used
or tried as needed.

Inoculated and control infants are hand-fed and kept in
modified germ-free isolators.  They are removed from isolators
at about 8 weeks of age and placed in filtered air cages for
months or years of observation.  The holding area now contains
approximately 1200 animals up to 5 years old.  Approximately
300 are culled every year at a rate of about 25 per month.
This is necessary to make room for young animals inoculated
with new or improved virus preparations.

New importance is being given to the New World species of
monkeys, including squirrel, marmoset, and spider monkeys.
Animals currently on study are being actively culled to reflect
this change.

Special emphasis has been placed on virological studies
characterizing the Mason-Pfizer monkey virus (M-PMV).  Seven
sublines established from chronically M-PMV-infected rhesus
foreskin cultures were shown to be releasing moderately high
titers of infectious M-PMV, and in addition seemed to have
undergone in vitro transformation.  Inoculation of cells of
these sublines into newborn rhesus monkeys produced palpable
masses at the sites of inoculation.  Biopsies performed on
these masses and on the regional lymph nodes of the same
animals revealed the presence of proliferating virus characteristic of M-PMV by both electron microscopic and cell culture

195

analysis. Proliferating M-PMV was found in the lymph nodes of monkeys inoculated with cell-free M-PMV preparations.

Chromatographic examination of transfer RNA's (tRNA's) from control and virus-transformed rat and mouse embryo cells demonstrated differences in phenyl-alanyl-tRNA's and aspartyl-tRNA's. No differences were noted in the elution profiles of seryl-, tyrosyl-, leucyl-, asparaginyl-, or glutaminyl-tRNA.

The effects of 11 rifamycin derivatives on viral reverse transcriptase and on DNA polymerases from human normal and leukemic blood lymphocytes were evaluated. Compound 143-483, 3-formyl rifamycin SV: octyl oxime showed the greatest potency and inhibited all DNA polymerases from both viral and cellular origins.

The contractor also engaged in collaborative studies involving the oncornavirus, RD-114, from a human sarcoma, isolated by Drs. McAllister, Gardiner, and Huebner. The virus is being produced and supplied by Dr. Gilden of Flow Laboratories. Another virus, a human papovavirus associated with progressive multifocal leukoencephalopathy, is being supplied by Dr. Duard Walker for inoculation into newborn monkeys.

Significance to Biomedical Research and to the Program of the Institute: Inasmuch as tests for the biological activity of candidate human viruses will not be tested in the human species, it is imperative that another system be developed for these determinations and. subsequently for the evaluation of vaccines or other measures of control. The close phylogenetic relationship of the lower primates to man justifies utilization of these animals for these purposes. Further study of altered transfer RNA and polymerase enzymes would determine their significance in neoplastic change and provide a basis for selection of therapeutic agents.

Proposed Course: The previously mentioned studies will be continued and expanded. Particular attention will be given to research on animals inoculated with candidate human cancer viruses, and investigations will be carried forward into the nature of neoplastic changes and their possible control at the cellular level. Collaborative efforts with other researchers within the SVCP will continue.

Date Contract Initiated: February 12, 1962

Current Annual Level: $2,153,850

196

218

"Robert, I forgot to check one thing. Give me a couple minutes and I'll call you right back."

In that time, Len reviewed the list of experiments reported to the NCI in 1971 by Litton Bionetics researchers. He looked for the name Gadjusek to see if his work on kuru was cited. Sure enough, there it was.

"Robert. I've got something for you. I'll fax it right through for you to see this with your own eyes." Len then faxed Robert Cohen the document shown in figure 7.4.

Indeed, the document showed, Rhodes's story was incomplete at best. The author of *Deadly Feasts* alluded to chimpanzee inoculation studies outside Washington, D.C., in 1963.[18] But he never mentioned Gadjusek had inoculated eight chimps, and maybe even humans, with minced human tissues containing kuru in 1966. Nor did Rhodes mention the most critical "Special Virus Cancer Program" ongoing at the NIH and NCI at that time. The cooperative study between Gadjusek, the NCI, and the bioweapons contractor Litton Bionetics, listed in this document, showed that four of the original eight "animals" inoculated died within one month—between April and May of that year. This indeed was remarkable given the fact that it generally takes years for prions to incubate and then cause brain damage. Had something else been done during the study to induce a faster kill?

Besides the use of chimpanzees, use of human subjects by Gadjusek is not out of the question. Particularly considering the period. That same year, again under U.S. Army contracts, Saul Krugman from the New York University Medical Center (another Army biological weapons contractor according to the U. S. *Congressional Record* as seen in figure 7.5.) injected hundreds of mentally retarded children with cancer causing hepatitis B viruses.[19] In 1969, as these studies concluded, the Director for the Centers for Disease Control and Prevention (CDC), David Sencer, ordered the infamous Tuskegee syphilis study of infected African American men to continue. Shortly thereafter, Sencer was rewarded with the top position in New York City's public health

# Fig. 7.3. Bionetics's Menu of Infectious Agents Under Study

transferred are real numbers. The dates present in the tabulations refer to the time the animals were placed on study.

1. Material inoculated

   a. Origin

      | | |
      |---|---|
      | A | avian |
      | B | bovine |
      | C | chemical |
      | E | equine |
      | F | feline |
      | G | guinea pig |
      | H | human |
      | M | murine |
      | O | ovine |
      | R | rabbit |
      | S | simian |

   b. Diagnosis

      | | |
      |---|---|
      | A12S40 | Adenovirus 12 + SV-40 |
      | A2S40 | Adenovirus 2 + SV-40 |
      | Ad2P | Adenovirus 2 + parainfluenza |
      | Ad 7 | Adenovirus 7 |
      | AL | Acute leukemia |
      | ALL | Acute lymphocytic leukemia |
      | ALL I | Acute lymphocytic leukemia + influenza |
      | ALL PI | Acute lymphocytic leukemia + parainfluenza |
      | AM BL | American Burkitt's lymphoma |
      | AML | Acute myelogenous leukemia |
      | AM MOL | Acute myelogenous leukemia + monocytic leukemia |
      | AMOL | Acute monocytic leukemia |
      | Arbo | Arthropod-borne virus |
      | AT MON | Atypical monocytosis |
      | Au Ag | Australia antigen |
      | Bac Agt | Bacterial agent |
      | BL | Burkitt's lymphoma |
      | BOL | Bovine leukemia |
      | CA | Condyloma acuminatum |
      | CCHy | Congenital cerebral hyperplasia |
      | CF | Control familial |
      | C-H | Chediak-Higashi |
      | Chondr | Chondrosarcoma |
      | CLL | Chronic lymphocytic leukemia |
      | CML | Chronic myelogenous leukemia |
      | CMV | Cytomegalovirus |
      | CSCL | Congenital stem cell leukemia |
      | DC | Disease control |
      | D Enc | Dawson's encephalitis |
      | Echo 9 | Echovirus 9 |
      | EL | Erythroid leukemia |

| | |
|---|---|
| Eosinp | Eosinophilia |
| Fibro | Fibrosarcoma |
| GB | Glioblastoma |
| H-1 | H-1 virus |
| Herp/G | H. genitalis |
| Herp/S | H. simplex |
| HD | Hodgkin's disease |
| HV | Herpesvirus |
| I | Influenza |
| IM | Infectious mononucleosis |
| Kuru | Kuru |
| L | Leukemia |
| Liposar | Liposarcoma |
| L lymph | Lymphocytic leukemia |
| LRL | Leukemoid reaction of the liver |
| LS | Lymphosarcoma |
| Lymph | Lymphoma |
| Mamm T | Mammary tumor |
| Mening | Meningitis |
| MH | Malignant histiocytosis |
| Misc L | Miscellaneous leukemia |
| Misc V | Miscellaneous virus |
| ML | Malignant lymphoma |
| MM | Multiple myeloma |
| MSV | Moloney sarcoma virus |
| MSV AV | Moloney sarcoma virus + arbovirus |
| MSV L | Moloney sarcoma virus + leukemia |
| MSV MT | Moloney sarcoma virus + monkey tumor |
| Osteo S | Osteosarcoma |
| P | Papilloma |
| PI | Parainfluenza |
| PIA C | Pia mater control cell culture |
| Plyctm | Polycythemia |
| PPLO | Mycoplasma |
| R | Rubella |
| Rau Vi | Rauscher virus |
| RCS | Reticulum cell sarcoma |
| Reo 1 | Reovirus 1 |
| Reo 3 | Reovirus 3 |
| ● Rhabd L | Rhabdomyosarcoma + leukemia |
| Rhabdo | Rhabdomyosarcoma |
| RTC | Rous transformed cells |
| S | Sarcoma |
| S20S40 | SV-20 + SV-40 |
| SA 7 | Simian agent 7 |
| SCL | Stem cell leukemia |
| Sq S | Squamous cell sarcoma |
| SV-5 | Simian virus 5 |
| SV-20 | Simian virus 20 |
| SV-40 | Simian virus 40 |
| T | Thrombocytopenia |

● = Possible Marburg predecessor

# Fig. 7.4. Gajdusek's Kuru (Prion) Study Report to the NCI

| | | Inoculum | Source | No. Inoc. | Dead or Transferred |
|---|---|---|---|---|---|
| 18. | Rauscher-Reisinger-Bowser, 4/67-5/67 | H; BL | 1 | 14 | 6 |
| | | Irradiation | | 1 | 1 |
| | | H; CML | 2 | 1 | 0 |
| 19. | Sarma-Huebner, 9/69 | F; Fibro | 1 | 3 | 0 |
| 20. | Shachat-Moloney, 8/65-11/66 | M&S; MSV MT | 1 | 2 | 2 |
| | | M; Rhabdo | 1 | 10 | 8 |
| 21. | Stewart, 4/62-6/68 | H; ALL | 1 | 56 | 24 |
| | | H; AML | 1 | 6 | 6 |
| | | A; S | 4 | 32 | 23 |
| | | H; GB | 1 | 2 | 2 |
| | | H; BL | 1 | 51 | 31 |
| | | H; CML | 1 | 2 | 2 |
| | | H; HD | 1 | 9 | 9 |
| | | H; Liposar | 1 | 4 | 4 |
| | | H; D Enc | 1 | 3 | 3 |
| | | H; Undiag | 1 | 2 | 2 |
| | | S; SV-5 | 1 | 3 | 3 |

### E. Terminated Studies

| | | Inoculum | Source | No. Inoc. | Dead or Transferred |
|---|---|---|---|---|---|
| 1. | Aisenberg-Zamecnik, 5/64-6/64 | H; HD | 2 | 8 | 5 |
| 2. | Blumberg-Moloney, 6/66-10/66 | M; Rhabdo | 4 | 1 | 1 |
| | | M; MSV L | 1 | 2 | 2 |
| 3. | Chirigos, 5/66-3/69 | C; pI:C | 6 | 8 | 7 |
| | | M; S | 1 | 6 | 6 |
| | | M; Arbo | 1 | 2 | 2 |
| | | M; MSV AV | 1 | 2 | 2 |
| | | M; MSV | 1 | 2 | 1 |
| 4. | Cohen, 3/68-1/69 | H; AL | 2 | 6 | 5 |
| | | H; BL | 1 | 3 | 3 |
| | | R; ALS | 3 | 7 | 6 |
| | | Control | | 2 | 2 |
| | | H; AML | 2 | 2 | 0 |
| | | H; CLL | 2 | 2 | 0 |
| | | H; EL | 2 | 2 | 0 |
| 5. | Dreyer, 9/64 | H; ML | 1 | 2 | 2 |
| 6. | Gajdusek, 1/67 | H; D Enc | 4 | 4 | 3 |
| *7. | Gajdusek-Gibbs, 4/66-5/66 | H; Kuru | 4 | 8 | 4 |
| 8. | Gazdar-Moloney, 7/69-8/69 | F; Fibro | 4 | 3 | 0 |
| 9. | Grace, 2/64-8/64 | H; MyL | 1 | 1 | 1 |
| | | H; AML | 1 | 10 | 8 |
| | | H; ALL | 1 | 2 | 1 |
| 10. | Grace-Horoscewicz, 5/67 | H; BL | 1 | 6 | 5 |
| 11. | Gross, 5/62-4/63 | M; L lymph | 4 | 12 | 7 |

*Study conducted by C.D. Gajdusek and C.J Gibbs on eight (8) primates—chimpanzees and possibly humans as well—whereby prion infected "minced tissues" extracted from human victims were inoculated into test subjects. In study number seven, half of the experimental subjects died within one month, highly atypical of traditionally slow growing prion infections. From: NCI staff. *The Special Virus Cancer Program: Progress Report #8*. Office of the Associate Scientific Director for Viral Oncology (OASDVO). J. B. Moloney, Ed., Washington, D.C.: U.S. Government Printing Office, 1971, pp. 286.

department. The assignment was just in time for Sencer to lend his support for the recruitment and inoculation of gay men with Merck's contaminated experimental hepatitis B vaccines. These vaccines, according to scientists worldwide, were hideously contaminated with viruses including those currently linked to chronic fatigue immune dysfunction (CFIDS), certain cancers, and the AIDS epidemic as well.[20]

## Szmuness and the Pope

Relating scientific and religious history to this period of prion research, another researcher should be considered besides Gadjusek—Wolf Szmuness, chief of the New York hepatitis B vaccine trials. Several scientists have argued that Dr. Szmuness's hepatitis B vaccine experiments contributed greatly to the spread of HIV to gay men in New York.[21] A decade prior to these suspected trials, in the mid 1960s, as Gadjusek was inoculating primates (and possibly humans) with kuru, and Krugman was injecting children with an assortment of cancer viruses, Szmuness sojourned from Communist Poland to United States where he "miraculously" secured a position as a "lab tech" at the Rockefeller-controlled New York City Blood Center.[21]

Ten years earlier, some authors alleged, he shared a room with a very unique Catholic priest. According to publications by infectious disease investigator and author Alan Cantwell, M.D., "'a remarkable friendship developed' between Szmuness and the clergyman. The two men corresponded 'for a long time thereafter' . . . The Polish priest eventually became the first Polish pope in Catholic history: Pope John Paul II."

In America, "within a few years, Szmuness was given his own lab and a separate department of epidemiology at the [NYC Blood] Center." Then, in "record time," Szmuness leapfrogged to full professorship at Columbia University's School of Public Health." By the mid-1970s, Cantwell wrote, "Szmuness became a world authority on hepatitis and 'transfusion medicine.' Szmuness's meteoric and unprec-

## Fig. 7.5. Army Biologial Weapons Contractors for FY 1969

Mr. Mahon. List for the record the major contractors and the sums allocated to them in this program in fiscal year 1969.
(The information follows:)

The following list contains the major contractors and amounts of each contract.

| Contractor | Fiscal year 1969 |
|---|---|
| Miami, University. of Coral Gables Fla | $645,000 |
| Herner and Co., Bethesda, Md | 518,000 |
| Missouri, University of, Columbia, Mo | 250,000 |
| Chicago, University, of Chicago, Ill | 216,000 |
| Aerojet-General Corp., Sacramento. Calif | 210,000 |
| Bionetics Research Laboratories, Inc., Falls Church, Va | 180,000 |
| West Virginia University, Morgantown, W. Va | 177,000 |
| Maryland. University of, College Park, Md | 170,000 |
| Dow Chemical Co., Midland, Mich | 158,000 |
| Hazelton Laboratories, Inc., Falls Church, Reston, Va | 145,000 |
| New York University Medical Center, New York, N.Y. | 142,000 |
| Midwest Research Institute, Kansas City, Mo | 134,000 |
| Stanford University, Palo Alto. Calif | 125,000 |
| Stanford Research Institute, Menlo Park, Calif | 124,000 |
| Pfizer and Co., Inc., New York, N.Y. | 120,000 |
| Aldrich Chemical Co., Inc., Milwaukee, Wis | 117,000 |
| Computer Usage Development Corp., Washington, D.C. | 110,000 |
| New England Nuclear Corp., Boston, Mass | 104,000 |

Source: Department of Defense Appropriations For 1970: Hearings Before A Subcommittee of the Committee on Appropriations House of Representatives, Ninety-first Congress, First Session, H.B. 15090, Part 5, Research, Development, Test and Evaluation of Biological Weapons, Dept. of the Army. U.S. Government Printing Office, Washington, D.C., 1969, p. 689.

edented rise to world prominence was halted by his death from cancer in 1982."

Pope John Paul II's history is likewise challenged. In *Behold a Pale Horse*, Naval Intelligence veteran and author William Cooper wrote that during World War II Karol Wojtyla worked for I. G. Farben—the infamous Nazi-linked Rockefeller partner. Towards the end of the war, he sought refuge, fled to Poland, and was protected there by the Catholic Church. Subsequently, and very uniquely, he was elected Pope.[22]

Expressing gratitude to his electorate, on November 27, 1983, as one of his first acts as the new "Holy Father," John Paul II lifted the Freemason excommunication order that had been pronounced in the "Codex Iuris Canonici."

"That today's pope knows the Masonic secret language is obviously proven by the Masonic handshake" he occasionally administers publicly, Jan van Helsing wrote in *Secret Societies: And Their Power in the 20th Century*. Moreover, on September 15, 1982, on the occasion of the death of

224

Lebanese president Gemayel, Pope John Paul II "spoke of Jerusalem, the City of God, and said: 'Jerusalem can also become the City of Man.' The 'City of Man' is a keyword of the Illuminati for world dictatorship."

In addition, on April 18, 1983, the Pope held audience with the entire Trilateral Commission—the secretive organization founded in 1973 by David Rockefeller and Zbigniew Brzezinski to help facilitate the development of "One World Government." As shown earlier in figure 3.6, the Trilaterals developed as a branch of the Committee of 300 controlled Royal Institute for International Affairs. Trilateral Commissioners commonly hold seats on the Council on Foreign Relations (CFR) which heavily influences U.S. Government policy and media propaganda. (See appendix figure A13.) According to van Helsing, the Trilateral Commission attracted "elite coming from different branches of Freemasonry . . . to give a broader political basis to the influence of the Bilderberger group. Most European members had long-term contracts with the Rockefellers."[23]

## Vaccines for "Public Health" and "Disinfection"

In the 1930s it was determined that scrapie—the mad cow-like disease of sheep—could be transmitted by injection and be one hundred percent fatal. Five years later Dr. William Gordon of the British Agricultural Research Council field station at Compton, Berkshire, England, began to test 44,000 doses of an experimental sheep vaccine he had developed to rid the animals of "louping-ill" disease. His vaccine consisted of "homogenized brain, spinal-cord and spleen tissue taken from sheep infected with louping ill, diluted in saline solution and inactivated by adding a small amount of formaldehyde. . . . In 1937, to Gordon's horror, the sheep inoculated . . . began developing scrapie. The vaccine was evidently contaminated."[17]

Dr. Gordon relayed in *Deadly Feasts*, "I visited most of the farms on which sheep had been vaccinated in 1935 . . . I shall not forget the profound effect on my emotions when I . . . was warmly welcomed because of the great benefits resulting from the application of louping-ill vaccine, whereas the chief purpose of my visit was to determine if scrapie was appearing in the inoculated sheep."[24]

Ten years later, scrapie appeared on American soil in Michigan where, according to Rhodes, purebred British sheep had been imported through Canada. Soon there were outbreaks of it in California and Ohio as well. That these outbreaks occurred by accident, or simple ignorance as Rhodes advanced, is highly uncertain. Given the *Deadly Feasts* author's funding sources and censored text, the first American outbreaks were as likely associated with vaccine trials much like the outbreaks in which doctors Szmuness and Gordon were implicated.

Therefore, given the social, political, religious, economic, and scientific history provided thus far, it is not inconceivable that today's physician's offices and public health units that offer "free vaccines" are like the concentration camps of yesteryear. And that Rockefeller controlled blood and vaccines are much like the gas.

"When you don't learn history," Len told Robert, "because of laziness, ignorance, or because the history itself was a major covert operation that never made it into the history books, history repeats.

"Today with AIDS, mad cow disease, chronic fatigue, and the rest, history is apparently repeating. In fact, even the message is the same. The millions of holocaust victims were told they were going into 'showers' for 'pubic health' and 'disinfection.' That's why we're being told to get vaccinated. Virtually nothing has changed, not even the message."

## "Family Planning" is Population Control is Genocide

> Once I found a woman who was 9 months pregnant, but did not have a [Chinese] birth-allowed certificate. According to the policy, she was forced to undergo an abortion surgery. In the operation room, I saw how the aborted child's lips were sucking, how its limbs were stretching. A physician injected poison into

its skull. The child died, and it was thrown into the trash can. . . .
I could not live with this on my conscience. I, too, after all, am a
mother.[25]

These words by Chinese "family planning" director and defector
Kiao Duan Gao, gave an insider's view of the extent to which "population control," as genocide, is practiced today. Genocide is defined as
the mass extermination of people for political motives. Easily rational-
ized and then dismissed as egalitarian policy, "family planning"
reaches worldwide. Its practices are not confined to developing nations, nor even overpopulated ones. Its finances are provided by the
United Nations Fund for Population Activities, and powerful Non-
Governmental Organizations (NGOs) dedicated to population reduction. Among the most active are: Zero Population Growth,
International Planned Parenthood Federation, Population Resource
Center, Population Communications International, Negative Population Growth, Inc., the Merck Fund, and most importantly the Rockefeller Foundation. Their efforts are not confined to abortion.
Vaccinations are also "mandated" in many countries, particularly for
women who enter "family planning" centers and "maternal and child
health clinics."[25,26]

In July, 1986, for example, an experimental contraceptive vaccine
developed by Dr. Vernon Stevens, Director of Reproductive Biology at
Ohio State's Department of Obstetrics and Gynecology in Columbus,
was tested on Australian women.[27] It contained the female pregnancy
hormone—HCG (short for human chorionic gonadotrophic hormone).
It caused the vaccine recipients to become sterile. The study was based
partly on earlier sterilization success using the same hormone injected
into women in tetanus vaccines.[28] Based on these early "trials," during
the 1990s, the sterilizing hormone was secretly placed in additional
tetanus vaccines given to more than 3.5 million women of child bearing age in the Philippines. With the aid of the Rockefeller-influenced
World Health Organization (WHO), similar contraceptive shots were
also administered to untold others in Nicaragua, Mexico, and North

America. All the women became unwitting victims of global depopulation policy.[27]

"During the 1920s," Len explained to Robert, "the Rockefeller family established the cancer industry along with a virtual monopoly over American medicine. The latter was secured through the Rockefeller's funding a fraudulent, allegedly 'scientific investigation' resulting in the 'Flexner Report' to the U.S. Congress that vilified traditional preventive and natural healing methods. Homeopathy, herbology, acupuncture, chiropractic, and naturopathy fell victims to the more lucrative, and far more risky, drug-based methods of disease care that the Rockefellers and their associates largely control to this very day.[29]

"Most people today have no idea what the term "eugenics" means," Len continued. "According to *Webster's Dictionary*, it is 'a science that deals with the improvement of hereditary qualities of a race or breed.' Another little known fact is that Rockefeller family members and their secret society friends, including Prescott Bush—George Bush's father, William Draper III, the Royal Family, and several other political notables, began funding this 'science' during the 1920s. Studies were initiated in the mid-Atlantic states whereby school children were required to take intelligence tests. If they failed to achieve a seventy-five percent score or higher they were sterilized.[30]

"In 1928 the Rockefellers again provided most of the money needed to build and run the Kaiser Wilhelm Institute for Anthropology, Eugenics, and Human Heredity in pre-Nazi Germany. Chief executive for the institute was the fascist psychiatrist Ernst Rudin. He later became Hitler's top racial hygienist."

## The Eugenic Roots of Planned Parenthood

Among Rudin's, Hitler's, and the Rockefeller's most ardent supporters was Margaret Sanger—the founder and chief promoter of "Planned Parenthood."

According to a review of Sanger's work by medical physician and author Stanley Monteith, as superficially described in Chapter 3, Sanger brazenly supported the Nazi eugenics policy during the 1930s. To further the genetically-engineered "super race," she argued that, "the extermination of 'human weeds' . . . the 'cessation of charity, . . . the segregation of 'morons, misfits, and the maladjusted,' and . . . the sterilization of 'genetically inferior races'" was a practical necessity. In her magazine, *The Birth Control Review*, she hailed the Nazi's "infanticide program," and championed Hitler's goal of developing the supreme white Aryan race.

Prior to WWII, Sanger commissioned Ernst Rudin, then the director of German Medical Experimentation Programs, to advise her colleagues at the fledgling Planned Parenthood.

George Grant, in his book *Killer Angel*, described Sanger's first birth control clinic in the "Brownsville section of New York . . . populated by newly immigrated Slavs, Latins, Italians, and Jews. She targeted the 'unfit' for her crusade to 'save the planet.'"[30]

In 1939, when the world went to war, Sanger began her "Negro project." The "masses of Negroes," she said, "particularly in the South, still breed carelessly and disastrously, with the result that the increase among Negroes, even more than among whites, is from that portion of the population least intelligent and fit. . . ."[30]

Sanger then revealed her intention to employ a few "Colored Ministers" to travel to Black enclaves to "propagandize" birth control. She wrote:

> The most successful educational approach to the Negro is through a religious appeal. We do not want word to go out that we want to exterminate the Negro population. . . . [T]he Minister is the man who can straighten out that idea if it ever occurs to any of their more rebellious members.[30]

"As Margaret Sanger's organization grew in power, influence, and acceptance," Dr. Monteith recalled, "she began to write of the necessity of targeting religious groups for destruction as well, believing that the 'dysgenic races' should include 'Fundamentalists and Catholics' in addition to 'Blacks, Hispanics, and American Indians'. . . . She became increasingly hostile to both Christianity and the American precepts of individual freedom under God."[30]

Around the time Margaret Sanger and Ernst Rudin were organizing their racial hygiene efforts, John Foster and Allen Dulles, representing the legal and financial interests of John D. Rockefeller's Standard Oil Company, negotiated a contract with the leading German company, I.G. Farben. For $35 million, the Rockefellers secured the patent rights over the synthetic fuel and rubber the holocaust victims were about to produce in factories adjacent Auschwitz and elsewhere. That contract made the Rockefeller family partners with the firm that developed the gas that killed the millions of Jews, Christians, Gypsies, Blacks, Gays and others deemed unfit for the "master race."[26] Again, Pope John Paul II, then named Karol Wojtyla, worked on behalf of I.G. Farben, according to reputable accounts.[22]

By 1944 Hitler knew he would lose the war. He summoned his chief financial officer, Martin Bormann, to a meeting. "Bury your treasure," Hitler ordered, "for you will need it to begin a Fourth Reich."[31]

Len relayed to Robert what had been detailed by CBS News correspondent Paul Manning in his book *Martin Bormann: Nazi in Exile* . That Bormann set in motion "the 'flight capital' scheme August 10, 1944, in Strasbourg. The treasure, the golden ring, he envisioned for the new Germany, was the sophisticated distribution of national and corporate assets to safe havens . . ." Chief among them was the Merck pharmaceutical company.[31]

"At the time, Merck's president, George W. Merck," Len recalled, was advising President Roosevelt as America's 'biological weapons industry director.'"[32]

"The Merck company, thus, received windfall 'profits' from the Nazi war chest." This cash transfer was specifically arranged to, according to Manning's evidence, "help actualize Hitler's proclaimed 'vision of a thousand-year Third Reich [and] world empire. This was outlined with clarity in a document called 'Neuordunung,' or 'New

[World] Order,' that was accompanied by a letter of transmittal to the [Bormann-led] Ministry of Economics. It declared that a new order for the chemical [and pharmaceutical] industry of the world should supplement Hitler's New Order. . . ."[31]

In essence, the partners decided that a world chemical and pharmaceutical cartel was needed to eliminate undesirable populations. Drugs and chemicals could be used most effectively to control minds, dull senses, and untraceably destroy unwanted populations.

## Modern Eugenics, Genetic Biotechnology, and Substitutes for War

Len continued to explain to Robert that following WWII, as Hitler's top Nazi scientists were secretly transported to serve NATO military, intelligence, and industrial positions, eugenics also moved its center to Cold Spring Harbor labs in New York where it was renamed "The Human Genome Project."[33]

During the late 1940s and early 1950s, while Watson and Crick were completing their DNA model for "The Human Genome Project" at the Rockefeller and Sloan-funded Cold Spring Harbor facility, Bertrand Russell was completing a related book. Russell, whose family held powerful British intelligence and aristocratic ties, wrote in *The Impact of Science on Society*:

> I do not pretend that birth control is the only way in which population can be kept from increasing. There are others, which, one must suppose, opponents of birth control would prefer. War . . . has hitherto been disappointing in this respect, but perhaps bacteriological war may prove more effective. If a Black Death could be spread throughout the world once in every generation, survivors could procreate freely without making the world too full. . . . The state of affairs might be somewhat unpleasant, but what of that? Really high-minded people are indifferent to happiness, especially other people's."[34]

As Russell was publishing and lecturing on his biological prescription for a genocidal pandemic, Henry Kissinger was at Harvard developing his "Meaning of History" doctoral thesis. In it, the CIA veteran laid out the need for ongoing small wars around the planet, to engage populations, and maintain the "economic alignment of the superpowers."[35]

After he received his doctorate in 1955, Nelson Rockefeller appointed Dr. Kissinger to chair the Council on Foreign Relations (CFRs) "Nuclear Weapons Study Group." His report, published in *Foreign Affairs*, the most prestigious political periodical published by the CFR, called for the deployment of nuclear weapons around the globe. Kissinger defended this policy by recommending, "A bomb shelter in every house" in America is the price Americans should be willing to pay for their freedom.[35]

Meanwhile, George Merck, during this period of the Cold War, continued to direct America's biological weapons (BW) industry. His company remained listed in the U.S. *Congressional Record* as being a major biological weapons contractor.

By the late 1960s, BW had been developed with several advantages over nuclear missiles. Aside from their reasonable cost, their deployment left attacked enemy property intact. BW developers for all the major super powers knew their germs might be used in future battles. Few fully comprehended, however, the public health implications of their work.

In 1969, Dr. Kissinger, as the new National Security Advisor under Richard Nixon, was informed about all of the above as well as a new highly classified report that later leaked. The report discussed several primary objectives of all New World Order enthusiasts—to create peace on earth, do away with military warfare, dissolve national boundaries, mentally control populations, and at the same time substantially depopulate the planet. The report focused on the principle objective advanced by Cecil Rhodes and subsequently the Rothschilds, Rockefellers, CFR members, and all Rhodes scholars to develop substitutes for war. It was required reading for Dr. Kissinger because of his philosophical bent as well as his premier role in addressing nuclear, chemical and biological warfare (CBW) options to "maintain the economic alignment of the superpowers." *The Report From Iron Mountain*, published by The *Dial* Press of New York, included lengthy sections on "The Functions of War" and "Substitutes For The Functions of War."

A few paragraphs from this section of the 1967 report pertained to Len's discussion with Robert concerning population control. Under "ecological" concerns the "Special Study Group" wrote:

War has not been genetically progressive. But as a system of gross population control to preserve the species it cannot fairly be faulted. . . There is no question but that a universal requirement that procreation be limited to the products of artificial insemination would provide a fully adequate substitute control for population levels. Such a reproductive system would, of course, have the added advantage of being susceptible to direct eugenic management. Its predictable further development—conception and embryonic growth taking place wholly under laboratory conditions—would extend these controls to their logical conclusion. The ecological function of war under these circumstances would not only be superseded but surpassed in effectiveness.

The indicated intermediate step—total control of conception with a variant of the ubiquitous "pill," via water supplies or certain essential foodstuffs, offset by a controlled "antidote"—is already under development. There would appear to be no foreseeable need to revert to any of the outmoded practices referred to in the previous section (infanticide, etc.) as there might have been if the possibility of transition to peace had arisen two generations ago.

The real question here, therefore, does not concern the viability of this war substitute, but the political problems involved in bringing it about. It cannot be established while the war system is still in effect. The reason for this is simple: excess population is war material. As long as any society must contemplate even a remote possibility of war, it must maintain a maximum supportable population, even when so doing critically aggravates an economic liability. This is paradoxical, in view of war's role in reducing excess population, but it is readily understood. War controls the *general* population level, but the ecological interest of any single society lies in maintaining its hegemony vis-a-vis other societies.[36]

"Six years after this report was prepared," Len explained, "Kissinger, in search of New World Order diplomatic leverage, called for a reassessment of America's biological weapons (BW) capabilities. When the BW report came in, the option to develop immune system ravaging viruses for germ warfare and population control was selected. Soon after, viruses descriptively and functionally identical to what the AIDS virus is and does were developed by Litton Bionetics.[26]

"With Kissinger now overseeing the CIA's top secret BW program—Project:MKNAOMI—on July 29, 1969, George (son of eugenics advocate Prescott) Bush chaired a House Republican research committee task force on earth resources and population. He cited the urgent need for population control activities to fend off a growing Third World crisis. Earlier in the week, their committee had heard from Prescott Bush's friend, General William H. Draper, III, the national chairman of the Population Crisis Committee, and Dr. William Moran, president of the Population Reference Bureau. Bush reinforced General Draper's call for additional WHO and Planned Parenthood World Population efforts to promote abortion and population reduction.[26]

The very next year Kissinger prepared *"National Security Memorandum 200"*—a document that called for massive depopulation of Third World countries. Then, in 1970, Litton Bionetics began to receive approximately $2 million annually for five years under NIH contract number 71-2025, to develop and test AIDS-like and Ebola-like viruses, and many others that might be used for biological warfare and population control including the protein prion linked today to Creutzfeldt-Jakob disease, or CJD.[37]

## Smoking Guns and Whistle Blowers

In 1986, the year Planned Parenthood distributed brochures saying they were "proud of their long history," Dr. Maurice Hilleman—President Clinton's 1998 Sabin Gold Medal of Honor Awardee—admitted, during a taped interview, that he had imported the AIDS virus into New York in contaminated monkeys shipped from Africa by Litton to Merck.[3]

More recently, the horror of Dr. Hilleman's admission was amplified by his esteemed colleague and coauthor, senior Merck scientist and vaccine investigator, Dr. Benjamin Sweet. Dr. Sweet stated during an interview published on the Internet that he and Dr. Hilleman didn't worry too much about the viruses they knew contaminated Merck's vaccines back then. But now, he lamented, "with the theoretical links to HIV and cancer, it just blows my mind."[38]

Another scientific insider, Dr. Eleanor Coletta, recalled studying viral-induced immune suppression and sarcoma cancers in young gay men in New York City between 1973-74. Her bosses, at Sloan's dermatology department, consistently kept the NCI's Dr. Robert Gallo, and others affiliated with Merck researchers, up to date on their progress with this new "gay disease."[39]

The 200,000 human doses of Merck's implicated "experimental hepatitis B vaccine" were administered at that exact time.[40]

The AIDS-related mortality which has peaked at approximately fifty-percent in populations including New York's gay men and several central African villages is suspicious in light of the following: 1) A 1994 U.S. Department of Commerce report[41] indicated such severe population reduction was warranted in many countries that have been ravaged by HIV/AIDS, and 2) A full page advertisement in *Foreign Affairs* journal called for a similar fifty percent population reduction in America.[42] Sponsored by the Negative Population Growth, Inc., of New Jersey, CFR members were alerted to the urgent need to reduce the U.S. population "in the range of 125 to 150 million," or about half its current size.[42] (See figure 7.6.)

"Indeed," Len told Robert, "Merck's 'experimental hepatitis B vaccine' is doing its job. Fifty percent of America's gay men are now dead, and the American AIDS epidemic has moved on to Blacks and Hispanics."

For decades, to the time of this writing, Dr. Kissinger—author of the definitive guide to world depopulation, that is, *National Security Memorandum 200*,[43] has played a leading role at the CFR, and has remained a principal consultant to the Board of Advisors of the Merck Pharmaceutical Company, or Merck, Sharp and Dohme.[35]

## Making Vast Fortunes While Reducing Targeted Populations

To say that Merck and the Rockefeller directed military–medical–industrial complex continues to make vast fortunes from humanity's suffering is an understatement. The grossest conflict of interest lies in the fact that as people die from their vaccines and drug related injuries, Merck's heavily funded population control program is additionally supported. The Merck Fund, after all, along with the Rockefeller Foundation, is among the leading agencies funding world depopulation as seen in figure 7.7.[44]

North Americans need to be reminded of the effects of hepatitis vaccines and contaminated blood. At the close of the twentieth century, class action lawsuits were pending in the United States and Canada as shown in figure 7.8. It was widely known that Rockefeller-directed blood bankers knew their shipments were contaminated with AIDS, hepatitis, and other viruses for decades. Suppressed was the fact that the international blood banking industry was, and still is, largely, if not completely, controlled by the Rockefeller family.

"While Merck's vaccines have remained heavily contaminated," Len told Robert, "extraneous viruses, bacteria, genetic fragments, foreign pieces of RNA and DNA, mercury, aluminum, formaldehyde, formalin, carcinogenic enzymes and more flow into human bloodstreams on behalf of those who seek to "control" world populations.[3]

"Margaret Sanger and Hitler's spin doctor, Josef Goebbels, would be proud. Today's eugenicists have figured out a way to defraud and depopulate the masses while literally making, with no pun intended, a 'bloody' fortune."

# Fig. 7.6. *Foreign Affairs* Journal Advertisment for Reducing the United States Population by Half.

*A message from Negative Population Growth, Inc.*

## Why We Need A Smaller U.S. Population
### And How We Can Achieve It

We need a smaller population in order to halt the destruction of our environment, and to create an economy that will be sustainable over the very long term.

We are trying to address our steadily worsening environmental problems without coming to grips with their root cause -- overpopulation.

**If present immigration and fertility rates continue, our population, now over 264 million, will pass 400 million by the year 2050 -- and still be growing rapidly!**

All efforts to save our environment will ultimately be futile unless we not only halt U.S. population growth, but reverse it, so that our population can eventually be stabilized at a sustainable level -- far lower than it is today.

### The Optimum U.S. Population Size

The central issue is surely this: **At what size should we seek to stabilize U.S. population?** Unless we know in what direction we should be headed, how can we possibly devise sensible policies to get us there?

The size at which our population is eventually stabilized is supremely important because of the effect of sheer numbers of people on such vitally important national goals as a healthy environment, and a sustainable economy.

We believe these goals can best be achieved with a U.S. population in the range of 125 to 150 million, or about its size in the 1940s. This optimum size could be reached in about three to four generations if we do two things now that are well within our grasp.

### How To Get There

1. **Impose restrictions on immigration** that would halt illegal immigration, and cap legal immigration at not over 100,000 per year, including all relatives, refugees and asylees. That alone would sharply slow our growth.

2. **Lower our fertility rate** (the average number of children per woman) from the present 2.0 to around 1.5 and maintain it at that level for several decades. We believe that non-coercive financial incentives will be necessary in order to reach that goal.

If almost all women had no more than two children, our fertility rate would drop to around 1.5, because many women remain childless by choice, or choose to have not more than one child. **We promote the ideal of the two-child maximum family as the social norm, because that is the key to lowering our fertility.**

### Incentives to Lower Fertility

NPG proposes these incentives to motivate parents to have no more than two children:

* Eliminate the present Federal income tax exemption for dependent children born after a specified date.

* Give a Federal income tax credit only to those parents who have not more than two children. Those with three or more would lose the credit entirely.

* Give an annual cash grant to low income parents who pay little or no income tax, and who have no more than two children. Those with three or more children would lose the cash grant entirely.

### Two Vastly Different Paths Lie Before Us

With the reductions in immigration and fertility we advocate, our nation could start now on the path toward a sustainable, and prosperous, population of 125 to 150 million.

Without such a program, we are almost certain to continue our mindless, headlong rush down our current path. That path is leading us straight toward catastrophic population levels that can only devastate our environment, and produce universal poverty in a crowded, polluted nation.

To learn more about NPG's recommendation for programs designed to halt, and eventually to reverse, U.S and worls population growth, write today for our **FREE BROCHURE.**

NPG is a national nonprofit organization founded in 1972. **We are the only organization that calls for a smaller U.S. and world population, and recommends specific, realistic measures to achieve those goals.**

### Negative Population Growth, Inc.

P.O. Box 1206, 210 The Plaza, Suite 7K, Teaneck, NJ 0766

From: *Foreign Affairs* journal, published by the Council on Foreign Relations, Volume 75, Issue 2, March/April, 1996.

## Fig. 7.7. Population Control Funding FYs 1993-95

### Carnegie Corporation
Planned Parenthood Federation of America .....................$25,000
Sex Information and Education Council of the US.........$325,000

### Clark Foundation
National Abortion Federation .........................................$120,000
National Family Planning and Reproductive Health........$110,000
Planned Parenthood Federation of America ...................$200,000
Sex Information and Education Council of the US.........$180,000

### Ford Foundation
Population Council ....................................................$1,749,194
Sex Information and Education Council of the US.........$255,000

### MacArthur Foundation
Population Council .......................................................$900,000

### Mellon Foundation
Population Council ....................................................$7,170,000

### Merck Fund
National Abortion Federation ..........................................$90,000
Planned Parenthood Federation of America ...................$160,000
Population Council .......................................................$180,000

### Mertz-Gilmore Foundation
Lambda Legal Defense and Education Fund ...................$90,000

### Mott Foundation
Planned Parenthood Federation of America ....................$35,006

### Pew Charitable Trust
Planned Parenthood Federation of America ...................$130,000
Population Council .......................................................$300,000
Zero Population Growth .................................................$150,000

### Rockefeller Foundation
National Family Planning and Reproductive Health..........$20,000
Planned Parenthood Federation of America ...................$130,000
Population Council ....................................................$1,877,170
Population Institute........................................................$20,000

## Fig. 7.8. Contaminated Blood Prompted Class Action Lawsuit

# WERE YOU INFECTED WITH HEPATITIS C AS A RESULT OF A BLOOD TRANSFUSION* IN BC BETWEEN AUGUST 1, 1986 AND JULY 1, 1990?

## If so, please read this information:

A class action lawsuit has been certified by the Supreme Court of British Columbia seeking compensation for persons who were infected with Hepatitis C through a blood transfusion. A trial date has been set for early in the year 2000. There are on-going discussions which may result in an out-of-court settlement.

**To be considered a class member, you must:**

- be a BC resident;
- have received a blood transfusion in BC between August 1, 1986 and July 1, 1990;
- have been infected with Hepatitis C as a result of your blood transfusion; and
- have tested positive to the antibody to the Hepatitis C virus.

Class members will be bound by the judgment of the Court **unless they have opted out of the class.**

If you fall within the definition of the class, but do not want to become a member of the class action, you must opt out of the class **by February 28, 1999.**

**In order to:**

- receive a copy of the Notice to Class Members;
- opt out of the class action; or
- learn more about the class action

**Please contact:**

Ms. Kim Graham
Camp, Church and Associates
4th Floor, Randall Building
555 West Georgia Street
Vancouver, BC V6B 1Z5

Telephone: (604) 689-7555
Facsimile: (604) 689-7554
Toll-Free: **1-888-236-7797**

(If you have already contacted the class action lawyers, there is no need to contact them again.)

*of whole blood or blood products, including packed red cells, platelets, plasma (both fresh frozen and banked) or white blood cells.*

BRITISH
COLUMBIA

Ministry of Health and
Ministry Responsible for Seniors

## References

1. Horowitz LG and Emory D. "The Nazi–American Biomedical Biowarfare Connection: Rockefeller, Kissinger, Bush and the Rise of the Forth Reich"—An audiotaped presentation. Rockport, MA: Tetrahedron Publishing Group. 1997.

2. Horowitz LG and Martin WJ. *Emerging Viruses: AIDS & Ebola—Nature, Accident or Intentional? Third Edition.* Rockport, MA: Tetrahedron Publishing Group, 1998.

3. Horowitz LG. "Horowitz 'On Vaccines'"—An audiotaped presentation. Rockport, MA: Tetrahedron Publishing Group, 1997.

4. Cohen R. *Milk The Deadly Poison.* Englewood Cliffs, NJ: Argus Publishing, Inc., 1997.

5. Rhodes R. *Deadly Feasts: Tracking the Secrets of a Terrifying New Plague.* New York: Simon & Schuster, 1997.

7. Horowitz and Martin WJ. *Op cit.* pp. 15-18.

8. Scott PD. How Allen Dulles and the SS preserved each other. *Covert Action Information Bulletin* (Winter)1986;25:4-14.

9. Hunt L. *Secret Agenda: Nazi Scientists, The United States Government, and Project Paperclip, 1945 to 1990.* New York: St. Martin's Press, 1991, pp. 4;145-147 (for information on General Bolling); 186 (for Naval Medical Research Institute's employment of Paperclip Nazis for biological weapons testing); and 256 (for Dow Chemical employment of convicted Nazi Otto Ambros);

10. Manning P. *Martin Bormann: Nazi in Exile.* Secaucas, NJ: Lyle Stuart Inc., 1981, pp. 29, 56, 64, 69, 113-118, and 134-135.

11. Loftus J and Aarons M. *The Secret War Against the Jews.* New York: St. Martin's Press, 1994, pp. 112-113, 142, 168-169.

12. Horowitz and Martin. *Op cit.* pp. 335-336; 494-496.

13. Robert Gallo is the alleged 1984 AIDS-virus co-discoverer, who falsely took credit as its sole discoverer. In fact, during the late 1960s and early 1970s he supervised the development of numerous immune system destroying agents functionally and descriptively identical to HIV and Ebola under a National Institutes of Health, National

Cancer Institute contract (NIH 71-2025) given to Litton Bionetics—the U.S. Army's sixth leading biological weapons contractor. In the book *Emerging Viruses: AIDS & Ebola* by Dr. Horowitz, Dr. Gallo is nailed as a fraud using his own publications.

14. A search through Sloan Foundation's annual reports, on file in Manhattan's New York Public Library, revealed nine ghastly and incriminating reasons that tied all the elements of Dr. Horowitz's investigation together. The Sloan Foundation: (1) supported black educational initiatives consistent with the COINTELPRO Black Nationalist Hate Group campaign; (2) administered mass-media-public-persuasion experiments completely consistent with the CIA's Project MKULTRA—efforts to develop brainwashing technologies and drugs to affect large populations; (3) funded much of the earliest cancer research involving the genetic engineering of mutant viruses; (4) began major funding of the National Academy of Sciences, Cold Spring Harbor Laboratory (for "neuroscience" and molecular genetics research), the Salk Institute (for viral research), and the Scientists' Institute for Public Information between 1968 and 1970; (5) funded population control studies by Planned Parenthood-World Population, New York, N.Y.; (6) funded the Community Blood Council of Greater New York, Inc., the "council of doctors" who established the infamous New York City Blood Bank; (7) maintained Laurence S. Rockefeller, the director of the Community Blood Council of Greater New York and the president of the Rockefeller Brothers Fund, as chairman of the board of the Memorial Sloan-Kettering Cancer Center, and a trustee for the Foundation; (8) gave in excess of $20,000 annually to the Council on Foreign Relations; and (9) maintained among its "marketable securities," 16,505 shares of Chase Manhattan Bank stock (in 1967, which it apparently sold by 1970 probably to avoid conflict of interest charges) along with 24,400–53,000 shares issued by Merck & Co., Inc. (which it maintained at least until 1973, the end of the investigated period).

15. Rhodes R. *Op cit.* pp. 134-5.

16. NCI staff. *The Special Virus Cancer Program: Progress Report #8.* Office of the Associate Scientific Director for Viral Oncology

(OASDVO). J. B. Moloney, Ed., Washington, D.C.: U.S. Government Printing Office, 1971, pp. 273-278.

17. Associated Press. American biologist is awarded Nobel Prize in Medicine. *International Herald Tribune*. Tuesday, October 7, 1997, p. 7.

18. Rhodes *Op cit.* p. 64.

19. Krugman S, Hoofnagle MD, Gerety RJ, Kaplan PM and Gerin JL. Viral hepatitis type B: DNA polymerase activity and antibody to hepatitis B core antigen. *New England Journal of Medicine* 1994;290;24:1331-1335; see also: Reich WT. "Human research and the war against disease." In: *Encyclopedia of Bioethics: Revised Edition, Vol. 4.* New York: Simon & Schuster Macmillan, 1995, pp. 2253-2254.

20. Horowitz and Martin WJ. *Op cit.* pp. 243-254; 326-328.

21. Cantwell A. *AIDS and the Doctors of Death: An Inquiry into the Origin of the AIDS Epidemic.* Los Angeles: Aries Rising Press, 1992, pp. 102-104.

22. Cooper W. *Behold a Pale Horse.* Sedona, AZ: Light Technology Publications, 1991, pp. 89-90.

23. van Helsing J. *Secret Societies: And Their Power in the 20th Century.* Gran Canaria, Spain: Ewertverlag S.L., 1995, p. 235.

24. Rhodes *Op cit.* p. 59.

25. Kuan Gao. K. Witness to the persecution: Family planning official defects, comes forward. *PRI Review*, May/June 1998, pp. 1-3. (Document available from http://www.pop.org/reports/rv069806.html)

26. Horowitz and Martin WJ. *Op cit.* pp. 153-188; for Roy Ash and Litton Bionetics information see pp. 206, 212.

27. Staff writer. Vaccine against pregnancy now being tested on humans. UPI New Service, Friday, June 11, 1986. As appeared in the *St. Louis Globe-Democrat*, p. 32; see also: Borraccia P. Vaccination, Inc. Part II. *Health Freedom News.* July/August, 1996 pp. 30-35. For this sterilization program conducted on 3.5 million Philippine women contact: Sister Mary Pilar Verzosa, RGS Pro-Life Philippines, Caritas

Bldg., 2002 Jesus Street Pandacan, Manila, Philippines. Phone or fax: 011-632-50-63-32.

28. Staff writer. Observations on the antigenicity and clinical effects of a candidate anti-pregnancy vaccine: B sub-unit of hCG linked to tetanus toxoid. *Fertility and Sterility*, Oct. 1980, pp. 328-335.

29. Starr P. *The Social Transformation of American Medicine.* New York: Basic Books, 1982, p. 118-127.

30. Monteith S. *The Population Control Agenda.* Soquel, CA: Radio-Liberty, pp. 1-11; see also Chaitkin A. Population Control, Nazis, and the U.N! Available from http://www.livelinks.com/sumeria/politics/eugenics.html; see also: Kuhl S. *The Nazi Connection: Eugenics, American Racism and German National Socialism.* Oxford: Oxford University Press, 1994.

31. Manning P. *Op cit.,.* pp. 29; 56; 134 and 148.

32. Covert N. *Cutting Edge: A History of Fort Detrick, Maryland 1943-1993.* Fort Detrick: Headquarters U.S. Army Garrison Public Affairs Office (HSHD-PA), 1993, pp. 17, 20 and 39.

33. Kuhl S., *The Nazi Connection: Eugenics, American Racism, and German National Socialism.* New York: Oxford University Press, 1994, pp. 15, 21 and 24.

34. Russel B. *The Impact of Science on Society,* 1953, p. xv.

35. Kissinger HA. *The Meaning of History: Reflections on Spengler, Toynbee and Kant.* Cambridge: Harvard University Library, Microreproduction Service, 1955; See also: Isaacson W. *Kissinger: A Biography.* New York: Simon & Schuster, 1992, pp. 64-67; for fall out shelter quote, p. 92; for connections to Merck, p. 734.

36. Lewin LC. *Report From Iron Mountain on the Possibility and Desirability of Peace.* New York: The Dial Press, Inc., 1967, pp. 73-74.

37. Horowitz and Martin WJ. *Op cit.* pp. 412, 422, 427-29.

38. Moriarty TJ. After thirty years, prominent polio vaccine researcher confirms suspicions about monkey-virus contamination. An interview with Dr. Benjamin Sweet. Available on the Internet from Chronic Illnet or in the FTP file at http://www.tetrahedron.org.

39. Personal communication, January 24, 1998.

40. Horowitz and Martin WJ. *Op cit.* p. 251.

41. Jamison E, Hobbs F, Way PO, and Stanecki KA. *World Population Profile: 1994: With a Special Chapter Focusing on HIV/AIDS.* Washington, D.C.: U.S. Government Printing Office; U.S. Department of Commerce, Economics and Statistics Administration. Bureau of the Census, February, 1994.

42. Negative Population Growth, Inc. Why we need a smaller U.S. population and how we can achieve it. *Foreign Affairs*, The Council on Foreign Relations, March/April, 1996.

43. National Security Council. *NSSM 200—Implications of World-wide Population Growth for U.S. Security and Overseas Interests.* Washington, DC: The White House, December 10, 1974. Declassified, July 3, 1989, NSIAD-ROX-89-4.

44. Staff writers. Conspiracy for global control: Special report, Expanded second edition—"Foundations pay the way." *The New American*, 1997, p. 56.

# Chapter 8.
# Prions and the Lords of Misrule

Following his weekend in Salt Lake City, and his heightened suspicions regarding prions and mad cow disease, Len decided to do some more research. He pulled from his library shelf his 1972 copy of *Synopsis of Pathology*—the standard reference text used by medical and dental students during the mid 1970s. Oddly, there were no entries regarding Creutzfeldt-Jacob disease, or CJD, or spongiform encephalopathies. Only kuru was listed under "Infections with slow viruses." Here it read:

> ... Because of the long incubation period, the virus is called a "slow virus." The diseases caused by slow viruses are prolonged degenerative disorders and include kuru (a disease among natives in the New Guinea Highlands), progressive multifocal leukoencephalopathy, and subacute sclerosing panencephalitis.[1]

"Interesting that back then kuru was thought to be caused by a 'slow virus,' not a protein fragment," Len thought. "It's also interesting that all the slow viruses were only associated with brain diseases."

The description continued:

> There are a number of other diseases in which there is a suspicion of a relationship with slow viruses but, at present, evidence of such a relationship is lacking. Among these diseases are multiple sclerosis, postencephalic parkinsonism, amyotrophic lateral sclerosis (ALS), and Alzheimer's presenile dementia.[1]

"Hmm," Len considered. "All of these are currently believed to be associated with vaccine injury related autoimmune disorders."

Then he referenced his old *Internal Medicine for Dentisty* textbook for a general overview of CJD. David Dunn, Associate Professor of Neurology and Anatomic Pathology at the Medical College of Pennsylvania, had this to say about CJD:

> ... a rare and fatal disorder that occurs throughout the world, mostly in middle-aged people. Dementia that progresses to death in usually less than 2 years is accompanied by other neurologic

deficits, especially rapid jerks of the trunk and limbs (myoclo-nus). The electroencephalogram usually shows a typical pattern. Brain tissue from patients has produced the disease months to years later in inoculated chimpanzees.[2]

"He's referring to Gadjusek's primate experiments reported in Litton's report to the NCI," Len realized, then read on:

. . . Vacuoles similar to those in scrapie and kuru are present in the brain cells. Because the cell vacuolation has a spongy appear-ance microscopically, these diseases are called subacute spongi-form encephalopathies.[2]

"That's interesting," Len considered. "Brain cell vacuolation." John Martin reported vacuole formation within the cells of chronic fa-tigue immune dysfunction (CFIDS) patients, particularly those in-fected with what he called 'stealth viruses.' He said they came from herpesviruses, including monkey cytomegalovirus (CMV) most likely derived from contaminated polio vaccines."[3,4]

## 'Stealth Viruses' and Cell Vacuoles

Dr. W. John Martin, a leading expert in vaccine contamination analysis, contributed the foreword to Len's earlier work, *Emerging Vi-ruses: AIDS & Ebola.* John had often mentioned similarities between the brain lesions he was seeing with what he termed "stealth virus" infections and those in CJD patients. A "stealth virus," much like the prion, had the remarkable ability to evade the immune systems of in-fected hosts and cause brain damage or "encephalopathy." Len began to wonder whether the protein prion associated with CJD and the "stealth virus" linked to CFIDS were one and the same, or at least linked somehow. A Professor of Pathology at the University of South-ern California, and Director of the Center for Complex Infectious Dis-eases in Rosemead, California, Martin had sent Len a number of his publications to digest.

"Let me pull Martin's papers to see what he said about this." A moment later Len read from the *Journal of Clinical and Diagnostic Virology*:

The CPE [cytopathic effect] induced by SCMV [simian (monkey) cytomegalovirus] is characterized by slightly enlarged rounded non-adherent cells. The CPE rapidly spreads to involve the entire culture. The CPE of the "stealth virus"-1 is characterized by a slower and more progressive enlargement of the adherent cells with prominent syncytia formation and *foamy vacuolated cytoplasmic changes*.[3] [Emphasis added.]

"Indeed, there are *vacuolated cytoplasmic changes* in "stealth virus" infected cells. Let me pull the paper Martin referenced."

Here is what it said about the "stealth virus" isolate:

The cultured virus is distinguishable from CMV [cytomegalovirus] . . . by the following criteria: growth in cells from multiple species; [and] the vacuolated, syncytial nature of the CPE . . . Isolation of the virus from CSF [cerebrospinal fluid bathing the brain and spinal cord] and the absence of an accompanying inflammatory response suggest that the *virus is neurotropic* [targets the brain and nervous system] *and yet noninflammatory. . . . It is conceivable that* the virus has arisen from CMV but that *portions of its genetic machinery have been deleted or mutated as a mechanism of avoiding immune recognition.*"[4] [Emphasis added.]

Len recoiled, "'*Portions of its genetic machinery have been deleted or mutated as a mechanism of avoiding immune recognition?*' I know that viruses have mutated over the ages, but it's odd that so many have mutated so much in that direction, that is, to have their immune recognizance genes suddenly disappear in the mid-twentieth century. It's far more likely, with the advances in molecular biology and recombinant genetics that began in the 1950s, that this virus, and perhaps the prion, was intentionally created in a lab to evade immune defenses."[6]

Len's concern was realistic considering the 1969 proposal by David Baltimore and/or others at the National Academy of Sciences National Research Council (NAS-NRC). They proposed to help the Department of Defense, and specifically the U.S. Army, develop "a new infective microorganism that could differ in certain important aspects from any known disease-causing microorganism. Most important of these is that it might be refractory to the immunologic and therapeutic processes upon which we depend to maintain our relative freedom from infectious diseases."[5] (See figure 7.1.) In essence, what Baltimore, or others on that council, had pledged to help create was a "supergerm." That word also appeared in the *Congressional Record*. An 'erst klassig' microorganism that could wipe out, or evade, human immunity against infectious diseases leaving people suffering symptoms like those seen in CFIDS, or even AIDS. Len wondered whether the NAS-NRC's effort might have initiated the genetic deletion or mutation to which Dr. Martin had referred, leading to the current array of epidemic encephalopathies and immune deficiency disorders. Perhaps not by chance the AIDS and CFIDS epidemics emerged simultaneously in North America in 1978 closely following hepatitis B vaccine trials.[7] Likewise, a surge in CJD cases ensued shortly thereafter.

Though the link between hepatitis B vaccines and AIDS was clearly established in *Emerging Viruses: AIDS & Ebola*, and other works by Drs. Horowitz, Cantwell, Strecker, and others, Len thought it odd that no one, to his knowledge, had drawn the link between this particular vaccine and CFIDS. That CFIDS, at first, predominantly struck women, teachers, and health care workers, those more inclined to get the earliest hepatitis B vaccines known to be contaminated with herpesviruses, including simian cytomegalo and Epstein–Barr, deserved additional consideration and research, Len realized.[7]

In another Martin paper, Len read that a "brain biopsy" from "a school teacher who had gradually lost her capacity for written and oral communication, showed "mild gliosis"—a condition marked by overgrowth or tumors of the "nerve cement," that is, the non-nervous cellular elements surrounding the nerve cells. Lacking was the white blood cell infiltration—the inflammation—that one would expect from traditional viral infections. Some of the virus infected cells showed "marked vacuolated changes and lipid accumulation," Martin wrote.[8]

"Brain cell vacuolation and lipid accumulation sounds like what researchers are also reporting with brain prion infections," Len noted. "Let me pull my 'mad cow' file and see."

He rummaged through a stack of mad cow articles. One was a reprint from *Scientific American* contributed by several authors responding to the question, "What is a prion?"

Mark Rogers, from the department of zoology at the Biotechnology Center at University College in Dublin, Ireland wrote:

> The term 'prion' was coined by Stanley B. Prusiner of the University of California School of Medicine at San Francisco in 1982 to distinguish the infectious agent that causes scrapie in sheep, Creutzfiedt-Jakob disease (CJD) in humans and bovine spongiform encephalopathy (BSE) in cattle from other, more typical infectious agents. The prion hypothesis postulates that these diseases are caused not by a conventional virus or bacterium but by a protein that has adopted an abnormal form.
>
> The process by which this change occurs is not clear and there is a great deal of work underway to establish the structure of the prion protein in both its normal and aberrant forms. Recently scientists have developed a molecular model of both variants and have published papers describing the structure of *prion proteins (as manufactured by E. coli bacteria that were altered through recombinant DNA techniques.)*[9][Emphasis added.]

## *E. coli*, Tyson, Hudson, Clinton, Industrial Espionage and Prions

"Interesting," Len reflected curiously. "Creating pathogenic prions by manipulating *E. coli* in a lab?"

His balk was based on knowledge that *E. coli* was one of the most commonly used bacteria for germ warfare research and development. The 157th strain of *E. coli* was associated with the deaths of children at the Jack-in-the-Box restaurants, as well as the recall of 25 million pounds of Hudson Beef Company meat before the company was purchased by Tyson Foods. *E. coli* 157, Len recalled, was probably prepared in a biological weapons lab. The Tyson takeover was likely an industrial espionage operation.[10]

How had Len drawn these seemingly outrageous conclusions?

Len's initial suspicions were based on a review of a U.S. *Congressional Record* that showed *E. coli* had been one of the principle germs manipulated by CIA and Army biological weapons contractors.[10] During the 1975 Frank Church Congressional Hearings into the CIA's illegal storage and utilization of biological weapons, long after the signing of the Geneva Accord by Richard Nixon that allegedly outlawed such activity, *E. coli* had often been cited as a useful experimental pathogen.

He wondered whether the CIA had taken a benign strain of *E. coli*, which they are most often, and engineered it to produce 157 more toxic varieties?

Later he read CIA Director James Woolsy's statement, "With the end of the Cold War, the CIA must enter the era of economic [or industrial] espionage." This function would be served, it was intimated, on behalf of American corporations that requested such CIA assistance.[10]

With that knowledge, the week the CDC announced an alleged outbreak of *E. coli* from Hudson,[11] Len told more than 700 people, during two lectures, of the likely "takeover of Hudson Beef by a large competitor. . . . You can't trust the CDC whatsoever," he warned.

One week later, newspapers heralded the takeover of Hudson by Tyson Foods. Hudson's stock had plummeted by a third following the fright and beef recall. Tyson took advantage of the business opportunity.[12]

Reuters reported that the "U.S. chicken processor Tyson Foods Inc., has agreed to buy Hudson Foods Inc. in a deal worth about $650 million, a week after Hudson Foods agreed to sell its only raw hamburger plant to IBP Inc. . . . Merrill Lynch & Co. Inc. analyst Leonard Teitelbaum was cited in one story as saying the acquisition will add to Tyson's earnings immediately and he called the deal favorable to both parties, although the value was at the "bottom end" of what he would consider a fair price for Hudson Foods."[12]

This occurred despite the fact that meat inspectors and public health officials never even confirmed the contaminations came from the Hudson plant.

Tyson, Len realized, had most likely gotten away with a ruse. Then it happened again a few months later, but this time it was a chicken influenza outbreak in Asia.[13] On December 23, 1997, the Associated Press reported that a 60-year-old woman had died of a "suspected bird flu." The U.S. Government immediately announced it would halt "all chicken imports from China in a move to curb the spread of the virus.

The virus—A H5N1—according to the report, "has long been known to infect birds but appeared in humans for the first time this year."[13]

"Oh come on!" Len protested. He knew that such cross-species transmission were extremely difficult and rare. Far likelier than a spontaneous cross-species leap, the chicken influenza viruses had, like *E. coli*, been mutated in a lab. This Len knew had been routinely done with chicken sarcoma viruses at the University of California under the direction of Dr. Peter Duesberg of AIDS-virus fame. Duesberg and other NCI colleagues had routinely cultured chicken viruses in human cells in an effort to get them to adapt their protein coat before jumping species.[14] All Len could do was shake his head as he thought, "This looks like another setup for some other ruse."

Days later it was announced the horrible outbreak required the slaughter of 1.2 million Asian chickens, and perhaps cats, dogs, and other animals as well! Asian chicken farmers were overwhelmed with concern and pressured to massacre their flocks.

Few knew that prior to these events, Tyson was vying to bring the Asian poultry industry into its worldwide monopolistic fold.[15] The emergency primarily targeted Tyson's Asian competition—mostly small chicken farmers. What was most likely a CIA-directed "outbreak" conveniently required the annihilation of Tyson's competitors. That would have been a very effective, albeit immoral, industrial espionage operation.

Morality, however, had not been one of Tyson's features. The Springdale, Arkansas-based company showered gifts upon Clinton administration policy makers like former Agriculture Secretary Mike

Espy.[16] Don Tyson, in fact, was one of Bill Clinton's "closest friends and biggest supporters," according to Arkansas state trooper Larry Patterson's testimony before the grand jury that investigated Tyson's unethical and illegal conduct.[17]

In fact, many Americans can recall the hoopla over Hillary Clinton's having made more than $100,000 virtually overnight in the commodities market in 1978. The cattle trading tip came from James Blair, chief counselor at Tyson Foods.

Don Tyson had also been Bill Clinton's top fund raiser during his Gubernatorial election. In return, the governor, and later president, eased regulations on Tyson's chicken industry. This allowed continued pollution of America's rivers and streams with chicken waste. Espy tidied up the meat packing industry, but killed the proposal to do the same for chicken processors, sixty-six of which, in America in 1998, were owned by Tyson. Thanks to Tyson and Clinton cronies, and their "environmental protection" efforts, in northwest Arkansas alone more than 500 miles of rivers were dangerously polluted and, at the time of this writing, were off-limits to swimmers.

In fact, given what Len was about to learn about prion transmission, Tyson's poultry industry was to become a prime suspect in the origin of America's mad cow problems and other TSEs including CJD.

## Pleomorphism and Terrain

Returning to the *Scientific American* article on prions, Susan Lindquist at the *Howard Hughes Medical Institute* in the department of molecular genetics and cell biology at the University of Chicago added:

> I and my colleagues have recently determined that a phenomenon much like prion infection exists in *yeast*. In the case of yeast, the phenomenon involves the passing of a particular genetic trait from mother cells to daughter cells . . . These genetic traits had been known for many years, but their baffling patterns of inheritance (for example, they can be passed along through a cell's cytoplasm, rather than the nucleus where the DNA resides) had eluded explanation. We now know that the genetic trait is

transmitted by proteins that are encoded in the nucleus but that can *change their conformation in the cytoplasm*. Once this change has occurred, the reconfigured proteins induce other newly made proteins of the same type to change their conformation, too. Molecular genetic research on *yeast* should speed up the resolution of fundamental questions about the workings of protein-folding chain reactions. . . . [9] [Emphasis added.]

"That's interesting," Len thought, "the proteins can *change their conformation*. That means they exhibit *pleomorphism*."

Author and lecturer Robert Young, Ph.D., D.Sc., had explained to Len about a year earlier the concept of pleomorphism. His presentation included a discussion of "mycotoxins,"* that is, fungus-related toxins. Dr. Young had studied this area extensively, and wrote a book called *Sick & Tired*. It covered the theory of "pleomorphism" advanced by Béchamp and Enderlein in the late 1800s and early 1900s. Their theory suggested that the end result of microbial pleomorphism or morphogenesis is fungus formation. Incredibly, Young wrote a section that dealt with the Catholic church's suppression of this information!

Dr. Young reported that the original "giants" in microbiology adhered to the "principle of pleomorphism (pleo=many; morph=form). 'Many-formism' is the idea that microorganisms, such as specific bacteria, can take on multiple forms during a life cycle," largely depending on the *chemistry of its environment*. The germs change form, function, and toxicity, the theory asserts, largely, if not entirely, due to the human terrain in which it exists. [18]

"The blood is not sterile," Young wrote. "It naturally contains tiny life forms" that can ultimately produce "disease symptoms if conditions are favorable. These Béchamp called "microzymas," and defined them as "living elements capable of fermenting sugar."

Young summarized the conditions that affect microzymas' growth in the blood, including oxygen content and electrical, that is spiritual, status this way:

---

*The word mycotoxin derives from the word "myco"—defined in *Steadman's Medical Dictionary*, as a "combining form relating to fungus;" while "fungus," is defined as "a member of the protein Fungi—a plantlike organism feeding on organic matter; such as mushrooms, yeasts, and molds."

[G]erms are symptoms themselves. In turn, they stimulate the occurrence of more symptoms (called diseases) as a result of thriving in an unbalanced terrain. Terrain is the internal environment of the body. It is primarily its pH, or acidity/alkalinity, its level of toxicity, and its nutritional status that determine a healthy or diseased condition. One symptom of diseased terrain is low oxygen. Still another is loss of electrical charge on the surface of red blood cells. This contributes to a condition called rouleau, sometimes also called "sticky blood."[18]

Enderlein, Young wrote, confirmed Béchamp's observation of pleomorphism, and "connected bacterial to fungal changeability." Likewise with viruses, though the original organizing structures were the microzymas, theory suggested these were likely RNA and DNA repair units, at least until they were genetically engineered in labs to produce diseases. This theory of pleomorphism, or at least the conditions that Béchamp, Enderlein and Young suggested determine illness, is particularly important in-so-far as prevention and healing is concerned. This will become more apparent in the next chapter.

## More Persecution and Suppression

Until prions were discovered to "change form," mainstream medicine shunned the notion of pleomorphism. Instead, Western medicine followed the dogma of French researcher Louis Pasteur (1822-1895)—the chemist who pioneered pasteurization of milk. Young explained:

Pasteur's main theory is known as the "Germ Theory of Disease." Also referred to as the "microbian theory," this doctrine says that external, fixed species of so-called microbes, invade the body and cause disease. It became the foundation of western medical microbiology—a scientific dogma of monomorphism. The concept of specific types of bacteria causing specific diseases became officially accepted . . . in the late nineteenth century. . . Abetting, if not creating, this reactionary atmosphere was the fact that ecclesiastic authorities at the University of Lille, where Béchamp had moved in 1875 to teach, in a mood of repressive ignorance quite similar to that which devastated Galileo, vigorously opposed the heresy of the microzymian view.[18]

Young went on to describe the irony of the situation Béchamp faced as a "devout Christian who felt his inquiries were merely revealing the Creator's modus. . . . Heightening the poignancy of this tragedy was the depth of ecclesiastic ignorance, which left it unable to realize that [Béchamp's] view was not heretical at all. . . .[It] is perversely awe-inspiring to see that such bias, and a supporting power structure in science, has persisted for a hundred more years so that Béchamp's principles have not yet been given fair examination in the mainstream."[18]

Given the information about the church discussed in previous chapters, Young's additions here were not particularly surprising to Len. It was, however, another example of how pervasive church power has been.

## Royal Raymond Rife

Dr. Young's book also advanced Len's knowledge about Royal Raymond Rife, the first to microscopically confirm Béchamp's theory using his innovative light refraction techniques.

Rife, an American microscopist, might have changed the face of modern medicine were it not for the ruthless persecution he received at the hands of the Rockefeller-directed medical–industrial complex. His story is best told in *The Cancer Cure That Worked!* by Barry Lynes.[19] It included a description of Rife's extraordinary microscope. Detailed in the *Journal of the Franklin Institute* (Vol. 237, No. 2, 1944), the Rife Universal Microscope had a 31,000 diameters resolution, weighed 200 pounds, stood two feet high, and consisted of 5,682 parts. It used natural light frequencies dispersed by glass or crystal prisms, rather than acid stains or electronic beams, to view *live* objects in extraordinary detail.

Based on Nikola Tesla's brilliant studies in frequency magnetics, Rife's microscopes and frequency-generating healing devices captured the attention of numerous members of the scientific, medical, and intelligence communities. One microscope was even developed to measure "crystal angles" at the cancer virus level.

As seen in figure 8.1, Rife had even invited the FBI to advance its analytical technology. Hoover refused his offer. Hoover had already developed a thick file on Rife's mentor Tesla.

A likely source of Hoover's trepidation was Rife's timing. He had researched microscopy and electronic treatments for disease beginning in the early 1920s—virtually the same time the Rockefeller family created the cancer industry. Rife's work was said to be a simple answer to cancer. The Rockefellers preferred a costly pharmaceutical approach.

Rife began by identifying radio frequencies that could irradiate and kill tubercle bacilli—the bacteria associated with tuberculosis. Using trial and error, he finally succeeded in killing the germ, but in the process the guinea pigs he used for the experiment died as well of "toxic poisoning."

Rife reasoned that viruses within the bacteria, that were not destroyed by the resonant frequency, had been released when the bacilli broke apart. To study the viruses, he needed to enhance his microscopic resolution. To do this, intuitively he conceived of a "method of staining the virus with light." Again the idea used resonant frequencies of light that both Béchamp and Rife knew were found inherent and specific to every microorganism. Rife demonstrated that light, rather than deadly chemicals, could be used to "stain" the subjects being studied, and thus observed them in their natural living condition.

Later, Rife observed the pleomorphic transformation of viruses in cancerous tissues. He observed them becoming fungi. Then, he planted these fungi in a plant-based medium. Spontaneously, a bacteria—bacillus coli, typically found in the human intestine, developed. He repeated the study with the same results several hundred times. Later, he used this knowledge to apply resonant frequencies to cure certain cancers.

Scientists and physicians from around the world hailed Rife's work and sojourned to observe for themselves its legitimacy. His list of

## Fig. 8.1. Letter From J. Edgar Hoover to Royal R. Rife Re: Invitation for Analytical Collaboration, 1941

Federal Bureau of Investigation,
United States Department of Justice
Washington, D. C.

July 21, 1941

Royal R. Rife
3655 Alcott Street
San Diego, California

Dear Mr. Rife:

Mr. Nathan in charge of the Bureau's San Diego Field Division has advised me of your kind offer to make available to the Federal Bureau of Investigation the facilities of your laboratory. This is indeed appreciated. At present the laboratory analysis of evidence in investigations is conducted in the Bureau's Laboratory at Washington, D. C. If at any time in the future the services of your facilities would be useful I will be glad to take advantage of your offer.

Sincerely yours,

J. E. Hoover

John Edgar Hoover
Director

respected colleagues and observers included: Dr. Edward C. Rosenow of the Mayo Clinic; Dr. Milbank Johnson, a member of the board of directors at California's Pasadena Hospital, and Dr. Arthur I. Kendall, Director of Medical Research at Northwestern University Medical School. Newspapers heralded Rife's progress. His favorable notoriety seemed so infectious that his enemies were moved to act.

Morris Fishbein, at the helm of the American Medical Association when the U.S. Supreme Court found the organization guilty of anti-trust violations during the late 1930s and early 1940s, persecuted Rife and personally organized an attack against him. Fishbein, while in Chicago, learned of Rife's successful resonant frequency method of treating cancer. He then approached Rife with a "buy in" offer that the microscopist refused. Fishbein then brought suit against Rife's company for practicing medicine without a license.[19,20]

## Prions Grow Like *Crystals*

Following his pleomorphism refresher, Len went back to his "mad cow file" of articles and selected one that dovetailed with Dr. Young's and Béchamp's work on fungus. The article reviewed a May 30, 1997 publication in the esteemed scientific journal *Cell*. It was entitled, "New type of DNA-free inheritance in yeast is spread by a 'mad cow' mechanism." Again, "yeast" is a form of fungus. Researchers, again, at the *University of Chicago's Howard Hughes Medical Institute,* reported that "a protein molecule able to transmit a genetic trait without DNA or RNA in yeast is able to string itself together into long fibers much like those found in the brain in 'mad cow' and human Creutzfeldt-Jakob diseases."

The scientists found that somehow a normal protein in the brain somehow became "twisted" and then corrupted other "healthy molecules of the same protein to do likewise in a process much like the *seeding of a crystal.* The improperly folded protein molecules seem to spin themselves together into fibers, which grow as other molecules are recruited."[21][Emphasis added.]

This best explained the growth of the prion agent in all the TSEs including the neurodegenerative diseases of mammals such as sheep scrapie, mad cow disease (or bovine spongiform encephalopathy) and kuru disease of the Papua New Guinea tribes.

The text said that the infectious protein prions' existence had been hotly debated for 30 years since researchers showed that diseased brain tissue remained infectious even after treatment with radiation that would have destroyed any DNA or RNA.

"Last year," the article continued, "the Chicago team led by Susan Lindquist, Ph.D., professor of molecular genetics and cell biology, showed that *prion-like proteins exist in yeast.* In the mammalian brain, whose cells do not divide, *prions pass between cells and function as infectious agents;* in yeast, they produce [in]heritable changes in metabolism from one generation to the next as the cells divide. . . ."[15] [Emphasis added.]

"They produce inheritable changes from one generation to the next without DNA or RNA, that is, without genetic material. Plus they are like crystals," Len considered. "I wonder if they transmit the heritable changes using frequency vibrations since crystals receive and transmit these signals very well?"

The article continued, "Even in the test tube, the purified yeast protein can knit together into fibers that have the same staining properties and molecular architecture as the amyloid plaques seen at autopsy in the brains of animals and humans that have died of transmissible spongiform encephalopathies. They also show that the formation of fibers from normal protein molecules is greatly speeded up by the presence of defective ones."[21]

Though the article stated that this yeast protein posed "no risk to consumers of bread or beer," Dr. Lindquist said that these mycotoxic particles relayed genetic inheritance through a mechanism associated with several devastating neurodegenerative diseases *including Alzheimer's.*

"Alzheimer's!" Len balked. "Slow viruses, stealth viruses, and mycoplasma infections have also been associated with Alzheimer's-like memory loss."

"From the molecular standpoint," concluded John Glover, Ph.D., lead author of the *Cell* paper, "this looks like the changes you get in the mammalian prion" disease.

Len looked up from the page and considered the message, "First of all, the work was done at the Howard Hughes Institute, affiliated with the University of Chicago—built with Rockefeller money and today it is still funded by the Rockefellers. Second, Robert Gallo graduated from that university. Third, *Deadly Feasts* author Richard Rhodes wrote the biography of Howard Hughes. What a 'coincidence.'"

"Regarding the science," Len considered, "it's all believable except for the disclaimer. There's no way they can assure 'no risk' to consumers of 'bread or beer.' First, they tell you that the *prion-like proteins* are found *in yeast*, and that they can pass toxicity and inheritable messages *from one generation of fungus to the next*. Prions are also close to indestructible. So that means if it's in the yeast used to make bread or beer, then like the other TSEs, they can likely be passed through infected foods. Then, once it gets into the blood, and gravitates to the brain, the *prions pass between cells, function as infectious agents,* and grow *like crystals*.

"The protein crystals seem to evolve from a pleomorphic infectious process reminiscent of Béchamp's microzymas theory. Especially the fact that the prions, initially in a fungus, can evolve from a benign form to a deadly type that can leave the yeast to *pass into human brains and function as infectious agents* without cell walls, or any RNA or DNA. This fulfills the "virino hypothesis" supported by all the experts.

"Plus it's crystalline in its growth pattern. That means that it can likely resonate like every other crystal in the world. Maybe that's why prions have an affinity for nerve tissues, especially the brain," he reasoned. "They might be attracted to the microcurrents that nerve cells emit."

## Spiroplasmas and Mycoplasma

To make matters more confusing, which might be expected given the pleomorphic process that prions pose, one article based on a presentation at an American Medical Association conference in the Spring of 1996, suggested a "spiroplasma" might be associated with CJD and TSEs. This caught Len's attention as the thesis seemed related to the hypothesis of fungal involvement as well as Dr. Young's theory of pleomorphism.

Dr. Frank O. Bastian, a professor of pathology at the University of South Alabama College of Medicine, cited research that showed brain biopsies of patients with CJD contained "spiroplasma-like inclusions" associated with "internal fibril proteins" identical to those seen in TSEs. These spiroplasma proteins were immunologically very similar to the TSE proteins, and when inoculated into rodents, they produced similar neuropathology. This according to three scientific papers published in esteemed periodicals.[22]

Spiroplasmas were only discovered in 1976. This suggested to Len that once again man had likely mixed two beasties together to gain another more pathogenic form. Such a unique combination, a spiroplasma, appeared to come from a spirochete—a spiral shaped bacteria that sometimes possesses a moving tail, and a mycoplasma—a jelly-fish-like bacteria that does not possess a cell wall. Mycoplasmas thus take many shapes including balls, rings, or curved filaments. Interesting enough, spirochetes most commonly grew in sewage and polluted waters. This related to the Tyson chicken waste problem mentioned earlier, and in greater detail in the next chapter. Also, in keeping with Dr. Young's theory of pleomorphism based on body chemistry or the "terrain," no one knew whether the pleomorphic mycoplasmas evolved into bacteria or whether bacteria evolved from viruses.

If this seems confusing, you're not alone. Even physicians and scientists find this area of microbiology troublesome. The reason is that mycoplasmas never became part of traditional medical training until the late 1950s when *Mycoplasma pneumoniae* was suddenly identified as a cause of atypical pneumonia.

Since then, mycoplasmas have been linked to a number of rapidly growing epidemics including chronic fatigue immune dysfunction syndrome (CFIDS), fibromyalgia, rheumatoid arthritis, Alzheimer's, multiple sclerosis, and Gulf War Syndrome (GWS). Dr. Harold W. Clark, former Director of Research for the T. McP. Brown Arthritis Institute, and founder of the Mycoplasma Research Institute, explained the association between mycoplasma infections and these autoimmune related disorders this way:

> [Mycoplasmas] have more recently been implicated as a cause of rheumatoid arthritis. These diseases are considered to be the result of immune complex (mycoplasma + antibody) and also the self destructive autoimmune reaction (mycoplasma + host protein). Recent studies are now supporting the role and mechanism of mycoplasmas as both immune complex and as an autoantigen. If this proves to be the case we may soon see mycoplasma associated with many other immunologic disorders besides rheumatoid, i. e., Alzheimer's, diabetes, multiple sclerosis, etc.[23]

Like "stealth viruses," Len realized that mycoplasma infections evade host immune surveillance. In other words, as Dr. Clark wrote,

> Mycoplasmas can attach to specific cells without killing the cells and thus their infection process can go undetected. No symptoms suggests no disease. In some people the attachment of mycoplasmas to the susceptible cell membranes acts like a living thorn, a persistent foreign substance, causing the host's immune defense mechanism to wage war.[23]

## Pathogenic Mycoplasmas in Gulf War Syndrome (GWS)

Len had closely followed the mycoplasma analyses performed by the Nicolsons during their investigations into GWS.[24] He had along with Dr. Garth Nicolson, director of the Institute for Molecular Medicine, in Irvine, California, Captain Joyce Riley, American Gulf War Veterans Association (AGWVA) Director, and Canada's leading GWS activist, Lt. Louise Richard, produced a three-hour videotape, *Gulf War*

*Syndrome: The Spreading Epidemic Cover-up.*[25] The tape presented suppressed facts about the mycoplasma and CFIDS-linked illness, and what to do about it.

The disease was associated with mycoplasma-poisoned vaccines the troops had received enroute to the Gulf. Soldiers spread it to their wives, children, healthcare professionals, and even pets. By 1995, it had spread massively throughout the civilian population causing many people to suffer from chronic fatigue and related neurological ailments.

Hugh McManners, a defense correspondent at the *London Sunday Times* wrote how British immunologists had linked the GWS to vaccines and the chemical exposures that followed their administration.[26] Their report, published in the prestigious *Lancet,* opened the door to massive compensation claims filed on behalf of ailing veterans. "For six years, former soldiers have battled to prove that the drug cocktails they were given to protect them against disease and chemical weapons were to blame for their illnesses," McManners reported. Professor Graham Rook and Dr. Alimuddin Zumla, who "made the breakthrough," also believed the knowledge could "lead to an effective treatment . . ."

The "devastating" effect of the vaccinations combined with insecticides were explained this way:

> The drug cocktails suppressed one part of the body's immune system, known as Th1, which combats viruses and cancers. At the same time Th2, a part of the immune system which normally reacts mildly against pollen or house dust mites, was made hypersensitive to outside irritants. This double effect meant that soldiers were more likely to succumb to common diseases, while also suffering extreme allergic reactions to harmless elements in the atmosphere."A systematic shift towards Th2 leads to patients developing more diseases, particularly chronic virus infections, as their Th1 protection is diminished," said Rook. "There is also an increase in allergic symptoms prompted by increases in Th2 reactions, and mood changes which we can attribute to the corresponding changes in their hormone and cytokine levels. This explains the extraordinary diversity of symptoms seen in the Gulf War veterans."[26]

"Many of the vaccines given to British and American troops in the Gulf, including cholera, anthrax and bubonic plague, are believed to cause the precise immune system changes described by Rook," thought Len. French troops, who did not receive the same vaccines and drug cocktails as their American and British counterparts, did not suffer the epidemic. British soldiers often received several vaccinations at once, without proper records being kept. Many erroneously received more than one dose of each.

This knowledge jibed with Dr. Nicolson's testimony before the United States House of Representatives' inquiry into GWS, except for one thing—mycoplasma was not mentioned despite the fact that Nicolson had detected this most common vaccine contaminant "deep inside the blood leukocytes (a form of white blood cell) of approximately one-half of the GWS patients examined, including 2 out of 3 British Desert Storm veterans with GWS.[27]

Furthermore, Dr. Nicolson (at the time the David Bruton Jr. Chair in Cancer Research, and Professor at the University of Texas M.D. Anderson Cancer Center in Houston, and Professor of Pathology and Laboratory Medicine at the University of Texas Medical School) told the investigating committee, "Dr. Steven Joseph, Assistant Secretary of Defense, has stated in letters to Congress that this type of infection is commonly found not dangerous and is not even listed as a human pathogen. These statements could not be further from the truth. The Uniformed Services University of the Health Sciences, the U.S. military's medical school, has been teaching for years that this type of infection, although rare in the U.S. population, is very dangerous and can colonize major organs and can lead to system-wide organ failure and death."[27]

Defense secretary assistant Joseph was apparently involved in a Pentagon-wide coverup that news sources said extended to the CIA.[28] Indeed, there was good cause for burying the truth. Not only had top Pentagon officials known that American-made biological and chemical weapons—weapons that had been shipped to Saddam Hussein from

264

the American Type Culture Collection (ATCC) of Rockville, Maryland, and several other American locations before the war—would likely be used against allied troops,[29,30] but officials knew that the vaccines given to the service men and women were potentially tainted and lethal![31] Medical intelligence sources might have even *predicted*, in advance of the war, the percentage of deadly mycoplasma infections that would result from the vaccination program.[32] Moreover, military medical authorities withheld their knowledge that a good percentage of the troops, perhaps as many as fifteen percent, had been used unwittingly as experimental subjects in vaccine studies, including AIDS-vaccine trials.[33] In fact, after lying before the Congressional investigating committee,[25] General Norman Schwarzkopf let the truth slip during a lecture in Las Vegas where he admitted that vaccines were the primary cause of GWS.[34] This news never made the national press.

In the final analysis, the Pentagon, pharmaceutical interests, and a Texas vaccine manufacturer said to be connected to George Bush and his secret cabal, had violated the FDA's AIDS vaccine testing requirements. The FDA had provided the Defense Department (DoD) with the protocols required to "assure" military safety, but they were not followed.[35]

"The deviations in Bosnia show that DoD has not corrected its procedures to prevent the recurrence of problems in the use of investigational products that arose during the Persian Gulf War," wrote Dr. Michael A. Friedman, the FDA's leading deputy commissioner, in a letter to Dr. Edward A. Martin, acting assistant secretary of defense for health affairs, dated July 22, 1997. "The deviations . . . do not give us confidence that DoD is, at present, capable of carrying out its obligations under investigational new drug applications for drugs and biologics [vaccines] that are intended to provide potential protection to deployed military personnel," Friedman continued. "We have previously discussed most of these concerns with various DoD personnel over the last several years. . . . We are concerned that a number of the lessons that should have been learned from the Gulf War have not led to corrections that should have been demonstrated in Bosnia. . . ."[36]

In fact, the mycoplasma germ(s) contaminating the experimental AIDS vaccine given to the troops may have been *intentionally developed and administered.* How so?

It is clear that mycoplasma research and development was ongoing at the University of Maryland—Robert Gallo territory (near Bethesda, the NIH, NCI, Pentagon and Fort Detrick—America's premier bioweapons testing center—and Rockville, Md., the home of the ATCC) in 1970. American citizens were then being used as experimental subjects according to documents obtained by Captain Joyce Riley, a registered nurse and AGWVA director. She reported:

> I have verified that mycoplasma was used as a research item on private citizens by the University of Maryland in 1970. I have the actual ad from the newspaper back in 1970 that says it was a vaccine safety test. It says, "If you would like to come to our pleasant surroundings and make $20 per day at the University of Maryland, etc." I have talked with participants in that test who are today very ill with GWI symptoms. . . .
>
> Scientists have been using mycoplasmas experimentally as a transmission agent because they are transferred very easily from man to man, woman to woman, throughout the population and it doesn't cause much of an immediate problem if you have a strong immune system.[35]

Figure 8.2 documents a certified patent on the most important "pathogenic mycoplasma." The developer was the Armed Forces Institute of Pathology (AFIP) "inventor" Dr. Shyh-Ching Lo. Lo assigned the rights and royalties on the patent to AFIP's American Registry of Pathology in Washington, D.C. As detailed herein, this lethal germ had been genetically engineered during the mid-1980s by Lo and colleagues. They initially isolated the germ from AIDS patients, then planned to use it to detect antibodies in HIV carriers as well as to develop vaccines against mycoplasma.

Mycoplasmas, for the reasons Capt. Riley described, and more—their "stealth virus"-like capacity to evade the immune system, thereby being very difficult to identify and treat—had been routinely used by

**Figure 8.2. U. S. Patent On "Pathogenic Mycoplasma" Linked to Autoimmune Diseases**

# United States Patent [19]

Lo

US005242820A

[11] Patent Number: 5,242,820

[45] Date of Patent: Sep. 7, 1993

[54] PATHOGENIC MYCOPLASMA

[75] Inventor: Shyh-Ching Lo, Potomac, Md.

[73] Assignee: American Registry of Pathology, Washington, D.C.

[21] Appl. No.: 710,361

[22] Filed: Jun. 6, 1991

**Related U.S. Application Data**

[63] Continuation-in-part of Ser. No. 265,920, Nov. 2, 1988, abandoned, which is a continuation-in-part of Ser. No. 875,535, Jun. 18, 1986, abandoned.

[51] Int. Cl.⁵ .............. C12N 5/00; C12N 5/02; C12N 1/00; C12Q 1/70

[52] U.S. Cl. .............. 435/240.2; 435/5; 435/872

[58] Field of Search ............. 435/870, 5, 872, 240.2

[56] **References Cited**

**PUBLICATIONS**

Marquart et al (1985) Mycoplasma-Like Structures ... Eur J Clin Microbiol 4(1):73-74.
Lo et al (1989) A Novel Virus-like Infectious Agent ... Am J Trop Med Hyg 40(2):213-226.
Lo et al (1989) Identification of *M Incognitus* ... Am. J. Trop-Med. Hyg 41(5):601-616.
Lo et al (1989) Association of the Virus-like Agent ... Am J Trop Med Hyg 41(3):364-376.

Lo et al (1989) Fatal Infection of Silvered Leaf Monkeys ... Am. T Trop Med Hyg 40(4):399-409.
Lo et al (1989) Virus-like Infectious Agent ... Am J Trop Med Hyg 41(5):586-600.
Marquart et al (Feb. 1985) Abstract Only Eur J Clin Microbiol 4(1):73-74.
Hu et al (1990) Gene 93:67-72.

*Primary Examiner*—Christine M. Nucker
*Assistant Examiner*—D. R. Preston
*Attorney, Agent, or Firm*—Venable, Baetjer, Howard & Civiletti

[57] **ABSTRACT**

The invention relates to a novel pathogenic mycoplasma isolated from patients with Acquired Immune Deficiency Syndrome (AIDS) and its use in detecting antibodies in sera of AIDS patients, patients with AIDS-related complex (ARC) or patients dying of diseases and symptoms resembling AIDS disease. The invention further relates to specific DNA sequences, antibodies against the pathogenic mycoplasma, and their use in detecting DNA or antigens of the pathogenic mycoplasma or other genetically and serologically closely related mycoplasmas in infected tissue of patients with AIDS or ARC or patients dying of symptoms resembling AIDS diseases. The invention still further relates to a variety of different forms of vaccine against mycoplasma infection in humans and/or animals.

2 Claims, 39 Drawing Sheets

top secret biological weapons researchers and genetic engineers. Moreover, mycoplasma infections are associated with some, if not all, of the symptoms and conditions associated with "stealth virus" and prion infections. Other mycoplasma-associated illnesses include Wegener's Disease, Sarcoidosis, respiratory distress syndrome, Kiuchi's disease, and the autoimmune diseases including Collagen Vascular Disease. According to Lo, "*Mycoplasma fermentans* incognitas," the primary strain Dr. Nicolson found infecting fifty-percent of vets with GWS, "may be either a causative agent of these diseases or a cofactor in these diseases."[37] In addition, according to Lo's report, this species of mycoplasma produced "cytoplasmic degeneration" and "vacuolization" of infected cells—virtually identical to that observed in "stealth virus" and prion infections.[37]

Len also learned from reading Lo's application, that Carlton Gajdusek, of prion fame, had actually been working intimately on AIDS projects essential to Robert Gallo's research, including HIV infection studies on chimpanzees during the early 1980s. Gallo allegedly discovered HIV, which was called HTLV-III at that time.[38]

Lo's patent filing also revealed a fascinating and important finding that, like Dr. Duesberg argued, "HIV does not cause AIDS," though it is associated with the infection. *Mycoplasma fermentans* (incognitas strain), in fact, may be the single most important agent "responsible" for the acquired immune deficiency syndrome! Here's how Lo explained it:

> The human retroviruses have not fulfilled Koch's postulates, i.e., producing transmissible AIDS-like diseases in experimental animals. HTLV-III/LAV (HIV) is not associated with the unusual malignancies such as B-cell lymphoma and Kaposi's sarcoma, commonly found in patients with AIDS. Shaw, G. M., et al., *Science* 226:1165-1171, 1984; Delli Bovi, P. et al., *Cancer Research*, 46:6333-6338, 1986; Groopman, J. E., et al., *Blood* 67:612-615, 1986. Furthermore, HIV infected patients often show a wide variation in times of disease incubation and speed of disease progression. It is not known whether any specific infectious agent other than HIV can be responsible for the complex pathogenesis often seen in this disease. One such candidate,

**Fig. 8.3. Letter From Dr. Nicolson to Huntsville Prison Official**

THE UNIVERSITY OF TEXAS
MDANDERSON
CANCER CENTER

Department Of Tumor Biology · 108
Telephone No.: (713) 792-7477
Fax No.:      (713) 794-0209

March 22, 1996

Hughes Unit
Route 2 Box 4400
Gatesville, TX 76597

current address!
P.O. Box 52470
Irvine, Cal. 92619

Dear

I do not have any information on the Palestine Unit of the TDCJ. We did, however, assist in an outbreak of mycoplasmal infections in Palestine that could have originated in the Palestine Unit. Most of our work has been with the inmates and guards at the Walls Unit in Huntsville where we have identified mycoplasmal infections associated with a vaccine development program supported by the US Army and conducted by Tanox Biosystems of Houston, a spin-off company of Baylor College of Medicine. We strongly suspect that Biological Warfare agents (weaponized mycoplasmas) were being illegally tested in the Walls Unit, but the evidence is circumstantial.

We have heard that other units were also involved in these tests, but we do not have any direct information on this. Our primary data comes from a TDCJ CFIDS support group that has an unusual frequency of mycoplasmal infections, and one of the microorganisms involved is a highly unusual mycoplasma that may have been engineered to make it more pathogenic and dangerous. Please be aware that there is a chance that you and your colleagues may be asked or coerced into a vaccine program. If this happens, it is my recommendation that you do not take part in any such program.

Sincerely,

Garth L. Nicolson, Ph.D.
David Bruton Jr. Chair in Cancer Research
Professor of Tumor Biology
Department of Tumor Biology (Box 108)
The University of Texas M. D. Anderson Cancer Center (use this address)
1515 Holcombe Blvd.
Houston, Texas 77030
and
Professor of Pathology and Laboratory Medicine
Professor of Internal Medicine
The University of Texas Medical School at Houston

Tel (713) 792 7481
Fax (713) 794-0209

TEXAS MEDICAL CENTER
1515 HOLCOMBE BOULEVARD • HOUSTON, TEXAS 77030 • (713) 792-2121

initially identified as a virus or virus-like infectious agent in patent application Ser. No. 265,920 [their earlier American Registry of Pathology assignment] has now been discovered to be mycoplasma *M. fermentans* (incognitas strain).[37]

If that's not bad enough, in a 1993 "Respiratory Distress Syndrome" report published by Lo and others in *Clinical Infectious Diseases*, the prognosis for those suffering from *Mycoplasma fermentans* was summarized thusly:

Although mycoplasmal agents are susceptible to antibiotics, eradication of the organisms from infected hosts is difficult. Antibiotic treatments of systemic *M. fermentans* infections may be difficult. Antibiotic therapy may relieve symptoms effectively but may leave a residual, persistent infection. Once treatment is stopped, the organisms may reactivate. Thus, "cure" of mycoplasmal infection may depend on an intact immune system in the host. Unfortunately, mycoplasmal infections alter the host's immune functions. . . .[39]

Moreover, they wrote, "We believe there is a wide spectrum of disease presentation following *M. fermentans* infection ranging from chronic debilitating illness to a fulminant course. . . . Continuing studies that focus on the development of more sensitive assays to detect *M. fermentans* infections and on increasing our understanding of the biology of this newly-emerging human pathogen are important."[39]

### Huntsville Virus and Vaccine Trials

It was, therefore, not surprising to insiders that Dr. Nicolson found the AIDS-virus envelope gene attached to *M. fermentans* incognitas in many Gulf War vets that came to him for treatment.[40] Nor was it surprising that their likeliest exposure to this agent came not from the war, per se, but from the "war on AIDS." Figure 8.3 shows a letter, submitted by investigators,[40] from Dr. Nicolson to a Texas Department of Corrections official advising against further participation in apparently lethal vaccination programs conducted on inmates by the U.S. Army and Tanox Biosystems of Houston—a "spin-off company of Baylor College of Medicine." Dr. Nicolson wrote, "We strongly sus-

# Fig. 8.4. Medical Experiments Done on Huntsville Prisoners

76

TABLE 1

Summary of Research Programs Conducted By
Baylor University School of Medicine

| Study | Number of Inmates | Date |
|---|---|---|
| Hong Kong flu program | 500 | 12-24-68 |
| Flu - influenza vaccine | 37 | 1  -69 |
| Rhinovirus 353 vaccine | 130 | 3-11-69 |
| Adenovirus vaccine | 43 | 7-22-69 |
| Adenovirus vaccine | 13 | 7-24-69 |
| A/Z Hong Kong flu | 9 | 7-26-69 |
| Equine flu study | 10 | 7-26-69 |
| Adenovirus 5 challenge | 58 | 9-27-69 |
| Influenza | 111 | 11-08-69 |
| Blood draw | 46 | 1-27-70 |
| Parainfluenza study | 55 | 5-29-70 |
| Mycoplasma pneumonia vaccine study | 46 | 9-10-70 |
| Rhinovirus type 15 plague pool | 55 | 9-10-70 |
| Parainfluenza | 37 | 3-17-71 |
| Mycoplasma pneumonia hall study | 116 | 5-19-71 |
| Adenovirus vaccine study | 15 | 5-19-71 |
| X-32 vaccine hall study | 4 | 6-13-71 |

TABLE 1  (Continued)

| Study | Number of Inmates | Date |
|---|---|---|
| Virus | 12 | 9-24-73/10-23-73 |
| Virus | 15 | 8-13-73/9-10-73 |
| Blood donor | 5 | 11-14-73 |
| Blood donor | 482 | 10-31-73 |
| Blood donor | 11 | 1-08-74 |
| Influenza/virus | 61 | 12-06-73/1-06-74 |
| Adenovirus | 77 | 12-16-73/1-13-74 |
| X-38 vaccine study | 16 | 11-09-73/12-07-73 |
| Blood donor | 11 | 2-01-74 |
| Virus study | 5 | 2-06-74 |
| Virus study | 419 | 2-07-74 |
| Blood donor | 55 | 2-14-74 |
| Adenovirus blood donor | 16 | 2-12-74 |
| Parainfluenza study | 29 | 3-11-74/4-07-74 |
| M. pneumonia | 20 | 3-11-74/4-14-74 |
| GCRC | 14 | 2-25-74/3-25-74 |
| Blood donor | 29 | 4-27-74 |
| Mycoplasma pneumoniae | 46 | 4-28-74/6-02-74 |
| Blood donor | 7 | 5-29-74 |
| GCRC | 10 | 5-06-74/6-03-74 |
| Adenovirus vaccine | 12 | 5-10-74 |

# Fig. 8.5. University of Texas Cholera Studies On Huntsville Prison Inmates.

TABLE 2

Summary of Research Programs Conducted By
University of Texas Medical Branch at Galveston

| Study | Number of Inmates | Date |
|---|---|---|
| Cholera H-3 | 180 | 4-67/4-68 |
| Cholera H-4 | 104 | 5-68/1-69 |
| Cholera H-5 | 171 | 9-68/1-69 |
| Cholera H-6 | 113 | 7-70/9-71 |
| Cholera H-7 | 74 | 10-70/2-72 |
| Cholera H-8 | 98 | 1-73/2-74 |
| Cholera H-9 | ---* | 10-73 |
| TOTAL   6 | 740 | 4-67/2-74 |

*Study in progress.

# Fig. 8.6. Baylor College of Medicine Cancer Contract

CONTRACT SUMMARIES

SPECIAL VIRUS CANCER PROGRAM
ETIOLOGY AREA, NCI
Fiscal Year 1971

DEVELOPMENTAL RESEARCH PROGRAM SEGMENT

Dr. Robert A. Manaker, Chief, VBB, Etiology Area, Chairman
Dr. Roy F. Kinard, VBB, Etiology Area, Vice Chairman
Dr. Jack Gruber, VBB, Etiology Area, Executive Secretary[1]

AICHI CANCER CENTER (NIH-69-96)

Title: Virus Rescue Studies in Human Leukemia/Lymphoma Cell Lines

Contractor's Project Officer: Dr. Yohei Ito

Project Officers (NCI): Dr. Jack Gruber
Dr. Virginia C. Dunkel

Objectives: (1) To establish cell lines in vitro from human neoplasms and
examine these for virus or antigens by electron microscopy, immunology and
transformation experiments. (2) To supply human embryonic cell cultures
and lymphoma-type tumor tissues available in the Far East.

Major Findings: Efforts to establish continuously growing cell lines from
human neoplastic tissues were resumed as one of the main lines of study in
the second year of the contract. In addition to the cultures from neoplasia
of the hematopoetic system, cell cultures from solid tumors such as naso-
pharyngeal carcinoma (NCP) were also attempted. This was done because of
the well established fact of high herpes-type virus (HTV) antibody titer
in the sera of patients with the disease. Among 13 NPC specimens cultured,
8 gave rise to monolayer culture, of which half showed morphological
alteration. From these cultures, one free-floating cell line was established.
The presence of HTV antigen in these cells was demonstrated by direct
immunofluorescence test.

To obtain an established cell line which grew in a floating state with less
or hopefully no HTV antigen, cultures from hyperplastic tonsils of children
were carried out. Of 136 specimens, 12 cell lines were established as free-
floating cells. The ratio of cells containing HTV antigen was relatively
small but HTV antigen was detected in all the cell lines.

Some 50 strains of cells were maintained in the laboratory and they served
as a procurement center for the supply of the cells for research workers
in the area. The procurement of human embryonic cultures was also continued
into the second year. About 40 human embryos in total were processed for
such culture. Human sera of high HTV antibody titer were also supplied to
colleagues of the SVCP.

[1] Replaced Dr. Roy Kinard as Vice Chairman on March 2, 1971.

Seroepidemiological studies using indirect immunofluorescence test have been continued to accumulate more data on the HTV antibody titer of individuals with various neoplastic diseases and normal subjects. However, a hope to reveal a new disease with high HTV antibody titer turned out to be fruitless so far.

Contacts have been strengthened with the institutes of the Asiatic area to provide access to the human tumor material and serum specimens which might be useful to the SVCP.

Significance to Biomedical Research and the Program of the Institute:
This project will supply supporting data from Far Eastern sources to supplement information obtained in the U.S. on the association of viruses with specific neoplastic diseases.

Proposed Course: In general, studies initiated previously will be continued. A new aspect of the work scope is the introduction of biochemical techniques to search for the presence of RNA-dependent DNA polymerase among the approximately 90 cell lines established from human neoplastic tissue during the past two years. Furthermore, fresh human cell materials from leukemic and lymphoma patients at the Aichi Cancer Center Hospital will be tested for polymerase activity. Such studies would provide new data on neoplastic cells from patients of oriental origin. Additionally, plans are to study the in vitro effect of various chemical carcinogens on established lymphoblastoid cell lines, and to initiate new investigations on other human neoplasms where virus activity is suspected.

Date Contract Initiated: May 2, 1969.

BAYLOR COLLEGE OF MEDICINE (PH43-68-678)

Title: Studies on Viruses as Related to Cancer with Emphasis on Leukemia

Contractor's Project Director: Dr. Joseph Melnick

Project Officers (NCI): Dr. Jack Gruber
                        Dr. Roy Kinard

Objectives: (1) To isolate, propagate and identify viral agents to provide evidence of association with human neoplasia and (2) to continue to hold and observe primates inoculated with suspected cancer viruses or cancer tissues.

Major Findings:

A. Viral etiology of leukemia and mononucleosis.

Propagation of selected lymphoblastoid (Ly) cell lines from patients with leukemia or mononucleosis and normal individuals is continuing, for use in immunological and biophysical studies.

101

Comparative chromosomal analysis of 16 lymphoblastoid cell lines cultivated up to 61 months revealed no specific association between the presence of EB virus and any of the chromosomal anomalies observed. Regardless of the source of cells or the presence of EB virus, cells with marker chromosomes or trisomies appear to have a selective advantage of growth in vitro, as documented by the increase in frequency of clones with these anomalies with progressive passage.

Studies were continued to search for antibody to possible tumor antigens in acute leukemia of childhood. Peripheral blood leukocytes are being reacted with serial autologous serum samples by indirect membrane immuno-fluorescence (IMIF). In autologous tests, cells from 20 of 25 children in remission have yielded negative results and 5 questionable. Cells obtained from 6 children during relapse were also tested for autoantibody. The IMIF assay has been uniformly negative for all sera and autologous relapse phase cells tested so far.

A 78 Al cell line of rat embryo fibroblasts that had been transformed by the murine sarcoma-leukemia virus (MSV-MLV) complex is being used as a model for characterization of RNA species obtained from various human Ly cell lines. The 68S RNA of MSV-MLV was found to dissociate after heating or dimethylsulfoxide treatment into 37S, 18S and 4S subunits, differing in base composition and buoyant densities in cesium sulfate. A double-stranded DNA with a sedimentation coefficient of 7S density was isolated from highly purified MSV-MLV. This DNA was complementary to the 18S subunit, but not to the 37S or 4S subunits of the viral RNA. Work is being initiated to follow infectious virus synthesis and macromolecular synthesis during de novo infection and transformation of cells by MSV-MLV.

B. Comparative studies on herpesviruses.

Studies continue on the distribution of complement-fixing (CF) antibody to EB virus-induced S antigen in groups with various disease entities and in normal individuals. The results are compared with those obtained in the immunofluorescence (IF) test with fixed EB3 cell preparations. Sera from 21 patients with sarcoidosis, kindly supplied by Dr. Phillip Glade, revealed both IF and S antibody to EB virus, a result similar to that reported earlier for patients with post-nasal carcinoma. A longitudinal study of the development of IF and S antibody starting with newborn children is being conducted. The results to date indicate that: (1) IF antibody to EB virus appears within several months after maternal antibody has disappeared, indicating an early infection with this agent. (2) There is a lag of several months between the appearance of IF and S antibodies. (3) Infection with the other three herpesviruses (herpes simplex, cytomegalo-virus and zoster virus) occurs much later than infection with EB virus.

Work continues to purify and characterize the soluble CF antigens extracted from two EB virus-positve (EB3 and P3J) and from one EB virus-negative (NC37) Ly cell lines. Ly cell line RPMI 8226, free of both EB virus and soluble CF antigen, is used as negative control. Studies on the non-serum-requiring complement-fixation (NSR-FCF) by EB virus-positive Ly cells indicate that the reaction may be measuring an EB virus directed antigen-antibody. Attempts are being made to identify antibody to EB virus in extracts of Ly cells.

The biochemical and biophysical properties of the DNA of HSV type 1 and type 2, infectious bovine rhinotracheitis (IBR) and Pseudorabies (Pr) viruses were compared. DNA-DNA hybridization was employed to investigate genetic relatedness between these four members of the herpesvirus group. Saturation and competition hybridizations demonstrated greater than 90% homology between three strains of HSV-1 and less than 5% homology between HSV-1, Pr virus and IBR virus. Saturation hybridization indicated at least 90% homology between two strains of HSV-2, but no homology between HSV-2 Pr virus and IBR virus. Preliminary experiments indicate that there is less than 50% homology between the DNAs of type 1 and type 2 HSV.

Further attempts to obtain additional BUDR-induced ts mutants of HSV have resulted in the isolation of 50 potential mutants. The 22 original ts mutants of HSV have been tentatively assigned to 8 complementation groups. Groups so far contain from 1-4 mutants. Before detailed characterization of representative members of complementation groups is undertaken, repeat tests are planned using both the 22 original mutants and the newly isolated mutants mentioned above.

The protein and glycoprotein synthesis by a HSV temperature-sensitive mutant (ts 343) and the wild-type virus has continued to be compared by polyacrylamide gel electrophoresis. Evidence was obtained that mutant ts 343 does not synthesize glycoprotein C5, a major envelope protein, at the nonpermissive temperature (40°). Studies are in progress on the glycoprotein synthesis of additional HSV ts mutants. Preliminary findings indicate that the glycoprotein profiles of mutants belonging to separate complementation groups may be significantly different.

C.  Role of herpes virus type 2 in cervical carcinoma.

Seroepidemiologic studies of women with invasive cervical cancer and controls from Uganda and Israel failed to reveal the same strength of association between antibodies to herpesvirus type 2 and malignancy, as previously observed in Houston, Atlanta, Baltimore and Brussels. Studies in different populations are continuing. Recently, 118 cervical cancer patients and 83 controls from Muslim and Christian women in Yugoslavia were studied. No difference in type 2 herpes antibodies was found between Muslim cases and controls, but the occurrence of antibodies among Christian women was twice that of control women. In New Zealand, the occurrence of antibodies was only slightly higher in the patients than in the control women. In the USA most of the studies that yielded a high incidence of antibodies were carried out among women of the lower socioeconomic group. Thus, in populations of different composition and different life styles, differences are found in the association between type 2 herpesvirus and cervical carcinoma.

Type 1 strains are susceptible to cytoside arabinoside and IUDR (iododeoxy-uridine), inhibitors of replication of DNA-containing viruses. However, type 2 strains are resistant to these DNA antagonists. This is apparently due to the low levels of thymidine kinase which are characteristic of type 2 strains in contrast to the high levels of this DNA-synthesizing enzyme found with type 1 strains.

D. Immunofluorescent cell surface antigens in human tumors.

Cell lines have been established from human melanoma and sarcoma tissue. Attempts are being made to separate tumor cells from the normal cells by (1) density gradient centrifugation, (2) by cloning out tumor cells, and (3) by injecting the mixture into immunosuppressed mice. With one of the two melanoma cell lines tested, the patient's serum reacted in the membrane fluorescence test. Sera from other melanoma patients reacted positively for antigen in the cytoplasm of the tumor cells. Lymphosarcoma cells reacted in the membrane fluorescence test with autologous sera, and cross reactions were seen with sera from other lymphosarcoma patients.

Significance to Biomedical Research and to the Program of the Institute: This contract provides a progressive comprehensive research program to determine the significance of viruses in human neoplasia. Techniques used are tissue culture, immunology, electron microscopy, primate inoculation, cytogenetics and nucleic acid homology.

Proposed Course: Investigations will continue to detect the presence of nucleic acid characteristic of the RNA tumor viruses in human tumor cells. Immunological studies with antigens associated with EB virus will be continued. Further serologic data will be acquired to aid in determining the relationship between the venereal herpes hominis type 2 virus and cervical carcinoma.

Date Contract Initiated: June 27, 1963

BIONETICS RESEARCH LABORATORIES, INC. (NIH-71-2025)

Title: Investigations of Viral Carcinogenesis in Primates

Contractor's Project Directors:   Dr. John Landon
                                   Dr. David Valerio
                                   Dr. Robert Ting

Project Officers (NCI):   Dr. Roy Kinard
                          Dr. Jack Gruber
                          Dr. Robert Gallo

# Fig. 8.7. Huntsville Civilians* Killed and Cited Cause of Death

1. Susan Baldy ............................................................................. ALS
2. James Brian, Esq. ................................................................. ALS
3. Georgia Stockman ................................................................ ALS
4. David Ward ............................................................................ ALS
5. James Selford ...................................................................... ALS
6. Jean Harold .......................................................................... ALS
7. Mary Ertz .............................................................................. ALS
8. Barbara Rango ..................................................................... ALS
9. Luther Antler ......................................................................... ALS
10. Ken Stalworth ...................................................................... ALS
11. Eula Andrew ......................................................................... ALS
12. Evelyn Baken ....................................................................... ALS
13. Saul Barr .............................................................................. ALS
14. Robert Carry ........................................................................ ALS
15. Velma Enver ......................................................................... ALS
16. Edwin Garrison ..................................................................... ALS
17. Katheryn Kravitz ................................................................... ALS
18. Gwen Robertson, RN ........................................................... Leukemia
19. Carolyn Wishert .................................................................... Cancer
20. Huston Carrie ....................................................................... Leukemia
21. Bernice Getty ....................................................................... ALS
22. Gracey Dunning .................................................................... ALS
23. Polly Langley ........................................................................ ALS
24. Wallace MacMillan ................................................................ ALS
25. Edward Naples ...................................................................... Brain Tumor
26. Thomas Green ...................................................................... ALS
27. Louis Pelling ......................................................................... Unknown
28. Helen Albert .......................................................................... Unknown
29. Joseph Cally, DDS ................................................................ Heart Burst
30. Eugene Akerly, MD ................................................................ Unknown
31. J.B. Sally .............................................................................. Brain Tumor
32. Sam Baldy ............................................................................ Unknown
33. Christine Angler .................................................................... Unknown

Total Dead ............................................................................. 42
Cause of Death Cited:
............................................................................... ALS    25
.............................................................................. Cancer    7
.................................................. Mycoplasma fermentans incognitis    1
............................................................. Cause Unknown    8
................................................................................. Heart    1

* Sample listing of forty-two (42) dead. All aliases cited.
  For more information contact attorney Northrop @ 405-946-8100; Fax 405-949-2172

# Fig. 8.8. Huntsville's Sick Plaintiffs*, Diagnosis, and Summary

| | |
|---|---|
| 1. Sally Meely | Mycoplasma |
| 2. Clarence Meely | Mycoplasma |
| 3. Julie Jackson | Mycoplasma |
| 4. Nancy Messler | CFIDS |
| 5. Marie Frankel | CFIDS |
| 6. Larry Ryan | Lupus |
| 7. Jerry Ryan | Lupus |
| 8. Jackie Clarry, RN | MS |
| 9. Robert Brandish | Cancer |
| 10. Cherry Hartley | Fibromyalgia |
| 11. Carol Derry | Crones |
| 12. David Derry | MS |
| 13. Mary Lou Perry | Mycoplasma |
| 14. Ken Perry | Mycoplasma |
| 15. Betty Curtan | Fibromyalgia |
| 16. Carol Chamas | Fibromyalgia |
| 17. Janice Selley | Cancer |
| 18. Charlie Spinney | Cancer |
| 19. Eugene Orlanda | Legionella |
| 20. Virginia Arder | Epstein Barr |
| 21. Dianne Nelly | Lupus |
| 22. Dorothy Merrie | Parkinson's |
| 23. Amy Ornstein | Fibromyalgia |
| 24. Mitchel Bates | MS |
| 25. Sheryl Horner | CFIDS |
| 26. Virginia Latley | CFIDS |
| 27. Jeanie Orders | CFIDS |
| 28. Jason Brownstein | Polymyositis |
| 29. Jackie Brownstein (Grandaughter) | Meningitis |
| 30. Earl Jenson (child) | Joint Disease |

Total Ill: 231

Diagnosis Cited:

| | |
|---|---|
| CFIDS | 71 |
| Mycoplasma | 13 |
| Fibromyalgia | 10 |
| Lupus | 8 |
| ALS | 4 |
| Cancer | 9 |
| MS | 13 |
| Various | 23 |
| Undiagnosed | 80 |

* Sample listing of 231 ailing. All aliases cited.

pect that Biological Warfare agents (weaponized mycoplasmas) were being illegally tested in the Walls Unit, but the evidence is circumstantial."

Figure 8.4 shows a table summarizing the research conducted by Baylor University School of Medicine on Huntsville Prison inmates beginning in 1968. Mycoplasma inoculation as well as vaccination studies were listed as having begun in 1970 under contract with the U.S. Army. Figure 8.5 shows cholera studies conducted on the same prison population.

One of several "cancer" contracts given to Baylor's School of Medicine beginning in 1968 is shown in figure 8.6. This contract funded "Studies on Viruses as Related to Cancer with Emphasis on Leukemia." One objective was "to continue to hold and observe primates inoculated with suspected cancer viruses or cancer tissues." The holding and observation functions could be readily accomplished in the Huntsville Prison where human primates were housed. Typically during these studies, when monkeys were used, the contracts stated "nonhuman primates." The absence of this clarification strongly suggests humans were the experimental subjects.

Interestingly, Litton Bionetics—the company with whom Dr. Gallo co-engineered numerous AIDS-like viruses, is cited on the adjacent contract.

Further raising the spectre of genocide, reflecting on Margaret Sanger and her Nazi-American collaborators, was Baylor's contract page number 103. It discussed herpes virus type 2 that was said to have been studied in different parts of the world where "Christian," "Muslim," Black, and Jewish women were investigated for cervical cancer tendencies. Other studies ongoing at the time included the herpes-type viruses, including Epstein Barr and cytomegalovirus currently associated with additional cancers and the CFIDS epidemic. Infectious CFIDS was virtually non-existent before 1968, that is, before these studies began.

## Bush, Baker and Genocide?

The evolution of "secret societies," including the Skull & Bones and CFR, foreshadowed the military and medical experiments that gave rise to several contemporary epidemics. Members of the cryptocracy, including George Bush and James Baker III, are implicated for their central roles in the contemporary eugenics movement.

For instance, based on reputable sources, George Bush's Secretary of State, James Baker III, was said to have owned part of the vaccine manufacturer against whom ailing Gulf War veterans have filed suit.[35] Moreover, Mr. Bush is said to have been a major shareholder in that company—Tanox Biosystems of Houston.[35]

In fact, Bush became a director of the Tanox affiliated Baylor College of Medicine after leaving his CIA director post.[43] Tanox is also closely linked to Dr. Lo's employer—The Armed Forces Institute of Pathology.

Further, what would seem inconceivable without the documents reprinted in figures 8.1 through 8.8, Tanox tested their mycoplasma vaccines on Huntsville prisoners. As a result, the prisoners developed Gulf War Syndrome long before the Gulf War. Thus, GWS could have been, and probably was, predicted and effected. Additional victims, as seen in figures 8.7 and 8.8, were those with whom the prisoners made contact. (This information derives from a class action lawsuit ongoing at the time of this writing. Due to the obviously urgent nature of this information bearing on public health, permission to reprint this documentation was granted.)[40]

Given the evolution of, in George Bush's words, "a New World Order," largely advanced by secret agents, and a history of genocidal practices involving "dispensible" populations, Gulf War Syndrome is reconcilable. The U.S. military, generally comprised of nationalistic, sovereign-thinking, patriotic individuals who pledged to kill and die to defend the U.S. Constitution against all foreign and domestic enemies, represented a risk to the evolving New World Order. Thus, the military needed to be culled, largely killed, defunded, "defanged," and demoralized—roughly where it stands today.

Lastly, the casualties borne initially by hundreds of civilians in Huntsville, and now millions of Americans at risk for mycoplasma and prion infections was additionally reconcilable in the eyes of this secret war-making cabal. Like billions of people worldwide who have been sacrificed over the centuries to promote "peace on earth," Huntsville, and America in general, has paid its share of the price. Again quoting from the *Report From Iron Mountain*, "War as a system of gross population control to preserve the species cannot fairly be faulted."

## Prusiner's "Stolen" Prize

The next article Len read was on the Internet posted by an anonymous author. It was largely an exposé on the Nobel Prize winner Stanley Prusiner, who, like Robert Gallo had done with AIDS, received the lion's share of misplaced credit for the theory in which protein prions extended their growth into surrounding tissues. Much like the scientific objections that followed the realization that Gallo had stolen glory for the first HIV isolations from Luc Montagnier, the author of this article expressed remorse that Prusiner received unwarranted credit for the prion thesis. His report was technically accurate and highly relevant to the politics at hand.

The article explained that the theory for which Prusiner took credit was primarily advanced by mathematician J. S. Griffiths and his predecessors.[41] Griffiths, it was abundantly clear, was not a normal mathemetician. Rather, he was an applied mathemetician/bioengineer whose work centered on *process control theory* The article explained:

> [T]he standard model of prion disease was explicitly and accurately introduced by . . . JS Griffiths in 1966 in his only publication in this area . . . [S]omehow SB Prusiner has stolen the credit for this notion.

> Most amusingly, Griffiths himself does not take credit for this idea, but clearly attributes it to a 1957 paper of the Penroses [published in *Nature* 1957;4571:1183], who are said to have elaborated on a 1922 paper by A. Gratia [published in the *British Medical Journal* 1922;ii:296.]. It can quickly be seen from a PubMed search that Griffiths's idea had no follow-up or support of any kind [until Prusiner].

The Gratia paper is . . . on the topic of 'bacteriophage.' [Bacteriophage is defined in *Steadman's Medical Dictionary* as "a virus with specific affinity for bacteria . . . " They have been routinely used to deliver viral genes, DNA, RNA, and other components into human cells through medically-induced infections currently called "gene therapy."] It consists of a few arguments regarding why bacteriophages need not be living organisms. One argument involves an analogy between the spread of fire and the reproduction of living organisms, and the other (the probable source of the "prion hypothesis" citation) discusses how a small fraction of thrombin [blood clotting factor] produced in one test tube can be used to cause plasma in another tube to clot, after which a small fraction of the second product can be used to clot another tube, ad infinitum.[41]

Len paused to consider how this bacteriophage thesis impacted the prion hypothesis. If a bacteriophage could spread viral infections and genetic material to humans, then bacteria or fungi could also carry prions as well, he reckoned, since prions are smaller than viruses.

Now Griffith should be credited more often than he is for writing a prescient mini-review article on protein 'self-replication' with possible application to the scrapie mechanism of replication. . . . Looking back at 1967 undergraduate biochemistry texts, we can confirm that Griffith's reaction chains, thermodynamic equations, and potential barrier theory of dimer conformational change were commonly taught to college students in that year. Griffith's free energy driving force, for example, is exactly that of a coupled ATPase.

In fact, Prusiner clearly and explicitly cited Griffith's paper in his landmark paper on prions (See: *Science* 1982 216:136-144; reference #32). Here Griffith was discussed only in connection to the "Hypothetical Structures of the Scrapie Agent," but not for the mechanism he advanced for the prion's spread. The passage reads:

". . . Hypotheses on the chemical structure of the scrapie agent have included: sarcosporidia parasite, 'filterable' virus, small DNA virus, replicating protein [Griffith cited], replicating abnormal polysaccharide with membrane. . . ."[41]

The original prion theory evolved from observations of Black people with sickle cell hemoglobin.[41] Len found this interesting considering the Illuminati's predilection for African eugenics and genocide. Sickle cell anemia was one of the earliest illnesses determined to be genetically linked. According to *Webster's Dictionary*, it primarily affected "individuals of African, Mediterranean, or southwest Asian ancestry." "Odd," he thought, "that the original theoretic work on prions began with such a potentially genocidal mechanism."

## Mind Blower

After skimming a technical portion of the *Scientific American* article Len had read earlier that day, he had an inkling to pick it up again. Shaun Heaphy from Leicester University's department of microbiology and immunology, actually explained prion pleomorphism and its possible link to viral reproductive mechanisms. He wrote:

> We now know that a normal cellular protein, called PrP (for proteinaceous infectious particle) and which is found in all of us, is centrally involved in the spread of prion disease. This protein consist of about 250 amino acids.

> Some researchers believe that the prions are formed when PrP associates with a foreign pathogenic nucleic acid [most likely provided by DNA or possibly RNA viruses, bacteria, or other infectious agents including fungi and mycoplasmas]. This is called *the virino hypothesis*. (Viruses consist of proteins and nucleic acids that are specified by the virus genome.) A virino would also consist of proteins and nucleic acids, but the protein component is specified by the host genome, not the pathogen genome. In support of the virino hypothesis is the *existence of different strains of prions that cause differing patterns of disease* and breed true; *the existence of strains in pathogens is usually the result of changes in the nucleic acid sequence of the infectious agent*. Scientists have not found any [complete] nucleic acid associated with a prion . . . Furthermore, prions appear to remain infectious even after being exposed to treatments that destroy nucleic acids.

285

This evidence has led to the now widely accepted prion theory, which states that the cellular protein PrP is the sole causative agent of prion diseases; there is no nucleic acid involved. The theory holds that PrP is normally in a stable shape (pN) that does not cause disease. The protein can be flipped, however, into an abnormal shape (pD) that does cause disease. pD is infectious because it can associate with pN and convert it to pD, in an exponential process—each pD can convert more pN to pD.

Prions can be transmitted, possibly by eating and certainly by inoculation either directly into the brain or into skin and muscle tissue. *Exponential amplification of the prion (converting pN into pD in the body) would then result in disease.* Occasional, sporadic cases of prion diseases arise in middle or old age, presumably because there is a very small but real chance that *pN can spontaneously flip to pD*; the cumulative likelihood of such a flip grows over the years. . . .

The prion theory has not been proved correct, but much evidence now supports it. We do not yet know why the pD structure of a prion would result in neurodegeneration, but we do know that prion protein accumulates in the brain tissue. *One part of the prion protein can cause apoptosis, or programmed cell death; perhaps this mechanism explains the pattern of disease.* [Emphasis added.][9]

"Programmed cell death? That's a frightening concept," Len thought. "I wonder what signals the program to turn on? Could it be electrical? The prion is, after all, a crystal—a microprocessor, receiver and transmitter of electromagnetic radiation.[42]

"Maybe a fungus, or even a mycoplasma, transmits the lethal prion into the host, after which prion infection is stimulated by microcurrents or vibrational frequencies."[42]

Then the word "apoptosis" drew his attention. "I've never heard of that word before. Let me look that one up."

He pulled his 1972 edition of *Steadman's Medical Dictionary* from the shelf and went through it. The word was nowhere to be found. "That's odd. It must be a new term. Let me try *Webster's.*

Again, nothing. The only close words Webster offered were eerily related to the metaphysical, creative, and religious subject matter that

## Fig. 8.9. Definitions of Words Derived From "Apo"

**apo-** *or* **ap-** *prefix* [ME, fr. MF & L; MF, fr. L, fr, Gk, fr. *apo* — more at OF] **1** : away from : off ⟨*aphelion*⟩ **2** : detached : separate ⟨*apogamy*⟩ **3** : formed from ; related to ⟨*apomorphine*⟩

**apoc·a·lypse** \ə-'pä-kə-ˌlips\ *n* [ME, revelation, Revelation, fr., LL *apocalypsis*, fr. Gk *apokalypsis*, fr. *apokalyptein* to uncover, fr. *apo-* + *kalyptein* to cover — more at HELL] (13c) **1 a** : one of the Jewish and Christian writings of 200 B.C. to A.D. 150 marked by pseudonymity, symbolic imagery, and the expectation of an imminent cosmic cataclysm in which God destroys the ruling powers of evil and raises the righteous to life in a messianic kingdom **b** *cap* : REVELATION **3** **2 a** : something viewed as a prophetic revelation **b** ; ARMAGEDDON

**apoc·a·lyp·tic** \ə-ˌpä-kə-'lip-tik\ *also* **apoc·a·lyp·ti·cal** \-ti-kal\ *adj* (1663) **1** : of, relating to, or resembling an apocalypse **2** : forecasting the ultimate destiny of the world : PROPHETIC **3** : foreboding imminent disaster or final doom : TERRIBLE **4** ; wildly unrestrained : GRANDIOSE **5** : ultimately decisive : CLIMACTIC — **apoc·a·lyp·ti·cal·ly** \-ti-k(ə-)lē\ *adv*

**apoc·a·lyp·ti·cism** \-tə-ˌsi-zəm\ *or* **apoc·a·lyp·tism** \ə-'pä-kə-ˌlip-ˌti-zəm\ *n* (1884) : apocalyptic expectation; *esp* ; a doctrine concerning an imminent end of the world and an ensuing general resurrection and final judgment

**apoc·a·lyp·tist** \ə-'pä-kə-ˌlip-tist\ *n* (1835) ; the writer of an apocalypse

**apo·chro·mat·ic** \ˌa-pə-krō-'ma-tik\ *adj* [ISV] (1887) : free from chromatic and spherical aberration ⟨an ～ lens⟩

**apoc·o·pe** \ə-'pä-kə-(ˌ)pē\ *n* [LL, fr. Gk *apokopē*, lit., cutting off, fr. *apokoptein* to cut off, fr. *apo-* + *koptein* to cut — more at CAPON] (ca. 1550) : the loss of one or more sounds or letters at the end of a word (as in *sing* from Old English *singan*)

**apo·crine** \'a-pə-krən, -ˌkrīn, -ˌkrēn\ *adj* [ISV *apo-* + Gk *krinein* to separate — more at CERTAIN] (1926) : producing a fluid secretion by pinching off one end of the secretory cell while leaving the rest intact ⟨an ～ gland⟩; *also* : produced by an apocrine gland

**apoc·ry·pha** \ə-'pä-krə-fə\ *n pl but sing or pl in constr* [ML, fr. LL, neut. pl. of *apocryphus* secret, not canonical, fr. Gk *apokryphos* obscure, fr. *apokryptein* to hide away, fr. *apo-* + *kryptein* to hide — more at CRYPT] (14c) **1** : writings or statements of dubious authenticity **2** *cap* **a** : books included in the Septuagint and Vulgate but excluded from the Jewish and Protestant canons of the Old Testament — see BIBLE table **b** : early Christian writings not included in the New Testament

**apoc·ry·phal** \-fəl\ *adj* (1590) **1** : of doubtful authenticity ; SPURIOUS **2** *often cap* : of or resembling the Apocrypha *syn* see FICTITIOUS — **apoc·ry·phal·ly** \-fə-lē\ *adv* — **apoc·ry·phal·ness** *n*

**apo·dic·tic** \ˌa-pə-'dik-tik\ *also* **apo·deic·tic** \-'dīk-tik\ *adj* [L *apodicticus*, fr. Gk *apodeiktikos*, fr. *apodeiknynai* to demonstrate, fr. *apo-* + *deiknynai* to show — more at DICTION] (ca. 1645) : expressing or of the nature of necessary truth or absolute certainty — **apo·dic·ti·cal·ly** \-ti-k(ə-)lē\ *adv*

**apod·o·sis** \ə-'pä-də-səs\ *n, pl* **-o·ses** \-ˌsēz\ [NL, fr. Gk, fr. *apodidonai* to give back, deliver, fr. *apo-* + *didonai* to give — more at DATE] (ca. 1638) : the main clause of a conditional sentence — compare PROTASIS

**apo·en·zyme** \ˌa-pō-'en-ˌzīm\ *n* [ISV] (1936) ; a protein that forms an active enzyme system by combination with a coenzyme and determines the specificity of this system for a substrate

**apog·a·my** \ə-'pä-gə-mē\ *n* [ISV] (ca. 1878) : development of a sporophyte from a gametophyte without fertilization — **apog·a·mous** \ə-'pä-gə-məs\ *adj*

Joey had described and the earlier chapters of this book relayed. (See figure 8.9.) Len began to read:

The syllable "**apo**" meant "formed from," as in the terms—

• **apocalypse** [from] ME [Middle English] revelation [and the] Gk [Greek] to uncover 1a: one of the Jewish and Christian writings of 200 B.C. to A.D 150 marked by pseudonymity, symbolic imagery, and the expectation of an imminent cosmic cataclysm in which God destroys the ruling powers of evil and raises the righteous to life in a messianic kingdom.

• **apocalyptic** . . . 2: forecasting the ultimate destiny of the world: PROPHETIC 3: foreboding imminent disaster or final doom : TERRIBLE 4: widely unrestrained: GRANDIOSE 5: ultimately decisive: CLIMACTIC—

Len wondered why all the terms in small caps were placed that way.

• **apochromatic** . . . free from chromatic and spherical aberration, an apochromatic lens.

• **apocrypha** . . . secret, not canonical, fr. Gk [Greek] *apokryphos* obscure, fr. [French] *apokryptein* to hide away, fr. apo- + kryptein to hide — more at crypt/ (14c) . . .

"What? What's that?" Len thought. "*More at crypt/ (14c)?* Maybe that's one of those 'hidden cross reference entries' Joey mentioned. I'd better check it out."

So Len turned the pages to find the word "crypt." But the first thing that *caught his eye* when he got close was "*(15c)*." It was located in the definition of "*crystalline*."

"Wow. I wonder if that's another hidden entry related to crystalline. *Prions are tiny crystalline proteins.*" He became obviously excited by the bizarre, seemingly serendipitous discovery. "Where's 'crypt' and '14c?'"

His eyes searched the word columns. Finally, there was the word "crypt." With great anticipation he read the definition looking for any reference to '14c.' "It's not here?" he questioned. "Where is it? It must

## Fig. 8.10. Cross Reference to "Crypt" Definitions

**crypt** \'kript\ *n* [L *crypta,* fr. Gk *kryptē,* fr. fem. of *kryptos* hidden, fr. *kryptein* to hide; perh. akin to Lith *krauti* to pile up] (1789) **1 a :** a chamber (as a vault) wholly or partly underground; *esp :* a vault under the main floor of a church **b :** a chamber in a mausoleum **2 a :** an anatomical pit or depression **b :** a simple tubular gland

**crypt-** *or* **crypto-** *comb form* [NL, fr. Gk *kryptos*] **1 :** hidden : covered ⟨*crypt*ogenic⟩ **2 :** CRYPTOGRAPHIC ⟨*crypt*analysis⟩

**cryp·ta·rithm** \'krip-tə-ˌri-t͟həm\ *n* [*crypt-* + *-arithm* (as in *logarithm*)] (1943) **:** an arithmetic problem in which letters have been substituted for numbers and which is solved by finding all possible pairings of digits with letters that produce a numerically correct answer

**cryp·tic** \'krip-tik\ *adj* [LL *crypticus,* fr. Gk *kryptikos,* fr. *kryptos*] (ca. 1638) **1 :** SECRET, OCCULT **2 a :** having or seeming to have a hidden or ambiguous meaning : MYSTERIOUS ⟨~ messages⟩ **b :** marked by an often perplexing brevity ⟨~ marginal notes⟩ **3 :** serving to conceal ⟨~ coloration in animals⟩; *also :* exhibiting cryptic coloration ⟨~ animals⟩ **4 :** UNRECOGNIZED ⟨a ~ infection⟩ **5 :** employing cipher or code *syn* see OBSCURE — **cryp·ti·cal·ly** \-ti-k(ə-)lē\ *adv*

**¹cryp·to** \'krip-(ˌ)tō\ *n, pl* **cryptos** [*crypt-*] (1946) **:** a person who adheres or belongs secretly to a party, sect, or other group

**²crypto** *adj* (1952) **1 :** CRYPTOGRAPHIC **2 :** not openly avowed or declared — often used in combination ⟨*crypto*-fascist⟩

**cryp·to·coc·co·sis** \ˌkrip-tə-(ˌ)kä-'kō-səs\ *n, pl* **-co·ses** \-(ˌ)sēz\ [NL] (1938) **:** an infectious disease that is caused by a fungus (*Cryptococcus neoformans*) and is characterized by the production of nodular lesions or abscesses in the lungs, subcutaneous tissues, joints, and esp. the brain and meninges

**cryp·to·coc·cus** \-'kä-kəs\ *n, pl* **-coc·ci** \-'käk-ˌsī, -ˌsē, -'kä-ˌkī, -ˌkē\ [NL] (ca. 1902) **:** any of a genus (*Cryptococcus*) of budding imperfect fungi that resemble yeasts and include a number of saprophytes and a few serious pathogens — **cryp·to·coc·cal** \-'kä-kəl\ *adj*

**cryp·to·crys·tal·line** \ˌkrip-tō-'kris-tə-lən\ *adj* [ISV] (1862) **:** having a crystalline structure so fine that no distinct particles are recognizable under the microscope ⟨~ quartz⟩

**cryp·to·gam** \'krip-tə-ˌgam\ *n* [ultim. fr. Gk *kryptos* + *-gamia* -gamy] (1847) **:** a plant (as a fern, moss, alga, or fungus) reproducing by spores and not producing flowers or seed — **cryp·to·gam·ic** \ˌkrip-tə-'ga-mik\ *or* **cryp·tog·a·mous** \krip-'tä-gə-məs\ *adj*

**cryp·to·gen·ic** \ˌkrip-tə-'je-nik\ *adj* (1908) **:** of obscure or unknown origin ⟨a ~ disease⟩

**cryp·to·zo·ol·o·gy** \ˌkrip-tə-zō-'ä-lə-jē, -zə-'wä-\ *n* (1969) **:** the study of the lore concerning legendary animals (as Sasquatch) esp. in order to evaluate the possibility of their existence — **cryp·to·zo·ol·o·gist** \-'ä-lə-jist, -'wä-\ *n*

**¹crys·tal** \'kris-t²l\ *n* [ME *cristal,* fr. OF, fr. L *crystallum,* fr. Gk *krystallos* — more at CRUST] (13c) **1 :** quartz that is transparent or nearly so and that is either colorless or only slightly tinged **2 :** something resembling crystal in transparency and colorlessness **3 :** a body that is formed by the solidification of a chemical element, a compound, or a mixture and has a regularly repeating internal arrangement of its atoms and often external plane faces **4 :** a clear colorless glass of superior quality; *also :* objects or ware of such glass **5 :** the glass or transparent plastic cover over a watch or clock dial **6 :** a crystalline material used in electronics as a frequency-determining element or for rectification **7 :** powdered methamphetamine

**²crystal** *adj* (14c) **1 :** consisting of or resembling crystal : CLEAR, LUCID **2 :** relating to or using a crystal ⟨a ~ radio receiver⟩

**crystall-** *or* **crystallo-** *comb form* [Gk *krystallos*] **:** crystal ⟨*crystallog*raphy⟩

**crys·tal·line** \'kris-tə-lən *also* -ˌlīn, -ˌlēn\ *adj* [ME *cristallin,* fr. MF & L; MF, fr. L *crystallinus,* fr. Gk *krystallinos,* fr. *krystallos*] (15c) **1 :** resembling crystal: as **a :** strikingly clear or sparkling ⟨~ air⟩ ⟨a ~ lake⟩ **b :** CLEAR-CUT **2 :** made of crystal : composed of crystals **3 :** constituting or relating to a crystal — **crys·tal·lin·i·ty** \ˌkris-tə-'li-nə-tē\ *n* be here!" He quickly turned back to the definition of "apocrypha" to verify Webster's apparent instruction. "'14c' was accurate," he confirmed.

"It's got to be here. It's got to be between "crypt" and "15c" in "crystalline."

So he returned to "crypt" and slowly scanned down the column seen in figure 8.10. At long last, there it was. Adjacent the word *"crystal"* was *"14c."*

"Holy dear Jesus! Could they have really done this? The Illuminati have got *crystals* linked to a biological *apocalypse* with prions in the middle of it all!"

His knowledge about prions being tiny crystals, electronic receivers and transmitters of resonant frequencies, and now its "hidden" link to "an imminent cosmic cataclysm" left him stunned. "Could prion crystals play a central role in a biological apocalypse? Could they be the 'little beasts' that Bible prophecy has linked to massive plagues and depopulation?"

## Divinely Guided Revelations

Later, after the shock of these possibilities subsided, Len searched the list of terms and definitions between "crypt," and "crystal." Almost all had to do with key subjects addressed in this book. These included:

• **cryptanalysis** . . . (1923) 1: the solving of cryptograms or cryptographic systems.

> • **cryptarithm** . . . (1943) : an arithmetic problem in which letters have been substituted for numbers and which is solved by finding all possible pairings of digits with letters that produce a numerically correct answer.

> • **cryptic** . . . 1: secret, occult 2 a: having or seeming to have a hidden or ambiguous meaning : mysterious . . . b: marked by an often perplexing brevity . . . 3: serving to conceal . . . unrecognized <a [cryptic] infection>5: employing cipher or code . . .

"A 'cryptic infection?'" Len questioned. "This is uncanny!"

• **crypto** . . . (1946) a person who adheres or belongs secretly to a party, sect, or other group

• **crypto** *adj* (1952) 1: cryptographic 2 : not openly avowed or declared—often used in combination <crypto-fascist>.

"'Crypto-fascist?' Isn't that perfect," Len realized.

• **cryptococcosis** . . . (1938) an infectious disease that is caused by a fungus (*Cryptococcus neoformans*) and is characterized by the production of nodular lesions or abscesses in the lungs, subcutaneous tissues, joints, and esp. the brain and meninges

"Boy do these symptoms sound familiar."

• **cryptococcus** . . . (ca. 1902) : any of a genus (Cryptoccus) of budding imperfect fungi that resemble yeasts and include a number of saprophytes and a few serious pathogens . . .

"Even fungal infections are defined here. I can't believe this. Am I losing my mind?"

• **cryptocrystalline** . . . (1862) : having a crystalline structure so fine that no distinct particles are recognizable under the microscope <[cryptocrystalline] quartz>

• **cryptogam** . . . (1847) : a plant (as a fern, moss, alga, or fungus) reproducing by spores and not producing flowers or seed . . .

• **cryptogenic** . . . (1908) : of obscure or unknown origin <a [cryptogenic] disease>

"This is outrageous!"

Then, intuitively Len thought, "I'd better go back and check out the word "apocalypse" for any other hidden entries. I might have missed it." So he did just that. (See figure 8.9.) Moments later, there it was. He had missed another cross reference to a hidden entry. Adjacent "apocalypse" read the words "fr. apo- + *kalyptein* to cover — more at HELL] (13c) . . .

"Okay. Here we go again," he thought.

Again, with great anticipation, now with his heart pounding, he looked up the word "hell" for any hidden entry or reference to "13c." The word and its definition is shown in figure 8.11. It reads: "hell . . .

## Fig. 8.11. *Webster's* Extraordinary Cross References to "Hell," "Heir," "Dial," "Loom," and the "Lords of Misrule"

¹**heir** \'ar, 'er\ *n* [ME, fr. OF, fr. L *hered-, heres;* akin to Gk *chēros* bereaved] (13c)  **1** : one who inherits or is entitled to inherit property  **2** : one who inherits or is entitled to succeed to a hereditary rank, title, or office ⟨~ to the throne⟩  **3** : one who receives or is entitled to receive some endowment or quality from a parent or predecessor — **heir·less** \-ləs\ *adj* — **heir·ship** \-,ship\ *n*
²**heir** *vt* (14c) *chiefly dial* : INHERIT
**heir apparent** *n, pl* **heirs apparent** (14c)  **1** : an heir whose right to an inheritance is indefeasible in law if he survives the legal ancestor  **2** : HEIR PRESUMPTIVE  **3** : one whose succession esp. to a position or role appears certain under existing circumstances
**heir at law** (1729) : an heir in whom an intestate's real property is vested by operation of law
**heir·ess** \'ar-əs, 'er-\ *n* (1607) : a female heir; *esp* : a female heir to great wealth
**heir·loom** \'ar-,lüm, 'er-\ *n* [ME *heirlome,* fr. *heir* + *lome* implement — more at LOOM] (15c)  **1** : a piece of property that descends to the heir as an inseparable part of an inheritance of real property  **2** : something of special value handed on from one generation to another
**heir presumptive** *n, pl* **heirs presumptive** (ca. 1737) : an heir whose legal right to an inheritance may be defeated (as by the birth of a nearer relative)

**hell** \'hel\ *n* [ME, fr. OE; akin to OE *helan* to conceal, OHG *helan,* L *celare,* Gk *kalyptein*] (bef. 12c)  **1 a** (1) : a nether world in which the dead continue to exist : HADES  (2) : the nether realm of the devil and the demons in which the damned suffer everlasting punishment — often used in curses ⟨go to ~⟩ or as a generalized term of abuse ⟨the ~ with it⟩  **b** *Christian Science* : ERROR 2b, SIN  **2 a** : a place or state of misery, torment, or wickedness ⟨war is ~ —W. T. Sherman⟩  **b** : a place or state of turmoil or destruction ⟨all ~ broke loose⟩  **c** : a severe scolding ⟨got ~ for coming in late⟩  **d** : unrestrained fun or sportiveness ⟨the kids were full of ~⟩ — often used in the phrase *for the hell of it* esp. to suggest action on impulse or without a serious motive ⟨decided to go for the ~ of it⟩  **3** *archaic* : a tailor's receptacle  **4** — used as an interjection ⟨~, I don't know!⟩ or as an intensive ⟨hurts like ~⟩ ⟨funny as ~⟩; often used in the phrase *hell of a* ⟨it was one ~ of a good fight⟩ or *hell out of* ⟨scared the ~ out of him⟩ or with *the* or in ⟨moved way the ~ up north⟩ ⟨what in ~ is wrong, now?⟩ — **hell on** : very hard on or destructive to ⟨the constant traveling is *hell on* your digestive system⟩ — **hell or high water** : difficulties of whatever kind or size ⟨will stand by her convictions come *hell or high water*⟩ — **hell to pay** : dire consequences ⟨if he's late there'll be *hell to pay*⟩

¹**loom** \'lüm\ *n* [ME *lome* tool, loom, fr. OE *gelōma* tool; akin to MD *allame* tool] (15c) ; a frame or machine for interlacing at right angles two or more sets of threads or yarns to form a cloth
²**loom** *vi* [origin unknown] (ca. 1541)  **1** : to come into sight in enlarged or distorted and indistinct form often as a result of atmospheric conditions  **2 a** : to appear in an impressively great or exaggerated form ⟨deficits ~ed large⟩  **b** : to take shape as an impending occurrence
³**loom** *n* (1836) : the indistinct and exaggerated appearance of something seen on the horizon or through fog or darkness; *also* : a looming shadow or reflection

**lord of misrule** (15c) : a master of Christmas revels in England esp. in the 15th and 16th centuries

[ME, fr. OE; akin to OE helan to conceal, OHG helan, L celare, Gk kalyptein] (bef. 12c) . . ." Again, in the definition there was nothing unusual and no reference to "13c," only "before 12c."

Len theorized "suppose this means to search the word columns 'before' the word 'hell'" to find any '13c' or '12c' references?" As seen in figure 8.11, the first "13c" followed the word "heir"—again a Middle English [ME] term that means "1 : one who inherits or is entitled to inherit property 2 : one who inherits or is entitled to succeed to a hereditary rank, title, or office <~to the throne> 3 : one who receives or is entitled to receive some endowment or quality from a parent or predecessor . . . ² heir *vt* (14c) *chiefly dial* : INHERIT."

"What the hell does that mean?" Len objected out loud. "'Chiefly dial'?" To him that meant to simply manipulate the telephone numbers. "Maybe I'm going crazy," he thought. "Maybe I'm just projecting this horrifying conspiracy *into Webster's* text? Let me read what Webster said these numbers mean. Then I'll look up "dial," then return to "heir" for related numbers or 'hidden entries.'"

So Len looked up what *Webster's Dictionary* explained the numerical references "(12c), (13c), (14c) and (15c) meant. They were simply described as "[T]he style that names only a century (as 14c) is the one used for the period from the twelfth century through the fifteenth century, a span that, roughly approximates the period of Middle English." The "Dark Ages," Len realized.

"But that wouldn't explain this outlandish series of 'coincidences'—word relationships all bearing on prion crystals and their role in a coming biological apocalypse," he considered.

Moments later he read the definition of "chiefly dial" from *Webster's*, which was described as meaning a *dialectical* usage of a word "too complex for summary," befitting a Babel-like confusion of languages, and:

¹**dial** . . . [ME dyal, fr. ML *dialis* clock wheel revolving daily, fr. L dies day — more at DEITY] (15c) 1 : the face of a sundial 2 obs : timepiece 3 : the graduated face of a timepiece 4 a : a face upon which some measurement is registered usu. by means of graduations and a pointer . . . b: a device that may be operated to make electrical connections or to regulate the operation of a machine <a radio ~> <a telephone~>

Len immediately noted the relevance. "This is completely uncanny! This can't be a simple 'coincidence,'" he realized.

₂**dial** . . . (1821) 1 : to measure with a dial 2 a: to manipulate a device (as a dial) so as to operate, regulate, or select . . . b : CALL 1m(1) . . .1 : to manipulate a dial 2 : to make a telephone call or connection . . .

"Now I have to look up 'deity (15c)' that was cross referenced in 'dial'."

*Webster's* provided:

**deity** . . . [ME *deitee*, fr. OF deité, fr. LL *deitatdeitas*, fr. L *deus* god; akin to OE *Tiw*, god of war, L *divus* god, dies day, Gk dios heavenly, Skt deva heavenly, god] (14c) 1 a : the rank or essential nature of a god : DIVINITY b *cap* : GOD 1, SUPREME BEING 2 : a god or goddess <the *deities* of ancient Greece> 3 : one exalted or revered as supremely good or powerful

And as for the (15c)s following the word "diety"—

₁**deject** . . . *adj*(15c) *archaic* : DEJECTED

₂**deject** . . . *vt* [ME, to throw down, fr. L *dejectus*, pp. of *deicere*, fr. *de-* + *jacere* to throw — more at JET] (1581) : to make gloomy

**delate** . . . [L delatus (pp. of deferre to bring down, report, accuse), . . . to bear — more at tolerate](15c) 1 : accuse, denounce 2 : report, relate . . .

**delegacy** . . . *n, pl* -cies (15c) 1 : a body of delegates : board 2 a : the act of delegating b : appointment as delegate

And as for the (15c)s preceding the word "diety"—

**deil** . . . [ME *devel, del*] (15c) *Scot* : DEVIL

Finally, going back to "heir" to search the columns for related "century periods" or "hidden entries," Len first saw what is reprinted in figure 8.11. As shown, the definition of "₂**heir**" includes "(14c)." Below this is "**heir apparent**" defined as ". . . (14c) 1 : an heir whose right to an inheritance is indefeasible in law if he survives the legal

**Fig. 8.12. Cover of the *Report From Iron Mountain***

# REPORT FROM

# IRON MOUNTAIN

## ON THE

# POSSIBILITY

### AND

# DESIRABILITY

### OF

# PEACE

WITH INTRODUCTORY MATERIAL BY

## LEONARD C. LEWIN

THE DIAL PRESS, INC. 1967 NEW YORK

Cover from the *Report From Iron Mountain on the Possibility of Peace*, a publication commissioned by an unknown government agency or "secret society" with links to the U.S. federal government. Although published in 1967 by The Dial Press, Inc., the actual study group began meeting in secret in 1963 and predated the "Committee on the Economic Impact of Defense and Disarmament," headed by Gardner Ackley, of the Council of Economic Advisers, in response to presidential order that year. To achieve peace on earth the group advised policy makers to develop "either a giant space-research program, a comprehensive social-welfare program, or a master program of eugenic control. . . ." Two other options the group deemed marginally acceptable, providing "credibility" issues could be overcome included: 1) "Development of an acceptable threat from "outer space," presumably in conjunction with a space-research surrogate for economic control . . ." and "The environmental-pollution model . . . [effective] through arbitrary acceleration of current pollution trends . . ." (pp. xix and 86-87.)

# Fig. 8.13. Freemasonry Promotion by Dial Company President, John W. Teets

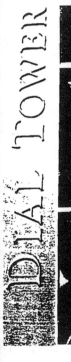

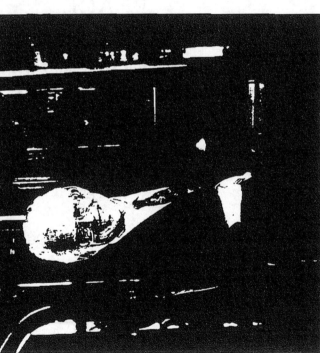

## JOHN W. TEETS

ACHIEVEMENTS IN EVERY FIELD OF HUMAN ENDEAVOUR THAT BENEFIT ALL MANKIND ARE NOT ONLY REWARDING FEATURES OF MASONRY. EQUALLY IMPORTANT ARE THE EFFECTS OF MASONIC IDEALS ON THE LIVES OF INDIVIDUALMASONS. THE TENETS OF THE CRAFT CAN AND DO INSPIRE AND ENRICH A MASON'S WHOLE LIFE – AS IS PERFECTLY EXEMPLIFIED IN THE CAREER OF JOHN TEETS, CHAIRMAN AND PRESIDENT OF AMERICA'S DIAL CORPORATION.

IN 1963 JOHN TEETS SUFFERED BOTH TRAGIC FAMILY LOSS, AND THE DESTRUCTION OF HIS THRIVING RETAIL BUSINESS. 'SUDDENLY,' HE RECALLED, 'AT AGE 30, I WAS A WIDOWED FATHER WITH TWO YOUNG DAUGHTERS AND OUT OF BUSINESS. IF EVER, HERE WAS A TRUE TEST FOR ONE'S EMOTIONAL AND SPIRITUAL FOUNDATIONS.' BUT HIS DEEP MASONIC COMMITMENT HELPED HIM TO REBUILD HIS LIFE. 'I'VE COME TO BELIEVE,' HE SAID, 'THAT MY PERSONAL TRIALS, ALONG WITH THE SENSE OF INDIVIDUAL RESPONSIBILITY INHERITED FROM MY FATHER AND TEMPERED THROUGH FREE-MASONRY, GAVE ME INNER STRENGTHS THAT PREPARED ME TO LEAD ONE OF AMERICA'S FORTUNE 500 FIRMS.'

From: *Freemasonry: A Celebration of the Craft.* Edited by John Hamill and Robert Gilbert, and published by Greenwich Editions in London, 1998.

ancestor 2 : heir presumptive 3 : one whose succession esp. to a position or role appears certain under existing circumstances."

Suddenly it dawned on him. "Dial—devil, the *Report from Iron Mountain*, the heir apparent of all the earthly possessions! *The Freemasons!*" Len flashed back to two documents, and spontaneously realized, "They're related!"

As shown in figures 8.12 and 8.13, *The Report From Iron Mountain* was published by "The Dial Press, Inc." Then, in the book *Freemasonry: A Celebration of the Craft* was John W. Teets, the "Chairman and President of America's Dial Corporation" was featured as a promoter of Freemasonry.

"Sure," Len considered. "The corporate crypto-fascists in secret societies create war and disease, 'hell' on earth, by 'manipulating,' 'confusing' and dividing the sheeple like the 'devils' they are—earthly 'dieties'—so they can inherit all the people's wealth and property. Makes total sense to me."

Then, two words down in *Webster's*, under the word "heirloom" which similarly involved inheritance, Len saw another cross reference to a hidden entry "— more at LOOM] (15c)" He flipped the pages to the word "loom." Then he saw the first definition of "loom" contained the "(15c)." It read, ". . . a frame or machine for interlacing at right angles two or more sets of threads or yarns to form a cloth."

"Like the 'fabric of society,'" Len considered. "'Frame' the masses of people and keep them interwoven in conflicting apposition so that you can steal their wealth and possessions."

Again he questioned his own sanity. "I need another 'reality check.' I might be just projecting all of this negativity into these definitions. Maybe it's just my blind bias that I'm exploring here. That could be. Dear God, let me know the truth. Guide me to the honest reality. All right," he thought. "Let me do just one more. I'll go to the next "(15c)" reference and see what it says." With that he reaffirmed, "God in heaven, help me learn the real truth here."

An instant later he saw it. As seen in figure 8.11 in bold black, a phrase that he had never seen or even heard of before. *Webster's* text read:

**lord of misrule** (15c) **:** a master of Christmas revels in England esp. in the 15th and 16th century.

## References

1. Anderson WAD and Scotti TM. *Synopsis of Pathology*: Eighth edition. St. Louis: The C. V. Mosby Company, 1972, p. 203.

2. Dunn DP. "Viral and slow viral infections of the central nervous system." In: *Internal Medicine for Dentistry*. Louis F. Rose and Donald Kaye, Eds. St. Louis: The C. V. Mosby Company, 1983, p. 828.

3. Martin WJ, Ahmed KN, Cheng Zeng L, et al. African green monkey origin of the atypical cytopathic 'stealth virus' isolated from a patient with chronic fatigue syndrome. *Clinical and Diagnostic Virology* 1995;4:93-103.

4. Martin WJ, Cheng Zeng L, Ahmed KN and Roy M. Cytomegalovirus-related sequence in an atypical cytopathic virus repeated isolated from a patient with chronic fatigue syndrome. *American Journal of Pathology* 1994;145;2:440-450.

5. Department of Defense Appropriations For 1970: Hearings Before A Subcommittee of the Committee on Appropriations House of Representatives, Ninety-first Congress, First Session, H.B. 15090, Part 5, Research, Development, Test and Evaluation, Dept. of the Army. U.S. Government Printing Office, Washington, D.C., 1969. The inclusion of David Baltimore as a chief suspect on the NAS-NRC is explained in Dr. Horowitz's previous text, on pages 404; 421 and 508-509.

6. According to those who defended against Dr. Horowitz's exposures in *Emerging Viruses: AIDS & Ebola*, concerning the genetic engineering of viruses that began at least in the 1960s during the "Special Virus Cancer Program," such gene manipulations could not have taken

place until 1975. This was falsely argued publicly by Drs. Robert Gallo and Anthony Fauci (Director of the National Institute for Allergies and Infectious Diseases) and *Coming Plagues* author Laurie Garrett. The fact is that crude, sloppy, and tedious methods of recombining bacteria and viruses were ongoing in the 1960s as definitively documented in Len's earlier works.

7. The link between herpesvirus contamination, including simian cytomegalovirus, and hepatitis B vaccines was made by Dr. Horowitz in conference with Dr. Martin when the former learned that the early 1970s hepatitis B vaccine was partially prepared at Merck-affiliated labs using viruses grown in rhesus monkeys and chimpanzees commonly contaminated with herpesviruses. Until then investigators had assumed the spread of simian cytomegalovirus was uniquely associated with polio vaccines derived partly from contaminated monkey kidney cell cultures.

8. Martin WR. "Stealth Viruses:" An oral presentation before the Twentieth Century Plagues symposia held at the Embassy Suites Hotel, Los Angeles, California, March 1-2, 1996. The document is available at URL# http://www.stealthvirus.com.

9. Contributing scientists. Ask the experts: Medicine—"What is a prion? Specifically, what is known about the molecular structure of prions and how they cause infections such as Creutzfeldt-Jakob disease? *Scientific American* Internet publication. Available from file:/// A/medicine14what is a prion.html.

10. Horowitz LG. *Emerging Viruses: AIDS & Ebola—Nature, Accident or Intentional?* Rockport, MA: Tetrahedron Publishing Group. 1998, pp. 313 and 509; for Woolsy's comments see p. 481.

11. CDC. Esceheria coli O157:h7 infections associated with eating a nationally distributed commercial brand of frozen ground beef patties and burgers. *MMWR*, August 22, 1997.

12. Staff writers. Tyson foods to buy rival Hudson foods. Reuters News Agency/UPI/AP, Chicago. September 4, 1997.

13. Kirsten-Tatlow D. Chicken imports halted due to bird flu death in woman. Associated Press News Service, December 23, 1997. (Available through the Internet at http://www.archive.abcnews.go. com/sections/living/fludeath1223/index.html.)

14. Horowitz L. *Op cit.*, pp. 120-125.

15. It is well known that Tyson is the chief supplier of chickens to the world. "Tyson Foods: Helping to Feed the World," an article on its website, explains from the company's "simple beginnings in 1931," they have grown to "become the largest and most-innovative poultry producer in the world. . . . Our universe nearly covers the globe. . . . Asia and the Pacific Rim countries" were relatively new acquisitions. "Today," their promotion stated on December 18, 1998, "we have established direct sales offices in Singapore, Hong Kong, Indonesia, Japan . . . and China."

16. Staff writers. Tyson Food's cornered, but top bosses go free. *Seattle Times*, Wednesday, January 7, 1998, pg. 1.

17. Crudele J. Probe inching toward White House. *NY Post*, August 28, 1997, p. 1.

18. Young RO. *Sick & Tired: Reclaim Your Inner Terrain*. Unpublished manuscript. Copyright 1997, by Dr. Robert O. Young, 134 East 200 North Alpine, Utah 84004, pp. 1-3; App. D., Sect. 1, p. 2.

19. Lynes B. *The Cancer Cure That Worked!* Toronto, Canada: Marcus Books, 1987, p. 127-136.

20. Starr P. *The Social Transformation of American Medicine: The rise of a sovereign profession and the making of a vast industry.* New York: Basic Books, 1982, p. 305.

21. Burton B. New type of DNA-free inheritance in yeast is spread by a "mad cow" mechanism. *Cell*, May 30, 1997. Press release from the University of Chicago. Available from: http://www.ucmc.uchicago. edu/news/1997/prionfibers.html.

22. Bastian FO. "Spiroplasma proposed as cause of Mad Cow Disease," an oral presentation before the American Medical Association's "Capital Conference," Washington, D.C., August 14, 1996. Related

citations provided by Dr. Bastian include: spiroplasma-like inclusions in brain biopsies from CJD patients (*Arch Pathol Lab Med.* 1979;103:665-6690; immunological cross reactivity study (*J Clin Biol.* 1987;25:2430-2431); and rodent inoculation neuropathology study (*American Journal of Pathology* 1984;114:496-514).

23. Clark HW. What is a Mycoplasma and how does it work? In: *The Intercessor*, Summer, 1993, published by The Road Back Foundation, 4985 N. Lake Hill Road, Delaware OH 43015-9249.

24. Nicolson GL and Nicolson NL. Diagnosis and treatment of mycoplasmal infections in Persian Gulf War illness—CFIDS Patients. *Int. J. Occupational Medicine, Immunology, and Toxicology.* 1996;5;1:69-78.

25. Horowitz LG, Riley J, Nicolson GL, and Richard L. *Gulf War Syndrome: The Spreading Epidemic Coverup.* Rockport, MA: Tetrahedron Publishing Group, 1997. (Available from the publisher by calling 1-888-50-VIRUS.)

26. McManners H. Scientists link GulfWar illness to vaccines and drugs. *London Sunday Times*, June 22, 1997. (A copy of the article is available from: Karin Schumacher, Vaccine Information & Awareness (VIA), 792 Pineview Drive, San Jose, CA 95117, 408-448-6658 (phone/fax) 408-397-4192 (voice mail/pager) via@ihot.com (email), and in the FTP Public access files through http://www.tetrahedron.org).

27. Nicolson GL and Nicolson NL. Written testimony of Dr. Garth L. Nicolson and Dr. Nancy L. Nicolson, Committee on Government Reform and Oversight: Subcommittee on Human Resource and Intergovernmental Relations, United States House of Representatives, April 2, 1996, p. 2-3.

28. Shenon P. Ex-CIA analysts assert cover-up on chemical risk to troops. *New York Times* News Service, Tuesday, Oct. 29, 1996.

29. *Washington Post* news staff. CIA knew of chemical weapons at Iraqi depot, agency reveals. *The St. Louis Post-Dispatch*, April 10, 1997, p. 1.

An extensive list of the biological weapons (BW) shipped from U.S. Government affiliated agencies and institutions to Iraq's leading biological weapons developers until just before the Gulf War was published in: *U.S. Chemical and Biological Warfare-related Dual Use Exports to Iraq and Their Possible Impact on the Health Consequences of the Persian Gulf War. A Report of Chairman Donald W. Riegle, Jr. and Ranking Member Alfonse M. D'Amato of the Committee on Banking, Housing and Urban Affairs with Respect to Export Administration.* United States Senate, May 25, 1994, pp. 38-47. Relatedly, this document provided knowledge that the CDC not only knew of these dangerous BW exports from the U.S. to Iraq, but apparently helped facilitate their transport. Included in the list of CDC cited exports was "West Nile Fever Virus," a relative of the incredibly deadly Ebola virus.

30. Associated Press. Officers suspected chemical [and biological] weapons but kept quiet. *North Virginia Daily*, February 26, 1997, p. A11.

31. Associated Press. Warning over Gulf War vaccine ignored: Soldiers not told drug unlicensed. *Press Democratic*, December 22, 1997, pg. 1.

32. Joint Hearing Before the Select Committee on Intelligence and the Subcommittee on Health and Scientific Research of the Committee on Human Resources, United States Senate, Ninety-fifth Congress, First Session, August 3, 1977. "Project MKULTRA, The CIA's Program of Research in Behavior Modification." Washington, D. C.: U.S. Government Printing Office, 1977 (Stock No. 052-070-04357-1), p. 388. The microbiology part of this overall "population and mind control" program, Project MKNAOMI, was reported here "To provide for the required surveillance, testing, upgrading, and evaluation of materials and items in order to assure absence of defects and complete predictability of results to be expected under operational conditions.

33. Rodriguez PM. Anti-HIV mix found in blood of Gulf War veterans. *The Washington Times*, National Weekly Edition, Aug 24, 1997,

p. 30. See also Rodriguez's excellent investigative reports in *Insight Magazine*, "Sickness and Secrecy," August 25, 1997, pp. 7-13, and "Gulf-War Mystery and HIV," November 3, 1997, p. 7.

34. Robiglio D. Gulf War ills blamed on inoculations: Retired Gen. Norman Schwarzkopf thinks some soldiers may be having adverse reactions to shots. *The Las Vegas Review Journal*, Saturday, Feb. 1, 1997, p. 19; See also Monday, Feb. 3, 1997, of the same paper for more on the story.

35. McAlvany DS. Special Report: Germ Warfare Against America: The Desert Storm Plague and Cover-up. *The McAlvany Intelligence Advisor*, (P. O. Box 84904, Phoenix, AZ 85071) August, 1996, pp. 1-40. For George Bush connections see p. 27.

36. Funk D. Pentagon slammed for testing drugs on troops / FDA still hasn't learned from Gulf War mistakes. *Navy Times*, October 27, 1997. p. 1.

37. Lo SC. Pathogenic Mycoplasma. United States Patent number 5,242,820, September 7, 1993. Assigned to the American Registry of Pathology, Washington, D.C. For cell cytoplasmic degenerative changes, including vacuolization, see p. 63.

38. It is well known that Robert Gallo and Carlton Gadjusek, a convicted pedophile, were good friends besides research colleagues. Gallo, in fact, paid a large share of Gadjusek's bail when he was initially arrested for sexually abusing his "adopted" children. See: Maass P. Colleague defends accused NIH scientist: Friend says law enforcement "setup" led to sexual abuse charges. *Washington Post*, April 8, 1996, p.1.

For Gajdusek's early chimpanzee studies using HTLV-III, see Gajdusek, D.C., et al., *Lancet* I, 1415 (1984), and *Lancet* I, 55 (1985).

39. Lo SC, Wear DJ, Green SL, Jones PG and Legrei JF. Adult respiratory distress syndrome with or without systemic disease associated with infection due to mycoplasma fermentans. *Clinical Infectious Diseases* 1993;17 (Suppl. 1):S259-63.

40. Materials submitted for publication by Candice Brown and lead investigator Will Northrop. See: Northrop W. and Migdall S. Re-

port of investigation: The TDC employee case, Huntsville, TX, Sept.-Oct. 1997 developed on behalf of two New York law firms—Goodkind Labaton Rudolf & Sucharow and Curtis V. Trinko, LLP. For Dr. Nicolson's report see: Nicolson GL, Hyman E, Korenyi-Both A, Lopez DA, Nicolson N, Rea W, and Urnovitz H. Progress on Persian Gulf War Illnesses—Reality and hypotheses. *International Journal of Occupational Medicine and Toxicology* 1995;4;3:1. Galley Copy.

41. Anonymous author. Prion creation theory myth. Internet: Mad Cow Home website, http://www.cyber-dyne.com/~tom/griff.html.

42. This theory, that prion crystals are activated by electromagnetic frequencies, was initially advanced without Dr. Horowitz's knowledge by a leading expert in bioelectrical medicine—Dr. Jacques Benveniste, at the University of Paris. Dr. Benveniste communicated his thesis in writing to French prion researchers and public health officials to no avail. Dr. Benveniste informed Dr. Horowitz of this fact during a clustered water conference sponsored by CellCore International Corporation in Irvine, California, on June 8, 1999.

43. According to Spanish investigative journalist Roman Ribera Canet, the Baker and Bush families "have deep roots in the eugenics movement . . . aligned with Harriman–Rockefeller interests. James A. Baker, grandfather of James Baker III, . . . started Rice University and created its biology department with the help of Julian Huxley in 1912. Years later, Huxley, as vice president of the British Eugenics Society, aided the Nazi Ministry of the Interior to develop "racial hygiene" programs.

James A. Baker III's major stock holdings include: Exxon, ARCO, Kerr McGee, and Merck, Sharp & Dohme, according to Mr. Canet.

Personal communication from Roman Ribera Canet, October 22, 1999.

# Chapter 9.
# The Fungus Among Us

The next day, Len called Joey.

"Joey, I'm coming over. I've got something unbelievable to share with you."

"Fine. I'll finish up with my last patient; then we'll spend some time together."

An hour later Len was at Joey's doorstep when the front door opened and out walked Joey with one of his patients. "Hey, Len! Great to see you. This is Marjorie."

After a brief introduction, Joey continued. "We've been treating Marge here with some herbs for her respiratory infection that she's had for weeks. She went to her medical doctor, but his antibiotics didn't work."

"That's right," Marjorie confirmed. "I had a miserable cough and was congested for two months. Now I'm rapidly improving."

"That's odd. That's exactly what Jackie, my wife, has been suffering with. What kind of an infection is it?" Len asked.

"It's a fungus," Joey replied. "We're almost certain of that."

"A respiratory fungus?"

"That's what I've got to tell you about. You're not going to believe what I've found," Joey challenged.

The two doctors said good-bye to Marjorie and retreated into Joey's house. They walked straight to Joey's office where Len was so interested and surprised at what Joey began to explain, that he momentarily forgot what he came to share. Len had been very concerned about Jackie who had been sick for about eight weeks with an upper respiratory flu—what they thought was a lingering virus.

Meanwhile, over the previous several months, and even more that week, Joey had an influx of similar cases—patients, family, friends, and neighbors too, who complained of similar symptoms. Various people with upper respiratory conditions were flocking to Joey's with malaise, fatigue, low body temperature, nasal congestion, and coughs. Most had tried and failed to respond to antibiotics. Even Joey's traditional antiviral and anti-flu naturopathic remedies failed at first. The only things that seemed to work, Joey said, were antifungal therapies. "'These people have fungal infections in their sinuses and lungs,' Jeshua told me. 'This isn't a flu, though it has flu-like symptoms. The infection is really a fungus.' But wait till you see what I dug up on the Internet. It's going to blow your mind."

"Before you blow my mind, just tell me what I can do for Jackie. It's not like her to be so sick for so long."

"I'll be right back. I'll get you some 'beta tea.'" Joey left the room and returned a minute later with a plastic bag filled with a remedy he had put together. He based it on his research of antifungal herbs, using the code charts provided in chapter six.

He told Len the story of how he came to develop and test the tea on his patients. Among the first to try the remedy was Dr. Dora Lofstrom, a Ph.D. and naturopathic physician, who had visited Joey from San Diego. She had followed Joey's recommendations with her patients who exhibited similar symptoms. They tried his antifungal tea, and experienced dramatic improvements. Realizing there was something special about his Bible code formulations, Dr. Lofstrom later brought her seventy-year-old mother to Joey for treatment, as well as further instruction in using the Bible codes.

Dr. Lofstrom's mother also had this strange respiratory disease for more than two months. After naturopathic treatments failed, she sent her mother to medical doctors whose antibiotics likewise failed. Then they informed her that her mother had an "infection of the myocardial sack," that is, the connective tissue envelope surrounding her heart. Along with this, the old woman experienced heart palpitations and a very strange acid indigestion that she never had before, with severe burping and acid reflux that worsened following her coughing spells.

So Joey began treatment with the beta tea, and another herb tonic that contained cayenne pepper that Joey knew would raise the Spanish woman's body temperature from subnormal to 98.6 degrees Fahrenheit—where it ought to be.

After four days of this treatment the woman began to improve. She ate without needing to take antiacid tablets, and no longer was getting heart palpitations. She even resumed cooking and eating her normal spicy Spanish meals, made with onions, peppers and tomatoes, that, to her chagrin, she was unable to eat for weeks. Within fourteen days Dr. Lofstrom's mother was completely healed. Even the infection around her heart disappeared.

## Fighting A Fungus

So Joey had been on the Internet for several months researching a suspected relationship between fungal infections and flu-like symptoms and much more.

"There were several news releases on the web last week that I downloaded this weekend," Joey said. "They talked about strange epidemics of flu-like illnesses that had filled health care centers in Los Angeles and elsewhere with patients. He handed a few of the downloaded reports over to Len. "And people keep coming to me with these symptoms.

"I'll bet the Los Angeles outbreak[1] is the same thing we're seeing here in Northern Idaho—a fungal infection. All of the symptoms are similar. The fluctuating and typically low body temperatures are unlike respiratory viral infections. The cough, chronic sinus congestion, lack of antibiotic response, digestive symptoms, are all most common. These cases are being reported around the country. And what I've noticed is that they all seem to pop up at the same time. I've gone for weeks with no one coming in with these symptoms, then suddenly, within 48 hours, I've got two dozen people on my antifungal regimen."

"That is odd," Len replied. "I know what Jackie's been going through. The funny thing is, no one else in our family got it, neither I nor the girls. And Jackie is typically the healthiest of all.

Besides the herbal remedies, how else have you been treating these people?"

Joey replied, "I told everyone to detox, deacidify, and boost immunity; to make dietary changes, including eliminating dairy products which form mucous, and sugars that exacerbate fungal infections. Patients did best and got better faster when they followed these recommendations. Oxygenation and bioelectric therapies have also been helpful.

"Sugars were particularly important to eliminate from their diet because they greatly changed body chemistry. Sugar-sweetened foods reduced blood pH [—the acid/base chemistry index—] and increase body acidity. This provided an environment ripe for fungal growth.[2] Also," Joey continued, "patients who increased their blood oxygen levels through various means, from exercise to dietary supplements, hastened their healing."

## A New CJD Transmission Theory

Joey grabbed the first of several articles he had stacked on his desk and handed them over to Len. "Are you ready to have your mind blown?"

"Sure," Len encouraged. "But that won't be so easy. Wait till you hear what I have to share with you. It's gonna knock your socks off."

"Here read this," Joey returned. "I found it while researching 'fungus' on the web." He handed the article to Len.

"You've got to be kidding! This is the same article I just read last night!"

"No."

"Yes!" Len exclaimed incredulously. "The *Cell* article that links the mad cow disease prion to yeast and crystals! I can't believe you're giving me this. You know I spent the weekend with Robert Cohen and Howard Lyman at BYU. I came back and investigated a few questions that Robert raised. I pulled this same article out of my mad cow disease file. I don't even know who sent it to me."[3]

Joey replied, "Well brother, we're off on the same track. Jeshua directed me to this on the Internet."

Len looked up from the page into Joey's serious brown eyes. "The concept of prions being crystals stunned me," he said. "Little receivers and transmitters of electromagnetic energies. That's possibly why prions go to the brain. They're likely attracted to the microcurrents the nerve cells generate."

"You're right," Joey concurred. "Did you see who's behind this work?"

"Yeah. I balked at that as well. The University of Chicago—Gallo and Rockefeller terrain, and the Howard Hughes Medical Institute funded the study. Do you recall that *Citizen Hughes*—a biography on the aerospace mogel—was written by *The Bible Code* disinformation specialist Michael Drosnin?" Len asked.

"Eerie."

"And I don't buy their disclaimer that people who eat bread or drink beer are not at risk," Len continued. "Not if you can't kill the prion at normal sterilization temperatures. And prion-like proteins spread through yeast!"

"I'll bet most of the prions are being passed through grains," Joey returned.

"Why do you say that?"

"Because yeast is a form of fungus. The prions can grow in fungus. Fungi grow in grains. That's how it's likely being spread all around the world. *Principally in grains.*"

Len probably would have put up some resistance to Joey's theory had he not discovered what he had the previous day. "If that's true, then the mad *cow* headlines are a distraction," he replied. "And that would make sense. Sure, the old magician's trick. 'Look over here, but don't look over there—look at the cows and meat, but don't look at how they really became infected.' That's what they did with AIDS and Ebola as well.[12] Gallo directed people to 'look at the monkeys in the African jungles,' but not at what he did to them in his labs with colleagues from Litton Bionetics. And Richard Preston did the same thing with Ebola in *The Hot Zone*. It fits the counterintelligence pattern.

"It never made total sense to me," Len continued. "Cows may have been infected by eating sheep brain in cattle feed, but that couldn't explain the entire epidemic, nor the other TSEs in deer, elk, mink, and chickens."[4,5]

Joey interrupted, "Fungal contaminated grains would explain it. Read the next two articles about wild animals getting sick." The areas Joey had highlighted read:

> The emaciated mule deer stares blankly into space. Then, stumbling in small circles, it falls over dead, another victim of chronic wasting disease.
>
> It is a grim sight for wildlife officials working in the Rocky Mountains on the border of Colorado and Wyoming . . . For health officials, a frightening question must be answered: Will this terrible illness cross over to the human population?
>
> The National Institutes of Health is investigating because mad cow disease, similar to the chronic wasting disease that has struck mule deer and elk, has been linked to a brain-wasting malady in humans—Creutzfeldt-Jakob disease. . . .[6]
>
> An illness similar to mad cow disease appears to have spread to a captive Nebraska elk herd from elk and deer in bordering states according to wildlife researchers.
>
> Chronic wasting disease (CWD) has been found already in herds of elk and deer in South Dakota, Wyoming, Colorado and Saskatchewan, Canada. The disease is a form of [transmissible] spongiform encephalopathy (TSE), connected to the so-called mad cow disease that recently has plagued the United Kingdom. . . .[7]

Finally, the report stated that this sudden expansive spread of TSE in wild animals was because "elk and deer chew on the bones of sheep that have been infected with scrapie."[7]

"I don't buy that," Len protested. "Maybe one or two cases here and there, but wild elk and deer are obviously not typically carnivorous, nor cannibalistic. They're reporting the spreading epidemic in wild herds covering virtually all of North America!"

"Here's my theory," Joey replied, "The prion is being passed through a fungus in grain. Fungi grow readily in corn, wheat, oats, and barley. The animals that are getting TSE in the wild are *not eating meat, nor even farm animal feed.* They are eating grains growing out in the wild or on fertilized farm fields.

"Moreover," Joey continued, "grains are being harvested and used to feed pigs, cows, and chickens. Pigs are also getting mad cow disease, but the government is largely avoiding the issue. Pig feces is being used to fertilize grain crops. Swine waste runs into rivers and streams where new neurological diseases are popping up in fish and humans. Like this new *Pfiesteria piscicida* infection of fish. It's causing Alzheimer's-like symptoms in humans. Many cases of CJD are being misdiagnosed in the United States as Alzheimer's disease. In Maryland and elsewhere, hog feces have been found to stimulate *Pfiesteria* toxicity. Just like in mad cow disease, some external protein, virus, 'stealth-virus,' or the like, suddenly stimulates this prion crystal to grow. Then the crystals destroy brain cells. I'll bet it's all coming from fungi infected grains. Here, read these reports too. . . ."

## Where's the Pork?

Indeed, Joey's theory, based on the supportive documentation he handed Len, seemed credible. A variety of fungi typically grew in grains including wheat, oats, corn, and barley.[8] Many fungi had in fact been genetically engineered in efforts to prevent a spectrum of plant diseases. As the *Cell* article[3] revealed, yeast, "a true fungi whose usual growth form is unicellular," according to *Steadman's Medical Dictionary,*[9] can carry the prion. This, researchers explained, transmitted the catalyst that made the protein prion crystallize and then grow in human and animal brains. The media largely overlooked the fact that potentially contaminated grains were being fed to cattle and pigs far more than infected sheep brains. Pigs had received little attention as far as

311

carriers and transmitters of prions and TSEs. Grain had received virtually no attention. Yet, Joey's documentation clearly showed an equal, if not more severe, risk of prion infection in swine populations as well as in cows. He produced documentation that showed that fungi-infected grains had been shipped to various areas where new neurological ailments were being reported in wildlife as well as domestic herds. Though not a definitive epidemiological study, Joey gave Len enough documentation to advance a definitive CJD transmission hypothesis beginning with agriculturally infected feed.

Figure 9.1 provides a map of the United States in which areas that received fungi infected grain shipments are highlighted. As reported by the U.S. Department of Agriculture, the map shows areas that correspond to these shipments and to overlapping areas of uncommon infectious disease outbreaks, mostly fungal in nature, including neurological illnesses like those seen in TSEs.

According to an Agricultural Department report on "Phase One Attack on Wheat Fungus" reported on August 21, 1996, the entire state of Arizona was placed on alert and quarantine for Karnal bunt infection. The wheat fungus and quarantine soon spread to areas of New Mexico, West Texas, and eastern California following wheat shipments to those areas, according to the government report. "Hot spots" of infection were, oddly enough, centered in the largely Native American counties of "Yavapai, Conconino, Navajo, Apache, Gila, Greenlee, and Santa Cruz, and from portions of Mohave and Pima counties in Arizona; from portions of Hidalgo, Luna, and Sierra counties in New Mexico; and from a portion of Hudspeth County in Texas."[10]

Three years later the U.S. Department of Agriculture, along with its Arizona state affiliate, were still scrambling to contain the wheat fungus outbreak. "Seeds carrying Karnal bunt spores," the Associated Press reported, "may have gone to fields free of the fungus."

An embarrassed Arizona Department of Agriculture director, Sheldon R. Jones, explained that his agency had inadequately tested some 232 tons of seeds that may have contaminated all of southern

# Fig. 9.1. Distribution of Infected Grain Possibly Associated With Neurological Disorders Including TSEs.

1—By March, 1996, the entire state of Arizona had been placed on quarantine for infected wheat (Karnal bunt), as well as areas of New Mexico, and west Texas. A "Declaration of Extraordinary Emergency" was declared by Secretary of Agriculture Dan Glickman.

2—Contaminated wheat was tracked to California and the quarantine was enlarged to include Imperial County and the eastern part of Riverside County, California.

3—Contaminated wheat shipments were soon tracked to Montana. The public believed that authorities had controlled the outbreak by destroying infected grain supplies, but prions could have easily survived. It is likely some of the processed wheat or protein prions were transmitted to Montana wastewaters and rivers subsequently infecting wildlife throughout the state. Besides dear and elk getting sick with TSEs, trout developed "whirling disease," at that time. In addition, herds of elk and deer in South Dakota, Wyoming, Colorado and Saskatchewan, Canada were reported affected.

According to U. S. Govt. reports, the infected wheat could have been processed into flour, or animal feed, or even shipped unprocessed to other countries.

4—Fungal infected wheat and other grains clearly made their way to the East Coast infecting swine diets and later river fish polluted with *Physteria piscicida* and related mycotoxins. "Whirling disease," with many similar symptons of neurological and immune system impairment as fungal and prion infections, occurred first in North Carolina in 1988 among laboratory scientists whose cultures had been contaminated from some "unknown" source. At virtually the same time infected wheat reached the Southwest, during the Mohave Desert outbreak, fishermen became intoxicated, and fell ill with similar symptoms by touching, eating, or breathing mycotoxins associated with their contaminated catch.

5—Whirling disease made its way from the mid-Atlantic and Gulf Coast states to Montana.

Adapted from: USDA Animal and Plant Health Inspection Service staff. Agriculture Department completes Phase One attack on wheat fungus: Actions protect wheat exports. August 21, 1996. U.S. Department of Agriculture. The six-page report is available through the Agriculture Department's website. See file:///A/et2_8-22 Wheat Fungus, htm

Arizona's wheat crop. "We are not pleased that our staff apparently misused filtering equipment and we are working to ensure this is an isolated incident," he promised.[10]

The Arizona Mohave desert area was likewise the site of a unique outbreak of a flu-like illness with neurological and gastrointestinal (GI) symptoms.[11] Suspiciously, this occurred *at the same exact time the fungal infected wheat was being identified* by Arizona Department of Agriculture seed analyst Ron Ykema. By Tuesday, March 5, 1996, Ykema had sent USDA plant pathologist Joel Floyd, with the Plant Protection and Quaranine (PPQ) program at Nogales, fungi infected wheat samples. At that time patients were coming into Dr. Donovan Anderson's office complaining of these symptoms along with immune suppression and chronic fatigue. In the weeks that followed, these cases were investigated by Dr. Anderson, 'stealth virus' expert W. John Martin, and several other health scientists.[11]

Likewise, at that time, public health authorities had issued warnings about possible Hantaan virus outbreaks in the Mohave Desert area, in Indian populations, allegedly linked to "rodent infections." The deadly Hantaan hemorrhagic fever virus, authorities said, had evolved suddenly in Bolivia from "deforestation." Trees had been uprooted to make way for cornfields and cattle farms. This most likely contributed to the sudden, inexplicable development of a bizarre human pathogen with no known original host, claimed world expert Karl Johnson.

Johnson had, by the way, become world famous for his heroics in Richard Preston's bestselling propaganda piece *The Hot Zone*. Preston's thesis advanced the same indefensible "deforestation" assertion—that as people cut down the African rain forest, deadly new viruses spontaneously jumped up their butts. Preston's "Kitum cave" in fact, in which the original African Ebola transmission was alleged to have occurred, concealed the Litton Bionetics lab operating in the same vicinity on behalf of the Pentagon.[12]

At the time Karl Johnson was, according to *The Los Angeles Times*, fishing near his Bozeman, Montana, retirement home, Dr. Anderson's patients were entering his clinic with the bizarre Mohave Desert disease. Johnson's problem at that time was that Montana's fish were dying before he could catch them. A strange "whirling disease" had suddenly made its way from twenty other mostly eastern states to affect prize rainbow trout—Johnson's fly-fishing game.[13]

"Whirling disease" in fish, said to be "caused" by *Pfiesteria piscicida*, was never known anywhere before 1988 when it suddenly emerged at the North Carolina State University's (NCSU) School of Veterinary Medicine in "a novel [fish] culture" sent from "origin unknown," according to a NCSU Aquatic Botany Laboratory report.[14] Most of the symptoms of intoxication, oddly enough, related to those seen in Mohave Desert patients as well as TSE cases. Thirteen NCSU researchers who initially worked with the "dilute toxic cultures of *Pfiesteria* sustained mild to serious adverse health impacts through water contact or by inhaling toxic aerosols. . . . " The effects included "a suite of symptoms such as narcosis (a 'drugged' effect), development of sores [on the contact sites of the skin, face and chest], uniform reddening of the eyes, severe headaches, blurred vision, nausea/vomiting, sustained difficulty breathing (asthma-like effects), kidney and liver dysfunction, acute short-term memory loss, and severe cognitive impairment (serious difficulty in being able to read, remember one's name, dial a telephone number, or do simple arithmetic beyond 1+2=3). . . . Some of these effects recurred (relapsed) in people following strenuous exercise, thus far, up to six years after exposure."[14] The NCSU news service added the symptoms of disorientation, mood swings, and impaired immune systems, followed direct exposure to the intoxicated fish. Later outbreaks, they said, had apparently been linked to *Pfiesteria* activated "by human sewage and swine effluent spills."[15]

So whirling disease, along with fungi infected wheat, and transmissible mycotoxicity, had found its way to Montana, according to the U.S. government. The U.S. Dept. of Agriculture reported that in Montana, just at the time of the Mohave Desert outbreak, contaminated wheat had been destroyed. They failed, however, to mention that the destruction process might have left prions, and possibly fungal mycotoxins, intact and transmissible.

Astonishingly, the authorities reported on what was to be done with the wheat infected with fungi, and potentially prions as well. They cited four options including: "(1) shipment to a flour mill within the quarantine area (flour can move freely once it is processed; mill by-products have to be heat-treated [the prion, remember, is heat resistant to well over 1000 degrees Fahrenheit] or moved under restriction); (2) use as animal feed provided it is subjected to heat treatment; (3) destruction [without mention of disposal]; or (4) movement to export if the country of destination will accept it."[10]

"Here's a situation where man is the culprit again," Karl Johnson lectured on the problem manifesting in Montana's fish. "The things we have done to nature have given us something we have all enjoyed, but we poisoned our own well," he admitted. "Almost all of these things that come at us from nature are our responsibility."[13]

Indeed, Joey's hypothesis was frighteningly credible.

## Vegetarian CJD Linked to British Water Supply

Early support for Joey's theory came from the *London Times* in a story written by Robin Young.[16] An investigation into a cluster of CJD cases in Kent, England had led to "fresh allegations that the domestic water supply could be a possible source of infection. . . . A former building contractor at a plant rendering the carcasses of slaughtered cattle which may have been infected with BSE claims that liquid waste was poured down a well. . . .

"Alan Colchester, consultant neurologist at Guy's Hospital in London, who has treated three of the new-variant CJD cases from Kent, has already voiced his concern over a possible link with infected water" leaked from the rendering plant's well. All new CJD cases, Young reported, "lived within 20 miles of the rendering plant."

New claims of prion contaminated water came only "days after the 22nd victim of new-variant CJD was identified. The case of Clare

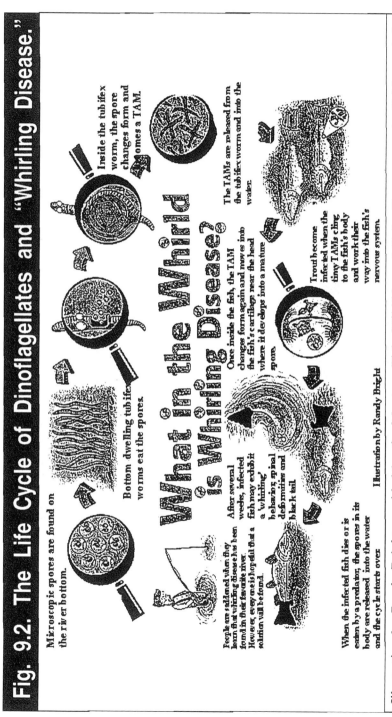

**Fig. 9.2. The Life Cycle of Dinoflagellates and "Whirling Disease."**

Microscopic spores are found on the river bottom.

Bottom dwelling tubifex worms eat the spores.

Inside the tubifex worm, the spore changes form and becomes a TAM.

The TAMs are released from the tubifex worm and into the water.

Trout become infected when the tiny TAMs cling to the fish's body and work their way into the fish's nervous system.

Once inside the fish, the TAM changes form again and moves into the fish's cartilage near the head where it develops into a mature spore.

After several weeks, infected fish may exhibit a "whirling" behavior, spinal deformities and black tail.

When the infected fish dies or is eaten by a predator, the spores in its body are released into the water and the cycle starts over.

People are saddened when they learn that whirling disease has been found in their favorite river. However, everyone is hopeful that a solution will be found.

**What in the Whirld is Whirling Disease?**

Illustration by Randy Bright

Illustration by Randy Bright provided by the Montana Fish, Wildlife, and Parks Department. Available on their website at http://btc.montana.edu/watercenter/docs/whirling/whirldwd.html

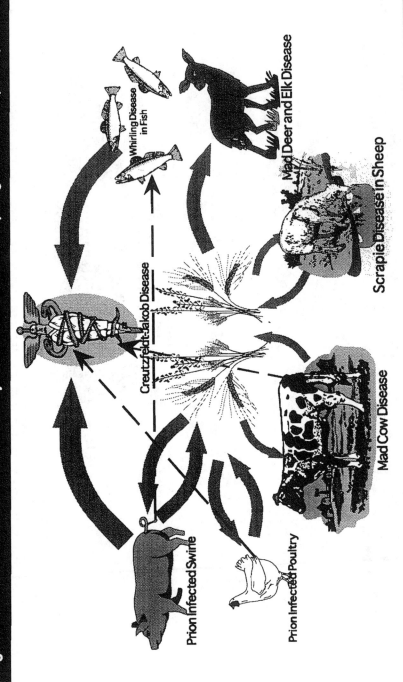

**Fig. 9.3. A New Transmission Theory for Transmissible Spongiform Encephalopathies**

In the United States, by 1999, an estimated 200,000 cases of Creutzfeldt-Jakob disease had been misdiagnosed as Alzheimer's disease. The rapid spread of this rare disease, transmitted by prion crystals that have been shown to transmit their inheritance in fungi, is most likely due to the infection routes diagramed above. Placing fungal infected grain at the center of the transmissible spongiform encephalopathies (TSEs) debate reconciles the rapid and widespread appearance of these new, yet clinically related, epidemics in various species and locations.

Tomkins, 24, from Tonbridge, in a different water area, . . . had raised fears about sources of infection because she has been a vegetarian since 1985, before the first case of BSE."

During subsequent interviews, Clare Tomkins's father said she had been a "strict vegetarian" since 1985. She even refused biscuits if they contained animal fats, and she avoided foods containing gelatin. The foods she consumed had to be made of "vegetable fats," Mr. Tomkins explained. The family often joked about how hard Clare was to feed.[16b]

Scientists questioned whether or not Clare might have "caught CJD from mechanically recovered food eaten before 1985," Mr. Tomkins said. "If my daughter was infected before 1985, then we have a CJD time bomb within the country."[16c]

In response to the news, John Pattison, the chairman of the British Government's Spongiform Encephalopathy Advisory Committee (SEAC), said that the case represented the longest incubation period seen with prion related CJD. "The fact that this woman was a vegetarian for such a long time is an unusual feature and we will think about what the implications for that are," he said.

Based on the evidence, scientists felt that other dairy products, including milk and cheese, were potentially risky for the spread of CJD. The article relayed Dr. Pattison's belief that these products needed to be "reassessed" as possibly prion vectors. Professor Richard Lacey, who first highlighted the BSE threat in England, cautioned scientists against dismissing the possibility that milk, with low concentrations of prion, over time, might be as deadly as eating highly infected beef and pork. "The experiments (using milk) are not satisfactory," Dr. Lacy explained. "It just means you can't pump enough infected milk into a mouse. But milk might be infectious if consumed over a long period."[16c]

Besides allegations that the cattle waste processing plant had dumped infected liquid into its well, the company was also reported to have "spread its effluent across fields above an aquifer from which drinking water" was taken. This was hypothetically linked to Ms. Tonbridge's CJD.

Mr. Skillet, a former contractor for the plant said: "Basically, they put down the well whatever they could get down it. They used an electrically operated pump . . . the well was used with everybody's knowledge to pump away materials they could not get rid of any other way."

Dr. Colchester was so "shocked" to learn that his patients possibly developed CJD because of this, he contacted the Department of the Environment to investigate further. A subsequent meeting with agency officials produced further shock and dismay when they were caught covering up incriminating evidence.

"I later discovered that, within hours of the meeting," Dr. Colchester said, "a key part of the evidence had, on the instruction of the Environment Agency, been removed by blocking off a pipe. The Environment Agency undermined my confidence in how thoroughly they were carrying out the investigation.

"In my opinion," Dr. Colchester concluded, "it is very likely that the new-variant CJD is BSE in man. . . . The route of infection has not been proven, but I think it is most likely by the oral route, which is the greatest risk. If it was through liquid, then it would probably be suspended particles within water."

## Consumers Petition the FDA

More support for Joey's grain fungus–cattle–pig connection to various forms of TSE came two days after Robin Young's article appeared in the *London Times*. The Consumers Union (CU) petitioned the U.S. Food and Drug Administration (FDA) regarding the prion risk posed by unregulated swine waste and swine products.[17]

To summarize, the union told the FDA to upgrade its rules concerning the use of swine tissues in animal feed. They wrote, on April 28, 1997, that the FDA's "draft rule is not adequate to protect public health, because it would continue to leave the door open for a porcine TSE to contaminate pork and other meat."

That year the FDA had proposed banning the use of ruminant and mink tissue protein in farm feeds. The CU noted that this did not cover the risks posed by infected pigs. Why exclude pigs "from the definition of 'any mammalian tissue?'" they asked the FDA.

Regarding the risks posed by the FDA's ill-conceived policy draft, and virtual neglect of the dangers associated with feeding prion contaminated pig meal to other animals, the CU wrote:

> [W]e think that this draft rule sends a particularly dangerous message. The draft rule suggests, that of all mammals, pigs are the safest and/or least likely to be infected with a TSE. We think this message is incorrect. Evidence from a number of sources suggests that pigs may already be infected with a TSE or TSE-like disease. The evidence comes from a 1979 USDA study of pigs and from two epidemiological studies that link consumption of pork to human TSE Creutzfeldt Jakob Disease (CJD).
>
> In brief, the 1979 study involved 106 pigs that exhibited similar clinical behaviors consistent with CNS symptoms. The study consisted of both clinical and pathological work. Known infectious diseases were ruled out. Thirteen of the affected pigs were filmed to document the subtle CNS symptoms. A pathological examination of the brains of these animals revealed no consistent patterns. The brain of one pig (#2709), however, had evidence suggestive of a TSE (vacuolation of neurons, astrocytosis). The Pathologist-in-Charge at the USDA's Eastern Pathology lab, who examined the brain, stated that the pathologic evidence was similar to that seen in scrapie and transmissible mink encephalopathy and diagnosed the case as "Encephalopathy and diffuse gliosis [astrocytosis] of undetermined etiology."
>
> Since BSE had not emerged in 1979, nothing came of the USDA work. However, the USDA inspector who did the 1979 study noticed that the symptoms displayed by cows with BSE were remarkably similar to the behaviors seen in the pigs in 1979. Indeed, virtually all the behaviors mentioned as characteristic of BSE in a USDA training video containing footage from BSE-affected cattle in the UK are also seen in the pigs from the 1979 study in the film of 13 affected pigs. . . .

In November, 1996, the USDA sent a single slide from pig brain #2709 to Dr. William Hadlow, a retired USDA researcher and one of the foremost veterinary pathology experts on TSEs in the world. He found evidence suggestive of a TSE, but felt that it would be useful to see sections from other portions of the brain.[17]

So the USDA sent Dr. Hadlow seven more slides containing other parts of the pig's brain. Unfortunately, the staining technique that they used had suddenly undermined his identification technique. "Surprise, surprise," Len complained to Joey. "Thus, Hadlow was forced to conclude, "Because of the extremely pale staining, neither spongiform change nor neuronal degeneration/loss is identified with certainty."[18]

Nonetheless the CU continued to describe Hadlow's disconcerting findings suggestive of TSE including diffuse astrocytosis characteristic of TSEs. . . ."

They reminded the FDA, "Should neurologic disease occur in swine exposed to that agent, conceivably it could be expressed microscopically mainly by astrocytosis, as is scrapie in some sheep, and as is the encephalopathy in cattle experimentally infected with the scrapie agent from American sheep."[18]

Moreover, the CU added to its knowledge that at least two epidemiologic studies in the scientific literature had addressed the issue of dietary risk factors for CJD. Both found links to pork. One research team compared 38 CJD patients with their healthy relatives. The authors concluded that "the practice [of eating brains] was more frequent among" CJD sufferers. These patients also had a greater preference for eating *hog* brains.[19]

In the second study, other coinvestigators found that their data also suggested for CJD victims "a dose-response relationship" for most of the processed meats. They found a positive association for smoked pork, deli ham/canned ham, hot dogs and scrapple."[16] This team concluded that, by 1985, there was already a good chance a TSE agent was in the nation's hog supply. They further wrote, "The present study indicated that consumption of pork as well as its processed products (e.g., ham, scrapple) may be considered as risk factors in the development of

Creutzfeldt–Jakob disease. While scrapie has not been reported in pigs, a subclinical form of the disease, or a pig reservoir for the scrapie agent, might conceivably exist."[20]

Besides the CU informing the FDA of the "very disturbing" fact that "evidence from a pig study and human studies both point to an unrecognized TSE in pigs . . . " they also related the growing epidemic of Alzheimer's disease to infected swine as well. "A number of studies," they wrote, "suggest that CJD may be misdiagnosed as Alzheimer's disease or other senile dementia and that a small percentage of the Alzheimer's cases are actually CJD.[17]

In one study at University of Pittsburgh, researchers found 5.5 percent of 54 Alzheimer's, or other dementia patients, had been misdiagnosed—they really had CJD.[21] A similar study conducted at Yale found more than twice that amount of misdiagnosed cases—13 percent.[22] Even at that small percentage rate, the CU concluded, with more than two million Alzheimer's cases in the United States today, there is likely a "hidden CJD epidemic" of approximately 200,000 cases!

## Swine Excrement and Deadly Fish

"Do you know what the histopathology [that is, microanatomy of diseased tissues] in pig encephalopathy described by Hadlow reminds me of?" Len asked Joey.

"What?"

"John Martin's 'stealth virus' associated encephalopathy slides. I reviewed those yesterday as well. The astrocytosis and the nerve cell vacuolation; all occurring with virtually no challenge by the immune system. The prion disease might be linked to Martin's 'stealth virus' research, and the 'stealth virus' might even be transmitted by a spiroplasma, a mycoplasma and/or a fungus like the prion is.

"In other words, we're likely dealing with co-infections or combinations of infectious agents that get into the body and, all tolled, induce a spectrum of neuroendocrine and immune-system related disorders that we are calling different names."

"I considered the fungus as a co-factor or delivery system for prion diseases," Joey replied. "Here, check this out." He rummaged through his desk drawers for another article. "Ahh, here it is."

The article's title was "Wheat Spindle Streak Mosaic Virus Disease Update." The article explained how a wheat virus that was transmitted by a fungus to a plant in the Fall, that is, the *Polymyxa graminis*, was found by Spring infecting the roots of growing wheat. It ultimately destroyed the crop.[23]

"So fungus can indeed carry viruses to contaminate grains," Joey reaffirmed. "Why don't you call John Martin and ask him about the possibility of fungi transmitting 'stealth viruses' as well."

"Sure, I'll be happy to. It seems plausible to me."

Len continued, "But tell me more about pig feces causing *Pfiesteria* disease in fish. You mentioned Alzheimer's to boot. What are you suggesting?"

"Not causing, but perhaps the fungus, or something in it, is *activating* the *Pfiesteria* with some sort of toxin, possibly even the 'stealth virus,' or protein, that tells the prion to start crystallizing. After all, what symptoms do the infected fish exhibit? Impaired memory, disorientation, learning problems, changes in brain metabolism.[24] Like you just said, there seem to be some remarkable similarities between the neuropsychiatric problems associated with TSE from prions and these other diseases that are said to be linked to other infectious agents including mycoplasmas, fungi, and other microbes. Prions, which are believed to exist harmlessly in yeast and in brain tissues, suddenly get activated by some unknown protein, chemical, or microelectric signal that triggers it to grow into a toxic crystal. The same is true for this *Pfiesteria* disease. Like the prion, *Pfiesteria* starts out harmless—a one-celled algae or dinoflagellate organism. Then suddenly something triggers it to emit a poison that is neurotoxic. Then those infected get chronic fatigue, headaches, and diarrhea, they lose weight and exhibit neuropsychiatric problems."[25] (See figures 9.2 and 9.3)

"But aren't we speculating a bit much? The unknown toxic substance that stimulates *Pfiesteria* might have nothing to do with the catalyst that causes the prion to begin replicating. It may be a completely unrelated pathogenic process."

"Well it may be," Joey replied. "But there seems to be a lot of 'coincidences' happening here. *Pfiesteria* disease in fish and man emerged around the same time that CJD emerged, that is, the mid-1990s. Similar neurological symptoms are exhibited between *Pfiesteria*, the TSEs in animals and humans, Alzheimer's, chronic fatigue, and the new Mohave Desert 'stealth virus' illness John Martin has been investigating."

"But you can't just lump them all into one related illness."

"Maybe they are, and maybe they're not. But consider these studies." Joey reached for another stack of articles. "These link fungus in swine feed to the pig feces run off into the rivers and streams that feed the *Pfiesteria*," he said. "Pig excrement in fertilizers are also being spread on the corn and wheat fields across America today. That would most rationally explain why so many wild deer and elk herds are becoming infected," Joey continued. "I think we're looking at the emergence of a new set of man-made plagues, TSE relatives, with various clinical and subclinical symptoms associated with varying degrees of infection, co-infection, and toxicity."

## A Second Opinion

Not long after this conversation, Len telephoned Professor John Martin, the Director of the Center for Complex Infectious Diseases in Rosemead, California, the leading expert in "stealth virus" research, to ask his opinion about the possibility of fungi delivered "stealth virus" and prions in the pathogenesis of mad cow disease and other TSEs.

"I can't comment about mad cow disease and the 'stealth virus,'" John Martin said. Nor would he say much about Garth Nicolson's work in mycoplasma and its possible relationship to AIDS, mad-cow disease, and/or Alzheimer's. "But the same general principles hold for all the viruses, the 'stealth virus,' and the scrapie agent," he said.

"Yes. We see reactive gliosis, or what is called astrocytosis, in 'stealth virus' infections. But there are all grades of astrocytosis. The term denotes a nonspecific change associated with any metabolic illness affecting the brain. Vacuolation of brain cells occurs similarly. It largely reflects a nonspecific change in cellular metabolism. . . . The vacuolation of brain cells appears similar in encephalopathies in general. Under the microscope it appears as spongiform cells.

"However, you can also see this in leukodystrophies where the white blood cells appear vacuolated when there is a metabolic illness of the white blood cells. So astrocytosis and vacuolation are pretty nonspecific."

In-so-far-as a possible relationship between fungal infections, "stealth viruses" and prion activation, Dr. Martin replied, "With 'stealth virus' infections we see primarily cognitive and immune system dysfunctions. . . . There might be a speculative connection between 'stealth virus' and these infections, and other illnesses including possibly cancers, but certainly neurocognitive and neurodegenerative diseases are associated with 'stealth virus' infections.

"No one knows yet what specific factor or factors initiate the soluble protein in TSEs to suddenly become insoluble and deadly. That catalyst is yet to be found. Somehow something prompts the aggregation or crystallization process to occur. The proteins then transit from their normal soluble form to the insoluble crystal prion structures. There may be some virus driving this aggregation process, although it may be some other factor. . . .

"A virus or viral component is a reasonable hypothesis as it appears that some protein acts as a nidus for crystallization. This could potentially include any viral fragment.

"But there is no evidence, really, linking 'stealth virus' infections to mad cow disease. The association is possible. But if you intend to advance that thesis, it's probably best to keep your theory relatively nonspecific."[26]

## Mycotoxins in Fungi and Salmonella in Pig Feed

In any case, Joey's concern that new neurodegenerative diseases may have evolved from fungi carrying viruses, viral particles (e.g., proteins or "stealth viruses"), mycotoxins, mycoplasmas, and/or prions that, through fertilizer and water runoff, infected other organisms including people, was valid.

Joey's theory was especially bolstered by the USDA's National Animal Health Monitoring System (NAHMS), and its "Swine 95 study." As part of this study the USDA asked 326 swine feed producers to submit "seven 100-gram samples of finisher diet" that they subsequently tested for mycotoxins using chromatographic methods. "Samples were sent to USDA:APHIS National Veterinary Services Laboratories (NVSL). Then they were tested for several types of fungi (i.e., aflatoxin, zearalenone, vomitoxin, and fumonismin B1, B2, and B3). Additionally, the USDA's National Animal Disease Center (NADC) tested 300 of these feed samples for the presence of Salmonella.

Many of the samples tested positive for stunningly high volumes of toxic chemicals—mycotoxins—associated with fungal contamination. Between five and twenty percent of the swine feed grains were positive for mycotoxins and/or Salmonella. In discussing their findings, the USDA investigators stated:

> The environment contains hundreds of different fungi that are able to infest crops and stored feeds. A few of these fungi (such as *Aspergillus* and *Fusarium*) have the capability, under the right conditions, to produce toxins. These mycotoxins can accumulate undetected in swine feeds and reduce feed intake and growth rate, cause multiple reproductive losses, or suppress the immune system making pigs more susceptible to infectious agents such as bacteria and viruses.[27]

The researchers concluded:

Many of the factors contributing to production of mycotoxins, such as humidity and drought-stressed corn, are beyond the control of a pork producer. However, producers can take preventive measures including placement of grain in dry storage and maintaining below 14 percent moisture. Frequent cleaning of feed storage bins, use of fungal inhibitors to prevent growth, and rapid use of ground feed are additional methods of preventing mycotoxin production.

The researchers also discussed Salmonella—a bacteria that causes disease in pigs, most animals in fact, and humans. "Salmonella," the authors stated, "can be introduced to a swine operation through carrier hogs which shed the organism. Other sources of salmonellosis include the environment, rodents, and feed contaminated with Salmonella. . . ." The Midwest region of the U.S. was determined to have the most Salmonella contaminated pig feed samples.[27]

## Antibiotic Overuse and Fungal Infections

One important aspect of fungal growth that the USDA researchers failed to mention was discussed in *The Lancet* by Dr. John Threlfall and his colleagues from the British Public Health Laboratory Service. In their report, these experts warned that lethal drug-resistant strains of salmonella were being produced because of antibiotic overuse particularly prevalent in the cattle, pig, sheep, and poultry industries.

Salmonella poisoning, they said, though rarely lethal, often caused stomach aches, diarrhea, and could lead to blood poisoning. This later illness occurred in 13 percent of salmonella infection cases in the United States and far less in the United Kingdom where mad cow disease occurred more frequently.

In a press statement simultaneously released with his *Lancet* publication, Dr. Threlfall addressed the agricultural overuse of antibiotics by saying, "These drugs are used legitimately for therapeutic purposes in animals, but at the same time they cause increasing [antibiotic] resistance."[28]

They also cause an increase in fungal infections that are antibiotic resistant as well. As farm animals receive antibiotics, their natural microflora is upset in favor of developing resident fungi. This partly explains why, for example, women who take antibiotics for bacterial infections, commonly develop fungal infections such as candidiasis. Such fungal infections can further upset the blood chemistry. As the fungi continue to grow, their fermentation products—acids—increase in the blood and tissues. This shifts body chemistry to more acidic supporting additional fungal growth and the production of mycotoxins. This additionally taxes the immune system and can leave people more susceptible to opportunistic infections and even certain cancers.

This mycotoxicity and acid production problem also directly impacted the fish that developed *Pfiesteria* disease in swine fungi contaminated waters.

## More on Swine Waste Water, Fungi and *Pfiesteria piscicida*

An executive summary of the "Interim Report of the Technical Advisory Committee" of the University of Maryland studying the Pocomoke River *Pfiesteria piscicida* outbreak was also relevant to the previously mentioned problem that raw swine waste had discharged into several mid-Atlantic rivers just prior to the toxic *Pfiesteria* blooms that caused fish to die and fishermen to become ill with neuropsychiatric conditions.[29]

In Maryland and North Carolina, between October, 1996, and August, 1997, eighteen technical advisors monitored and studied these problems for the benefit of a highly alarmed public. They related the appearance of skin lesions, on the affected fish, to bacterial and fungal infections and "certain other toxic chemicals" released by the previously benign *Pfiesteria*. Other *dinoflagellates* "which are similar to *Pfiesteria piscicida*, but do not belong to the same species," the experts reported, had been cultured from the polluted rivers and diseased fish as well.[29]

"The fish lesions," they wrote, "began to be observed following a period of unusually heavy precipitation and runoff through 1996. Salinity was lower in the estuary, waters were more acidic, and concentrations of organic nutrients were higher than previously observed during ten years of water quality monitoring."[29]

They said that though evidence was inconclusive, the possibility that the fish lesions were directly related to the organic pollution, largely attributable to the swine waste, merited further study. Moreover, they said that "runoff and groundwater seepage of nutrients, including organic nutrients, from fields on which fertilizers and animal wastes are applied, requires most attention."[29]

The fish lesions were unusual, the technical committee reported. Ulcerative lesions were found "in as many as 20–40% of fish caught." Many species of fish were affected. The species most injured were "white perch, striped bass, croaker, menhaden, white catfish and weakfish."[29]

Summarizing the environmental conditions that promoted the outbreak they wrote:

> 1996 was one of the wettest years on record and an unusual incidence of lesions began to be noticed in October, 1996 following high river discharge. Increased runoff not only lowered salinity, but also lowered the pH of tidal-fresh and brackish zones and added large amounts of dissolved organic matter, including organic P and N to the estuary. Salinity, pH, and dissolved organic carbon all fell outside of the range observed over the previous ten years in the estuary. Although these estuarine fish should not have been unduly stressed by lowered salinity, pH levels could have been low enough to induce stress and skin exfoliation. Furthermore, the organic enrichment could have been conducive to growth of microbes, both infectious agents and *Pfiesteria*. . . . Although there is, at this time, no demonstrable cause and effect linkage, non-point source inputs from agricultural activities could be implicated. These include inorganic and organic nutrients, microbial pathogen, and pesticides and herbicides. This should be a primary focus of further investigation.[29]

In simple terms, the acidity in the waters, mostly produced by the fermentation of organic nutrients by fungi, seemed directly linked to the skin lesions in which additional infectious fungi were found. The most likely source of the entire outbreak was the agricultural use of fungal infected fertilizers as well as fungal infected pig manure draining into the rivers.

That's why Joey was so certain about the swine–fungus–*Pfiesteria* –and possibly TSE associations. Obviously, with a significant percentage of pigs infected with prions, which could be spread by fungi through hog feces, this might be critical to the *Pfiesteria* disease issue. The neuropsychiatric symptoms of the infected fishermen, for instance, might possibly be linked to prion disease along with mycotoxicity from fungi infected pigs.

Those who might question the rapid onset of generally chronic prion-related pathology need only examine Gadjusek's studies on chimpanzees. Again, these noted rapid onset prion morbidity and mortality as seen in figure7.4.

And besides prion infected swine, sheep, cattle, and elk, similar concerns might be raised regarding fungi and chickens, chicken feed, and poultry manure.[5]

## Pfiesteria Hysteria in the News

Following the release of the University of Maryland's scientific advisory committee's findings on the strange *Pfiesteria* disease, the national press, without focusing on the central issue of fungi and prion diseases, had a field day. A number of local newspaper reporters in the heavily affected areas dove into the toxic wastewater issue. Stuart Leavenworth of the Raleigh, North Carolina *News and Observer* questioned the life cycle of *Pfiesteria*. (See figure 9.2) "What causes it to change form and become toxic?" he asked readers to consider. "To what extent is it stimulated by sewage, animal waste, and other pollutants?"[30]

Likewise, another North Carolina newspaper reported that, according to scientists, the "stupified" fish and people may be directly "generated by sewage, animal waste, and fertilizers flushed into rivers and streams."[31]

Months later, Earth Changes Television broke a story concerning the effects of Hurricane Bonnie on escalating *Pfiesteria*. The Internet was again flooded with related replies. One well circulated response came from an on-the-scene North Carolinian. John Hunter commented on the remarkable difference between mainstream media coverage of the *Pfiesteria* outbreaks, and the real facts as experienced by residents. He wrote:

> Here is some info most people aren't aware of. After at least 20 inches of rain dumped onto eastern North Carolina where about 9,000,000 hogs live on factory farms, all of the cheap hog waste lagoon dams will break again dumping about 500,000,000 gallons of raw swine waste into *Pfiesteria* dominated rivers, setting off a feeding frenzy from this plague-like microbe that will start to produce a cloud of aerosol toxins the size of the Pamlico sound. These toxins have been proven by doctors at Duke and John's Hopkins to cause a neurological syndrome in animals and humans! It affects the brain. This cloud of toxins will continue to be produced for weeks and possibly months thereafter. Big agriculture runs North Carolina and the state's propaganda newspapers that don't print anything [in depth] about *Pfiesteria* "the cell from hell."[32]

## The Fertilizer Industry

On a related note, with relevance to chemical co-factors in the spread of TSEs and their resilient prion agents and probable fungus vectors, 271 million pounds of *toxic waste* were used as farm fertilizer between 1990 and 1995 according to a report issued by the Washington-based Environmental Working Group (EWG). Although "no proven health risks were attributable" to this practice, some health scientists felt the practice was extremely risky.

Dr. William Leibhardt of the University of California, Davis, said, "It doesn't make sense to spread toxic materials at whatever level out on the land that is producing our food and fiber."

The EWG's study[33] found that toxic wastes were shipped along with other substances that fertilizer makers used such as zinc, which is an important corn nutrient. Other toxins (besides fungi and prions) that ended up in fertilizers included methanol, lead, cadmium, arsenic, and dioxin.

"Yet there are no federal regulations on [these and other toxic] substances, nor are there any labeling requirements on fertilizer for them—only for the beneficial ingredients," the report stated.

"You've got all these toxic riders coming along [in the fertilizers] and nobody has a sense of how much, or what form they're in, whether they move up [or, as with prion infected swine waste, up and down] the food chain," Leibhardt said. "We know very little about this."

The EWG found that "600 companies in 44 states shipped 69 kinds of toxic waste to farms or fertilizer companies over a six-year period beginning in 1990." The steel industry provided the greatest offenders including Nucor Steel of Norfolk, VA. Alone they contributed 26.2 million pounds of toxic waste to fertilizer makers. Other leading sources were electronics manufacturers and the chemical industry."

"Will you look at that?" Len recoiled as he and Joey reviewed the EWG report. "'Nucor Steel of Norfolk, Virginia.' Do you remember them?"

"No."

"I wrote about them in *Emerging Viruses: AIDS & Ebola.* You remember Richard Preston—the award-winning CIA propagandist, and author of the bogus book *The Hot Zone*? He promoted Nucor Corporation for its 'revolutionary' steel industry innovations."[34]

"How nice," Joey replied then paused. "But speaking of electrical waste, covert operations, and the CIA, I haven't even told you the worst yet!"

"Nor have I told you what I've found," Len returned. Then begrudgingly he invited, "All right, you go first. What have you got?"

"You see that other pile of research articles on the bookshelf?" Joey pointed to the stack.

"Yeah."

"That contains evidence that fungi, prions, genes, and even diseases react dramatically to varying electromagnetic frequencies, just like we talked about with the Solfeggio—creation and destruction is a matter of *vibrational frequencies*. The prions are *crystals*. You said it yourself. They're like little radios—little receivers and transmitters of electromagnetic energy. Man-made or not, they've been in the grains, beef, pork, fish, chickens, and now they're in us—virtually everyone— meat eaters and vegans alike. They are in our brains. And they have the capacity to receive and transmit wave frequency signals. They can even be used to transmit certain diseases to certain populations. The people at the very top of medical intelligence, the population con- trollers, have known about this bioelectric technology for a long time. Since the time they censored Keely's and Rife's discoveries, they've been working on it."

Len looked at Joey stunned. "Guess what?"

"What?"

"That's precisely what I wanted to tell you."

"Your kidding."

"I wish I was. If you don't believe me, just look up the word 'apo- ptosis'—the programmed cell death associated with prion disease, and see where the cross references and period codes take you."

## References

1. Saar M and Sharon K. Flu-like illnesses filling care centers: Influenza, croup and rotavirus are hitting the elderly and youngsters hard. The *Orange County Register*. December 30, 1997, p. 1.

2. Crook, WG. *The Yeast Connection*. Jackson, TN: Professional Books, 1986.

3. Burton B. New type of DNA-free inheritance in yeast is spread by a "mad cow" mechanism. *Cell*, May 30, 1997. Press release from the University of Chicago. Available from: http://www.ucmc.uchicago. edu/news/1997/prionfibers.html.

4. This information about prion diseases spreading in wild animals including deer and elk was posted on August 2, 1998, "Prions" website of the Internet in file:///A/Prions.html. Other such references follow.

It should also be noted that the sheep brain transmission theory of "mad cow disease" has been consistently questioned and often rejected by many reputable authorities. Leading alternative theories include changes in agricultural techniques including the "drenching of cattle with organophosphate pesticides to eliminate warble fly." See: Cookson C. Mad cow disease: Where did it come from? *The Financial Times*. Distributed by Scripps Howard News Service. Available on the internet at http://www.community-care.oaktree.co.uk/news bse0001.txt.

5. Preston J. Cheap meat said cause of mad cow disease in humans. Reuters News Service, March 12, 1998. (Available on the web from "SIGHTINGS" website, file:///A/cheapmeat.html.)

6. Staff writers. Deer Dropping Dead From Mad Cow In Colorado/Wyoming. Associated Press New Service, January 24, 1998. (Available on the web from "SIGHTINGS" website, file:///A/mccowdeer.html.)

7. Hoffman E. Mad Elk Disease Spreading—Now Found In Nebraska. Discovery News Briefs, June 3, 1998. (Available on the web from http://www. sightings.com/health/madelkspread.htm; and from www.discovery.com.)

8. McCoy T.J. and Wiese M. 1995 Managing Plant-Microbe Interactions in Soil to Promote Sustainable Agriculture. In: *Annual Report of Cooperative Regional Project W-147*. U.S. Department of Agriculture. File on "Plant and Seed Engineering" available through the Department of Agriculture, or through their website under file:///A/w14795Plant and Seed Engineering.htm; See also: Bryant J. Sorghum fungus hits high plains. *Agricultural News*. August, 26, 1997. (Available through: http://agnews.tamu.edu/stories/SOIL/Aug2697a.htm); Graebner L. Rice farmers fear fungus will kill crops. *Sacramento Business Journal*, October 28, 1996. (Available through: http://cgi.amcity.com/sacramento/stories/102896/story/7.html.)

9. The complete definition of "yeast" in *Steadman's Medical Dictionary* is:

Y.'s are true fungi whose usual growth form is unicellular. Used properly the term y. refers to ascomycetes which possess a unicellular thallus, reproduce asexually by budding or transverse division and sexually by ascospore formation originating from a zygote or parthenogenetically from a somatic cell. The Saccharomycetaceae contain the y.'s Saccharomyces cerevisiae is a common species. As the name implies, the y.'s are active fermenters of carbohydrate. The term y.-like fungus is often applied to fungi which are not known to form ascospores, but otherwise possess the characteristics listed above: such forms include members of the genera Candida, Geotrichum, Cryptococcus, etc. Such asporogenous y.-like fungi are properly placed with the Fungi Imperfecti unless methods of sexual reproduction are known.

10. USDA Animal and Plant Health Inspection Service staff. Agriculture Department completes Phase One attack on wheat fungus: Actions protect wheat exports. August 21, 1996. U.S. Department of Agriculture. The six-page report is available through the Agriculture Department's website. See file:///A/et2_8-22 Wheat Fungus, htm; Sheldon R. Jones's statements to the Associated Press may be found on: http://www.earthchanges TV.com in its posting—AP. Government testing may have contaminated wheat fields with fungus. Earth Changes Television, February 27, 1999.

11. Anderson D. CFIDS Epidemic Conference, March 9, 1997. Lecture by Dr. Donovan Anderson and Dr. W. John Martin on "Stealth Virus Encephalopathy. Text of lectures are available through Dr. Anderson's website at file:///A/1donovan. htm.

12. Horowitz LG. *Emerging Viruses: AIDS & Ebola—Nature, Accident or Intentional?* Sandpoint, ID: Tetrahedron Publishing Group, 1998, pp. 385-400; 412-114.

13. Manning R. The meddling disease. *The Los Angeles Times Sunday Magazine*, December 16, 1998. The Internet copy was relayed to Dr. Horowitz devoid of a website address. It's source was listed only as "Whirling Disease in Trout" file:///A/000294Salmonella Invection Whirling fish disease. htm.

14. Springer J. NCSU Aquatic Botany Laboratory Pfiesteria piscicida Page Report, June 26, 1998. pp. 1-6. (Available from http://www2.ncsu.edu/unity/lockers/project/aquatic_botany/pfiest.html.)

15. Lucas T. NC State scientist studies role of toxic algae in fish, human health. NCSU News Services. A release heralding Dr. JoAnn Bujrkholder's 1998 AAAS presentation. (Call 919-515-3470 for copies of the report, or e-mail: tim_lucas@ncsu.edu.)

16. Young R. Allegations about a rendering plant have raised fresh fears: New claims link CJD to water supply. *London Times*, August 26, 1997, pg. 1; See also: 16b. Arthur C. Interview with Clare Tomkins' family. *Independent Newspaper*, August 26, 1997, available through http://www.mad-cow.org/~tom/drink.html; and 16c. Bowcott O. Fear emerges in Britain of disease time bomb. *The Guardian*, August 27, 1997.

17. Consumers Union staff. Consumers Union comments to FDA on feed ban (Docket No. 96N-0135), Substances Prohibited for Use in Animal Food or Feed; Animal Proteins Prohibited in Ruminant Feed, Draft Rule. (Available through the Consumers Union, or the "Mad Cow Home" page, "Prions" Section, file:///A/collagen.html.)

18 . Hadlow WJ. Letter to Patrick McCaskey, USDA/FSIS/Eastern Lab, dated April 10, 1997.

19. Bobowick AR, Brody JA, Matthews MR, Roos R and Gajdusek DC. Creutzfeldt-Jakob disease: A case-control study. *American Journal of Epidemiology* 1973;98:381-394.

20. Davanipour Z, Alter M, Sobel E, Asher DM and Gajdusek DC. A case-control study of Creutzfeldt-Jakob disease: Dietary risk factors. *American Journal of Epidemiology* 1989;122:433-451.

21. Boller F, Lopez OL and Moossy J. Diagnosis of dementia: Clinicopathologic correlations. *Neurology* 1989;39:76-79.

22. Manuelidis L. Suggested links between different types of dementias: Creutzfeldt-Jakob disease, Alzheimer disease, and retroviral CNS infections. *Alzheimer Disease and Associated Disorders* 1989;2:100-109. See also: Manuelidis EF, Kim JH, Mericangas

JR and Manuelids. Transmission of Creutzfeldt-Jakob disease from human blood. *The Lancet* 1985:2:896-897.

23. Hart P. Disease update: Wheat spindle streak mosaic virus. Michigan State University Extension. Field Crop CAT Alert 1993-97–05099608, March 25, 1998.

24. This information is based on a scientific report published in *The Lancet*, Aug 15, 1998. See: Morgan D. Pfiesteria found in east coast fish now linked to memory disorder. Reuters News Service, August 14, 1998, for a review of the article.

25. Associated Press Wireservice. Mental impairment linked to Pfiesteria in Pocomoke River, Aug 15, 1998. This information was also based on a scientific report that appeared in *The Lancet*, Aug 15, 1998. (Available through the SIGHTINGS website at http://www.sightings.com/health/pfi.htm)

26. Personal communication with W. John Martin, M.D., Ph.D., Nov. 29, 1998.

27. Centers for Epidemiology and Animal Health, USDA:APHIS:VS, attn. NAHMS. Presence of mycotoxins and salmonella in swine finisher diets. The Swine '95 study. (For reprints of "Mycotoxins and Swine Performance" fact sheet [6/92] in the University of Illinois at Urbana-Champaign Pork Industry Handbook, contact: USDA: attn. NAHMS 555 South Howes, Fort Collins, CO 80521; [970] 490-7800; E-mail: nahms web@aphis.usda.gov)

28. Rense J. Salmonella multi-drug resistant superbug on the rise. SIGHTINGS website news from *The Lancet*, July 24, 1998. (Available through the Internet at URL#: http://www.sightings.com/health/supbugh.htm.)

29. Boesch DF, Anderson R, Burkholder J and Burreson et al. Interim report of the technical advisory committee on Pocomoke river fish health. University of Maryland, August 14, 1997. (Document available on the Internet at URL# http://www.mdsg.umd.edu/fish-health/pfiesteria/tac/pokomoke. html.)

30. Leavenworth S. Research team on trail of key Pfiesteria toxin. *The News and Observer*, Wednesday, August 27, 1997.

31. Staff reporter. Pfiesteria killing fish in North Carolina—River closings coming. *The Nando Times*, Wednesday, July 29, 1998. (Available through the Internet at URL#: http://www.sightings.com/earthchanges/pf.htm.)

32. Hunter J. Hurricane Bonnie may have escalated Pfiesteria. Reply to Earth Change Television/breaking news. Sunday, August 30, 1998. Copy of circulated e:mail on file.

33. Nando Media News. 271 million pounds of toxic waste used as farm fertilizer. A report by The Environmental Working Group of Washington, D.C. *The Nando Times*, August 2, 1998. (Available through the Internet at URL#: www.nando.net and also http://www.sightings.com/earthchanges/A/271.htm.)

34. Horowitz LG. *Op cit.,* p. 394.

# Chapter 10.
# Frequency Vibrations
# and the Biological Apocalypse

A s Joey retraced Len's steps through *Webster's Dictionary*, from prion "apoptosis," that is, programmed cell death," to the "lords of misrule," he caught the "more at JET" cross-reference in the definition of "deject," as seen in chapter 8. "Did you follow that lead?" he asked his co-investigator.

"Yeah. Wait till you see where that takes you."

Joey turned *Webster's* pages rapidly to the word "jet." As seen in figure 10.1, it was just below "Jesus—the Jewish religious teacher whose life, death, and resurrection, as reported by Evangelists, are the basis of the Christian message of salvation."

The term "jet" was followed by a "14c" code and not only referred to a "black-color" and "jewel," but also to "a narrow stream of material (as plasma) emanating or appearing to emanate from a celestial object (as a radio galaxy)." Next to this was "b: a nozzle for a jet of fluid 2: something issuing as if in a jet <talk poured from her in a brilliant~—*Time>*."

The italicized *Time*, commonly understood to denote *Time* magazine caught Len's attention as a CFR member directed purveyor of propaganda. (See appendix figure 13, and the appendix section titled "*Time*ly Propaganda in the Herbal Industry Takeover.")

The "narrow stream of material emanating from a celestial object" tweaked both men's recollection that high flying jet "contrails" or "chemtrails" had been seen over northern Idaho, and virtually every other state, in unique, noncommercial airline patterns. In fact, reports had been circulating that only military aircraft that used "JP8" fuel, allegedly containing the carcinogenic chemical ethylene dibromide, issued the puffy white polluted jet-stream. The trails these jets left behind were routinely observed, hours later, to cloud entire skies. By day's end a gloomy grey overcast condition had evolved over what had been previously clear blue sky. Research and mounting evidence eventially accumulated linking these poisonous chemtrails to upper respiratory infections, amples of *Pseudomonas aerogenosa*, fungal and myco-plasma droppings, aluminum oxide, and bizarre condition now called Morgellons disease.[1]

Curiously, in the word column immediately adjacent the term "jet" was the "Jewish calendar." The "Jewish Years 5754-5773 were listed therein including the year of this writing and century's end— 1999, the "Hebrew year" 5760. This, according to Pythagorean analysis, yielded 18 or 9—completion—and equaled 666 (6+6+6=18=9), the biblical "mark of the beast."

A few words above this was another cross reference to "more at JET" adjacent a "15c" in the definition of the word "jettison." This word was only defined as "a voluntary sacrifice of cargo to lighten a ship's load in time of distress."

Thus, it was time to consider the most horrifying possibility. Could those who buried, and for centuries applied, the sacred knowledge of resonant frequencies and related technologies be using this ancient arcana, as well as the current "cryptocrystalline" epidemics of TSEs, to "jettison" unwanted populations at a chosen time in history? In other words, could prion crystals be the quintessential "mark of the beast?" Could the Masonic-Nazi-linked "New World Order" governors have planned to transmit infectious agents, and then "dial" the morbid elec-tromagnetic frequencies to control and cull the population at large?

## Background on Vibrational Frequencies and Their Impact on Physical Reality

Of all the review articles on the powerful influence vibrational fre-quencies have on all physical forms, a German investigator, Peter Pet-tersson, provided one of the best. In "Cymatics: The Science of the

# Fig. 10.1. Definitions and Cross References of "Jet" to "Jettison" Adjacent Jesus and Jewish Calendar Year 5760

**Je·su·it** \'je-zu-ət, -zhü- also -zyü-\ n [NL Jesuita, fr. LL Jesus] (1559) 1 : a member of the Roman Catholic Society of Jesus founded by St. Ignatius Loyola in 1534 and devoted to missionary and educational work 2 : one given to intrigue or equivocation — **je·su·it·ic** \,je-zu-'it-ik, -zhü-, -zyü-\ or **je·su·it·i·cal** \-i-kəl\ adj, often cap — **je·su·it·i·cal·ly** \-i-k(ə-)lē\ adv, often cap — **je·su·it·ism** \'je-zu-ə-,ti-zəm, -zhü-, -zyü-\ or **je·su·it·ry** \-ə-trē\ n, often cap

**Je·sus** \'jē-zəs, -zəz also -zəs and -,zəz\ n [LL, fr. Gk Iēsous, fr. Heb Yēshūa'] 1 : the Jewish religious teacher whose life, death, and resurrection as reported by the Evangelists are the basis of the Christian message of salvation — called also Jesus Christ 2 Christian Science : the highest human corporeal concept of the divine idea rebuking and destroying error and bringing to light man's immortality

¹**jet** \'jet\ n [ME, fr. MF jaiet, fr. L gagates, fr. Gk gagatēs, fr. Gagas, town and river in Asia Minor] (14c) 1 : a compact velvet-black coal that takes a good polish and is often used for jewelry 2 : an intense black

²**jet** adj (1716): of the color jet

³**jet** vb **jet·ted**; **jet·ting** [F jeter, lit., to throw, fr. MF, fr. L jactare to throw, freq. of jacere to throw; akin to Gk hienai to send] vi (1692) : to spout forth : GUSH ~ vt : to emit in a stream : SPOUT

⁴**jet** n (ca. 1696) 1 a (1) : a usu. forceful stream of fluid (as water or gas) discharged from a narrow opening or a nozzle (2) : a narrow stream of material (as plasma) emanating or appearing to emanate from a celestial object (as a radio galaxy) b : a nozzle for a jet of fluid 2 : something issuing as if in a jet (talk poured from her in a brilliant ~ —Time) 3 a : JET ENGINE b : an airplane powered by one or more jet engines 4 : a long narrow current of high-speed winds (as a jet stream) — **jet·like** \-,līk\ adj

⁵**jet** vi **jet·ted**; **jet·ting** (1949) 1 : to travel by jet airplane 2 : to move or progress by or as if by jet propulsion

**jet-bead** \'jet-,bēd\ n (ca. 1930) : a shrub (Rhodotypos scandens) that has black shining fruit and is used as an ornamental

**jet-black** \-'blak\ adj (15c) : black as jet

**je·té** \zha-'tā\ n [F, fr. pp. of jeter] (1830) : a springing jump in ballet made from one foot to the other in any direction

**jet engine** n (1943) : an engine that produces motion as a result of the rearward discharge of a jet of fluid; specif : an airplane engine that uses atmospheric oxygen to burn fuel and produces a rearward discharge of heated air and exhaust gases — see AIRPLANE illustration

**jet·ti·son** \'je-tə-sən, -zən\ n [ME jetteson, fr. AF getteson, fr. OF getaison action of throwing, fr. L jactation-, jactatio, fr. jactare — more at JET] (15c) : a voluntary sacrifice of cargo to lighten a ship's load in time of distress

²**jettison** vt (1848) 1 : to make jettison of 2 : to get rid of as superfluous or encumbering : DISCARD 3 : to drop from an airplane or spacecraft in flight — **jet·ti·son·a·ble** \-sə-nə-bəl, -zə-\ adj

**nephelus itajara**) that are usu. dusky green, brown, or blackish, thick-headed, and rough-scaled

**Jew·ish** \'jü-ish\ adj (ca. 1546) : of, relating to, or characteristic of the Jews; also : being a Jew — **Jew·ish·ly** adv — **Jew·ish·ness** n

**Jewish American Princess** n (1979) : a stereotypical well-to-do or spoiled American Jewish girl or woman — called also Jewish Princess; often used disparagingly

**Jewish calendar** n (ca. 1888) : a calendar in use among Jewish peoples that is reckoned from the year 3761 B.C. and dates in its present form from about A.D. 360 — see MONTH table

## JEWISH YEARS 5754–5773

| JEWISH YEAR | | A.D. | | JEWISH YEAR | | A.D. | |
|---|---|---|---|---|---|---|---|
| 5754 | begins | Sept. | 16, 1993 | 5764 | begins | Sept. | 27, 2003 |
| 5755 | begins | Sept. | 6, 1994 | 5765 | begins | Sept. | 16, 2004 |
| 5756 | begins | Sept. | 25, 1995 | 5766 | begins | Oct. | 4, 2005 |
| 5757 | begins | Sept. | 14, 1996 | 5767 | begins | Sept. | 23, 2006 |
| 5758 | begins | Oct. | 2, 1997 | 5768 | begins | Sept. | 13, 2007 |
| 5759 | begins | Sept. | 21, 1998 | 5769 | begins | Sept. | 30, 2008 |
| 5760 | begins | Sept. | 11, 1999 | 5770 | begins | Sept. | 19, 2009 |
| 5761 | begins | Sept. | 30, 2000 | 5771 | begins | Sept. | 9, 2010 |
| 5762 | begins | Sept. | 18, 2001 | 5772 | begins | Sept. | 29, 2011 |
| 5763 | begins | Sept. | 7, 2002 | 5773 | begins | Sept. | 17, 2012 |

**Jew·ry** \'jü(-ə)r-ē, 'jü-rē\ n (14c) 1 pl **Jewries** : a community of Jews 2 : the Jewish people

**Jew's harp** or **Jews' harp** \'jüz-,härp, 'jüs-\ n (1595) : a small lyre-shaped instrument that when held between the lips gives tones from a metal tongue struck by the finger

**Jez·e·bel** \'je-zə-,bel\ n [Heb Izebhel] 1 : the Phoenician wife of Ahab who according to the account in 1 and II Kings pressed the cult of Baal on the Israelite kingdom but was finally killed in accordance with Elijah's prophecy 2 often not cap : an impudent, shameless, or morally unrestrained woman

**JHVH** var of YHWH

**jiao** \jē-'au\ n [Chin. (Beijing) jiǎo] (1949) : a monetary unit of the People's Republic of China equal to ¹/₁₀ yuan

## Fig. 10.2. Plate Oscillation Produced Chladni Figures

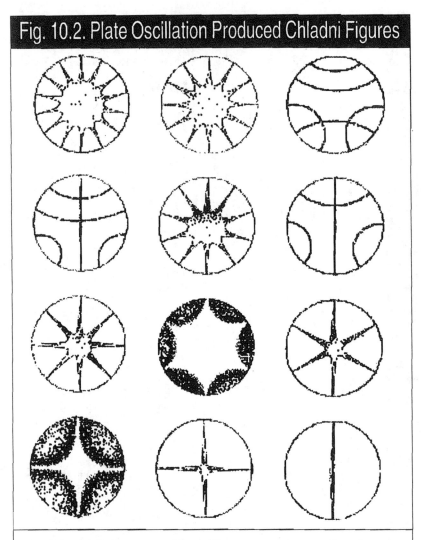

The Chladni figures seen above illustrate areas on a flat plate that are and are not vibrating. This causes sand, or some other material, to move into specific shapes and patterns depending on the frequency of the vibrations. The plates are made of elastic material. Parts of the plate vibrate more than others. The "node lines" on the plate, here seen in black, do not vibrate. Thus, the black material, sand in this case, collects in those specific locations. The oscillating areas of the plate become and remain empty. The opposite has been observed to occur with water or other liquids. Courtesy of: http://www.alphaomega.se/english/chladnifig.html

Future?"[2] he summarized the creative connection between sound, vibrations, and physical reality as he reviewed the work of the field's top researchers.

He began with Ernst Chladni, the first observer of the "Chladni figures" that Joey referred to at the end of Chapter 2.

Chladni was, not surprisingly, a musician and physicist. Born in 1756, the same year as Mozart, he laid the foundations for the discipline within physics called acoustics—the science of sound.

Coincidentally, Chaldni died in 1829, the same year as Beethoven. It may be recalled that Mozart, a Freemason, heavily influenced Beethoven with the mathematics of music, and likely influenced Chaldni as well.

In 1787 Chaldni published *Entdeckungen über die Theorie des Klanges,* or *Discoveries Concerning the Theory of Music.* "In this and other pioneering works he explained ways to make sound waves generate visible structures. With the help of a violin bow which he drew perpendicularly across the edge of flat plates covered with sand," Pettersson wrote, Chaldi "produced those patterns and shapes which today go by the term Chladni figures." As seen in figure 10.2, this was significant because it demonstrated that sound actually affected physical matter. It held the power to create geometric forms in substances.

Later, in 1815, Nathaniel Bowditch—an American mathematician who followed up on Chladni's work—studied "the patterns created by the intersection of two sine curves whose axes are perpendicular to each other, sometimes called 'Bowditch curves' but more often 'Lissajous figures' . . . after the French mathematician Jules-Antoine Lissajous, who, independently of Bowditch, investigated them in 1857-58. Both concluded that the condition for these designs to arise was that the frequencies, or oscillations per second, of both curves stood in simple whole-number ratios to each other, such as 1:1, 1:2; 1:3 and so on. In fact, one can produce Lissajous figures even if the frequencies are not in perfect whole-number rations to each other. If the difference is insignificant, *the phenomenon that arises is that the de-*

*signs keep changing* their appearance."[2] This, as you will soon see with regard to prions, is significant.

Such figures, empowered by fluctuating frequencies, move. What created the variations in the shapes of these designs was "the phase differential, or the angle between the two curves. In other words, the way in which their rhythms or periods" coincided.

Lissajous also observed that curves that had different frequencies and were out of phase with each other formed intricate weblike designs. "These Lissajous figures are all visual examples of waves that meet each other at right angles."[2]

This, Pettersson noted, reinforced the concept that existed in many societies around the world along with their mythologies. For instance, to the Mesoamerican people the universe was a dynamic web produced by "spinning and weaving." Cecilia Klein related this concept to the Aztecs and Mayans who believed that fertility goddesses were the great "weavers."[3, 3a]

Likewise, Lissajous figures were produced when a number of waves crossed each other at right angles. The effect looked like a woven pattern. The waves met at 90-degree angles which triggered Len and Joey to recall the definitions of "loom," "heirloom," and "heir" that they read in *Webster's Dictionary*. (See figure 8.11.)

In 1967 Hans Jenny, a Swiss physician and researcher, published in his native language *The Structure and Dynamics of Waves and Vibrations*. Jenny, like Chladni two-hundred years earlier, showed what happened when one took various materials like water, sand, iron filings, spores, and viscous substances, and placed them on membranes and vibrating metal plates. Shapes and patterns in motion appeared that varied from "perfectly ordered and stationary" to those that were chaotic.[2]

Pettersson acknowledged Jenny for originating the field of "cymatics" that allowed people to observe the physical results of voice, tones, and song. Here's how:

Jenny made use of crystal oscillators and an invention of his own
by the name of the tonoscope to set these plates and membranes
vibrating. This was a major step forward. The advantage with
crystal oscillators is that one can determine exactly which frequency and amplitude/volume one wants. It was now possible to
research and follow a continuous train of events in which one
had the possibility of changing the frequency or the amplitude or
both.

The tonoscope was constructed to make the human voice visible
without any electronic apparatus as an intermediate link. This
yielded the amazing possibility of being able to see the physical
image of the vowel, tone or song a human being produced directly. Not only could you hear a melody - you could see it, too![2]

Jenny applied the name "cymatics" to this area of research, from
the Greek term "kyma," meaning "wave." Thus, cymatics could be
defined as: "The study of how vibrations, in the broad sense, generate
and influence patterns, shapes and moving processes."[2]

Pettersson provided a more detailed description of the Chladni and
Lissajous figures produced by Jenny as follows:

He vibrated a plate at a specific frequency and amplitude—
vibration, [and] the shapes and motion patterns characteristic of
that vibration appeared in the material on the plate. If he changed
the frequency or amplitude, the development and pattern were
changed as well. He found that if he increased the frequency, the
complexity of the patterns increased, the number of elements
became greater. If on the other hand he increased the amplitude,
the motions became all the more rapid and turbulent and could
even create small eruptions, where the actual material was
thrown up in the air. The shapes, figures and patterns of motion
that appeared proved to be primarily a function of frequency,
amplitude, and the inherent characteristics of the various materials. . . .

When Jenny experimented with fluids of various kinds he produced wave motions, spirals, and wavelike patterns in continuous circulation. In his research with plant spores, he found an
enormous variety and complexity, but even so, there was a unity
in the shapes and dynamic developments that arose. With the

help of iron filings, mercury, viscous liquids, plastic-like substances and gases, he investigated the three-dimensional aspects of the effect of vibration.[2]

In addition, using his tonoscope, Jenny "noticed that when the vowels of the ancient languages of Hebrew and Sanskrit were pronounced, the sand took the shape of the written symbols for these vowels." Modern languages, including English, failed to generate these patterns.[4]

American researcher Dan Winter reported reproducing these effects using the Hebrew alphabet; whereas Stan Tenen expanded on the understanding of Hebrew in "The Meru Project" discovering geometrics in hand signs demonstrating mathematics fundamental to whole systems, physics, and cosmology. Both investigators, despite many differences, concluded that Hebrew is, indeed, a "sacred language."[35]

Another interesting phenomenon appeared when Jenny vibrated a plate covered with liquid, and then tilted it. Pettersson recalled that, "The liquid did not yield to gravitational influence and run off the vibrating plate, but stayed on and went on constructing new shapes as though nothing had happened. If, however, the oscillation was then turned off, the liquid began to run, but if he was really fast and got the vibrations going again, he could get the liquid back in place on the plate." This, the authors wrote, demonstrated the antigravitational effect caused by vibrations on physical matter.

Jenny concluded that, "In the living as well as nonliving parts of nature, the trained eye encounters widespread evidence of periodic systems. These systems point to a continuous transformation" of matter by electromagnetic energy.[5]

In other words, there were examples of cymatic elements everywhere—"vibrations, oscillations, pulses, wave motions, pendulum motions, rhythmic courses of events, serial sequences, and their effects and actions"—and they affected everything including biological evolution. The evidence convincingly demonstrated that all natural phenomena were ultimately dependent on, if not entirely determined by, the frequencies of vibration. "He speculated that every cell had its own frequency and that a number of cells with the same frequency created a new frequency which was in harmony with the original, which in its turn possibly formed an organ that also created a new frequency in harmony with the two preceeding ones."[2] Essentially Jenny argued that physical healing could be aided or hindered by tones. Different frequencies influenced genes, cells, and various structures in the body, he claimed.

In the last chapter of *Cymatics*, Jenny summed up these phenomena in a three-part unity. Likewise John Beaulieu, American polarity and music therapist, in his book *Music and Sound in the Healing Arts*, reached a similar conclusion based on subatomic particle science. "There is a similarity between cymatic pictures and quantum particles," Beaulieu wrote. "In both cases, that which appears to be a solid form is also a wave. They are both created and simultaneously organized by the principle of pulse. This is the great mystery with sound: there is no solidarity! A form that appears solid is actually created by a an underlying vibration."[6]

The entire field of quantum physics evolved largely to reconcile the unity in this dualism between wave and form. Here, Beaulieu asserted, vibration is understood as one true reality—the particle or form, and the wave or motion, are two polar manifestations of the one contextual element—what might be called God.

Cathie E. Guzetta, a poet, perhaps summarized this science best when she wrote, "The forms of snowflakes and faces of flowers may take on their shape because they are responding to some sound in nature. Likewise, it is possible that crystals, plants, and human beings may be, in some way, music that has taken on visible form."[7]

## Early Research in Vibrational Medicine

Even if one discounted the works of Chladni, Jenny, Tesla, Keely, and Rife etc., other scientists have proven the critical biological impact of electromagnetics and frequency vibrations.

In 1923, for instance, a Russian anatomy professor, Dr. A. G. Gurvich, advanced a theory that ultraviolet light was essential to one of life's greatest mysteries—cell division. He had pointed the root tip of a growing onion toward the side of a second proliferating onion root. He noticed that the cells of the latter in the area of the root tip divided much faster. He theorized that ultraviolet light, or some other electromagnetic "mitogenetic radiation," was likely responsible for the biological change later called the "Gurvich Effect."[8]

During the following decade teams of mostly German and Russian scientists attempted to confirm the "Gurvich Effect" without success. After more than 500 research papers were published in this field of study, the subject was dropped. Then it was resurrected in the 1950s with the development of the photon-counter photomultiplier. This technology, aided by cryogenic techniques, enabled photodetectors to be cooled to very low temperatures, and allowed researchers to confirm the "Gurvich Effect"—the effect of mitogenetic radiation on cells.[9]

Central to the biological apocalypse, by 1974 Dr. V.F. Kaznachayev and his associates showed that *ultraviolet light frequencies could transmit viral induced infections between cell cultures.* These researchers arranged "pairs of sealed glass tubes containing healthy cell cultures end to end separated only by a sheet of quartz." After inoculating a single culture with a deadly virus, the investigators were surprised to learn the adjacent sterile culture had also become ill.[9,10]

When the quartz sheet separating the two cultures was removed, then the sterile culture adjacent to the infected one remained unaffected. The glass tubes alone could not transmit the electromagnetic frequencies required to communicate the disease.[10,11] *The transmitter was found to be the quartz crystal.* In other words, special disease frequencies were transmitted by the crystal and these alone were sufficient to infect the sterile cell cultures!

After repeatedly reproducing these results, the Russian team surmised that when the infected cells in culture died, they emitted UV light which was transmitted through the quartz to the adjacent cell cultures. These electromagnetic frequency transmissions then induced, like progressive crystal growth, progressive cell death in the initially healthy cultures.

Kaznachayev's team also showed that with the introduction of a virus into cell cultures a change in the photon emission of the cells was seen even before cell degeneration and death occurred.

Then, as the cell cultures died, they were observed to change their UV frequency radiations again. This suggested to Kaznachayev et al., that disease processes could possibly be altered by determining the dying cell frequency emissions and intercepting or neutralizing them before they had a chance to kill adjacent cells or tissues within their energy field. Additional support for this theory came from the observation that yeast cell reproduction could be slowed using specific UV light frequencies.[9,10]

Given these observations, they concluded, "We feel we may then learn to affect healing by altering the photon flux before it contaminates neighboring systems."

Clearly, Joey and Len realized, these findings could have profound implications on treating and preventing prion and other diseases.

Also in 1974, the esteemed scientific journal *Biochemistry Biophysics Research Communication* published a study by two Western scientists who detected a "weak chemiluminescence" coming from yeast UV frequency emissions. They, like Kaznachayev's group, recommended additional research into the mitogenetic phenomenon.

Ultra-weak UV emissions and visible light in the range of 200-800 nanometers have since been shown to come from a variety of organisms and cells during mitosis.[11-15] *These radiation frequencies were found associated with cellular DNA. Stored photon energy is apparently associated with the nucleic acids, that is the nucleotides, that comprise the genetic double helix.* Scientists proposed this model might best explain a wide array of biological observations.[3a, 16-20]

Estimates indicate *only 0.1-2 percent of DNA functions as genetic material.*[3] *The vast majority of the helical strand not involved in coding for protein synthesis is believed to function electromagnetically.* The six-sided crystal clustered water molecules structurally support-

351

ing the nucleotide strands, and protein enzymes, apparently play a primary role in regulating every aspect of cellular metabolism.[3a] Additional evidence for this comes from the fact that when cells die, they release stored photons as "coherent, monochromatic, energy sources with properties similar to laser light. . . . UV radiation from a laser has been shown to stimulate DNA synthesis and change the permeability of cell membranes."[9,21]

A Norwegian doctor has suggested that viruses might emit lethal electromagnetic (EM) radiations, and thus kill cells in culture. Dr. Schjelderup added that viral infections might thereby transmit disease by specific frequency emissions besides physical or genetic contact.[9]

Relatedly, much experimental evidence has accumulated to support the notion that a spectrum of EM fields cause illness. In most cases, very weak signals were found to have the greatest effects whereas strong signals produced none at all. Therefore, the toxic effects of frequency vibrations are most commonly associated with only very tiny specific EM amplitudes and wave frequencies.

## Prions and Light Waves

Joey and Len immediately noted the relevance of this early research to Joey's prion hypothesis, and after reading the most salient papers, the two investigators recorded the following discussion:

**Joey:** DNA nucleotides, and/or clustered water molecules, contain light energy that is released during viral and prion infections, and subsequent cell death. This might explain a number of observations, including the sparks seen coming off the infected nerve cells in the area of prion infections. Electron microscopists have reported this but haven't explained it. The high energy laser-like photon release associated with prion infections might best explain the areas of brain damage surrounding prion crystals that histologically simulate areas of electocauterization with rampant "gliosis—astrocytosis," "vacuolization," and cell debris surrounding the infected lesions. This energy mechanism might even explain the phenomenon of crystallization and prion crystal growth."

**Len:** Elaborate.

**Joey:** Electromagnetic (EM) energy from some exogenous [that is, external] source could be the missing factor in prion disease. It might explain Dr. Heaphy's theory of prion pleomorphism and potential link to viral reproduction. The normal 250 amino acid sequence prion protein (PrP) suddenly changes. Odds are it's a frequency vibration that flips its physical form to the abnormal and lethal (pD) form. Although it appears that the normal protein "(pN) can spontaneously flip to pD," it's probably unobserved energy that initiates this chain reaction while more EM waves keep it going."[22]

**Len:** That would also support the "virino hypothesis" whereby a DNA virus or "stealth virus" would supply the energy and electromagnetic signal to start the ball rolling. The DNA could naturally release its potential nucleotide/clustered water energy and, as a result, the kinetic spark or energy emitted might cause the pN to convert to the pD associated with prion disease. That would explain why "different strains of prions" have been found to "cause differing patterns of disease." Numerous scientists have found that "the existence of strains in [prion] pathogens is usually the result of changes in the nucleic acid sequence of the infectious agent" believed to be "DNA or possibly RNA viruses."[22] Slightly different nucleotide sequences would naturally release different wave forms of energy—different frequency emissions. This might explain the slightly different prion crystallization patterns called prion "strains."

**Joey:** I repeat, it might also explain how "spontaneous" and "exponential" amplification of the prion (converting pN into pD in the body) occurs.

**Len:** Exactly! Like "Chladni figures" formed in response to varying frequencies of sound, which is electromagnetic energy. The physical patterns formed are highly organized patterns commonly simulating crystalline structures like snowflakes. These reflect an intelligence, an organization, inherent in, communicated by, and changed by, the specific wave frequencies broadcast. Much like God said, "Let there be light, Earth and seas" and then it happened "spontaneously" from the *sound* of his voice. The idea that prion protein conversion of pN to pD happens "spontaneously" is similar. Yet remarkably, scientists have not advanced this prion hypothesis. They've remained focused on the physical aspects of the disease heedless of the spiritual, that is, the electromagnetic.

**Joey:** Additional research that supports this EM prion thesis includes the work of Clarence Ryan, at Washington State University. Ryan, a member of the National Academy of Sciences, led a team of four WSU scientists at the Institute of Biological Chemistry in the Department of Biochemistry and Biophysics. They discovered UV light's profound impact on gene expression and gene repair in both plants and animals. Their study, published in the October 31, 1996 issue of *Nature*, showed that UV light activated the expression of more than fifteen defense proteins. So specific frequencies of color and light can undoubtedly impact DNA and its nucleotides, as well as cellular proteins. Therefore, it shouldn't be a surprise that prion proteins might "spontaneously" transform from benign human proteins to lethal ones when struck with certain EM frequencies, and visa versa.

"That's also likely related to the pleomorphic theory Béchamp advanced. [23]

"Additionally germane to prion disease, one colleague of Ryan's, coauthor Antonio Conconi, went on to study 'the effects of ultra violet light on DNA repair linked to gene transport in frogs and in yeast cells.' [22] The fact that yeast cells carry prion crystals that, like the quartz in Dr. Kaznachayev's studies, might transmit ultraviolet EM radiation to cause cell damage should be investigated.

"In fact, this destructive mechanism should also be investigated in-so-far-as the mysterious illness killing frogs. Apparently, scientists have found an 'unnamed fungus,' thought to be related to the earth's earliest fungi, linked to the massive frog death and disease happening all around the world. They have even published their suspicion that

## Fig. 10.3. Symptoms Related to Mycotoxicity

### Digestive System
- Diarrhea
- Vomiting
- Intestinal hemorrhage
- Liver necrosis and fibrosis
- Liver cancer (aflatoxin)
- Mucous membrane damage
- Anorexia
- Vomitoxin
- Esophageal cancer

### Respiratory System
- Respiratory distress
- Lung hemorrhage due to tricothecene toxicity
- Nasal irritation
- Asthma

### Nervous System
- Anxiety
- Depression
- Confusion
- Toxic encephalopathy
- Headaches
- General stress

### Neuroendocrine System
- Corticosteroid release
- Catecholamine release

### Skin Disorders
- Rashes
- Burning
- Sloughing
- Photosensitive

### Urinary System
- Nephrotoxicity

### Reproductive System
- Infertility
- Menstral problems

### Immune System
- T-cell suppression
- Repeated yeast and viral infections
- Frequent colds, flu
- Inflammatory response to damaged tissues

### Musculoskeletal Effects
- Severe Pain
- Headaches
- Chronic Fatigue (CFIDS)
- Tremors
- Multple Sclerosis (MS) related disorders

Fungi have been implicated for many years in a number of outbreaks. More recently, fungi such as *Stachybotrys atra*, *Aspergillus* and *Penicillinin*, have been linked to many contemporary illnesses including those seen above. Many of these ailments are linked to fungal-produced intoxication with the chemical trichothecene. Trichothecene was responsible for infant mortality and morbidity in 10 Cleveland cases, 8 Chicago cases, 32 Ohio cases, and 47 more in other parts of the country in 1994-95. (See: *MMWR* 1995;44:67-74.)

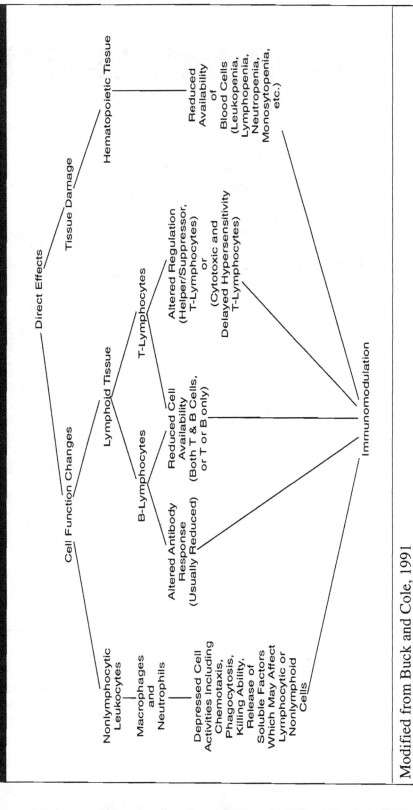

# Fig. 10.4. Immunological Affects of Trichothecene Exposure

Modified from Buck and Cole, 1991

'ultraviolet radiation penetrating the atmosphere' may be a cofactor in this fungus transmitted plague. According to a recent report, researchers aren't sure if the frogs, which breathe through their skins, are suffocating because of the fungus, or if the fungus is releasing a lethal mycotoxin that is suppressing their respiration. It may be that we're looking at a similar prion-linked illness that is killing the nerve and brain cells required for respiration.[24]

"The same may be true, or similar mechanisms at work, in the infections of thirty-four Cleveland infants, ten of whom died of a strange fungal infection between 1993 and 1997. The lungs of the infected children suddenly began to hemorrhage. The fungi, *Stachybotrys atra*, one of a number of black molds, was reported to have grown in water-soaked cellulose, typical in homes with water damage from flooding, plumbing leaks, or roof leaks that soak building materials such as insulation, gypsum board and ceiling tile. The spores of the fungus contained very potent mycotoxins that were particularly toxic to the rapidly growing infants' lungs.[25]

**Len:** It's also interesting that scientists have been using ultraviolet light to kill and mutate fungi, but new strains are apparently more resistant, and some fungi may even be activated by UV light. One study I read concerned fungi residing in wheat and wheat seeds. It was posted on the Internet by researchers from McGill University's Department of Agricultural and Biosystems Engineering. They discussed certain advantages of using radio frequencies, with longer EM wavelengths than microwaves, to effectively penetrate larger quantities of seed.[26] Another study of an anaerobic fungus, *Neocallimastix frontalis*—a common cell-destroying fungus in ruminants at high risk for prion diseases—proved the fungus was susceptible to "chemical and irradiational mutagenesis." But unlike most fungi that are killed by UV light, the researchers found this and other related fungal strains were "capable of photoreactivation"—meaning they were virtually able to raise this fungus from the dead by *exposing it* to ultraviolet light![27]

"Regarding that Cleveland fungus that killed the infants, I recently read an interesting series of articles by William Sorenson, an immunologist at the University of Texas, and one of the world's leading experts in the field of mycotoxin research. He reported new findings to the National Institute for Occupational Safety and Health (NIOSH) that grain dust is often contaminated with fungi and mycotoxins.[28] He showed that spores of several fungi that were commonly found in agricultural dust were linked to several outbreaks of "organic dust toxic syndrome," or ODTS. He and his colleagues found that the ODTS-associated dust stimulated the production of blood chemicals and immune system altering agents (e.g., leukotriene, KC, MIP-la, and complement). Sorenson's group found suggestive evidence linking the inhalation of these fungal spores to the deaths of the Cleveland infants. [The cause of death was listed as "ideopathic hemosiderosis."] (See figures 10.3 and 10.4 for more information regarding *Stachybotrys atra* infection and related symptoms from tricothecene mycotoxicosis.)[28]

**Joey:** If anyone thinks that prion disease develops independently of bioelectric phenomena, particularly during the transformation of the affiliated benign protein pN to the lethal pD, they would be enlightened to read *Protein Science*. Here, investigators who study prions routinely reference measurements of "rotational-resonance distances," "cross-polarization phenomena," and even "magic-angle spinning conditions" associated with prion proteins."[29]

## Prion Crystals Compared to Medical "Biochips"

Given the historic realities and stunning revelations provided thus far, the concept that modern biotechnologies, including man-made infectious agents, might be "inoculated" into the masses for population control is solidly evidenced. Support for this thesis not only comes from scientific papers and government documents, but also revelations from the King James Bible, *Webster's Dictionary*, the *Protocols of the Elders of Sion*, *The Report From Iron Mountain*, Baylor College's

Huntsville Prison documents, and Dr. Horowitz's earlier book *Emerging Viruses: AIDS & Ebola*. This evidence propels a rational concern that prions, much like the infamous "mark of the beast," might be the quintessential agents for mind and population control. While even mainstream periodicals and national news broadcasts have heralded forthcoming "biochip" technologies, the widespread presence of prion proteins in human brains potentially provides the cryptocracy with more insidious capabilities.

"Biochips," in fact, have long been regarded as a worthy technology for development by military and intelligence contractors, as well as for private corporations. A recent feature story circulated by Reuters, for example, hailed the creation of "new 'biochips' aimed at medicine [and] agriculture."[30] Motorola, Packard Instrument, and the U.S. government's Argonne National Laboratory had "teamed up to mass-produce 'biochips'—devices akin to computer chips," that had widespread applications.

Argonne and the Russian Academy of Science's Englehardt Institute of Molecular Biology in Moscow had already developed nineteen "biological microchip" inventions that contained "chemical compounds" that could analyze, affect, or attack "biological targets" including DNA sequences, genetic variations, gene expressions, protein interactions, and human immune functions.[30]

During a telephone news conference, Reuters reported, "U.S. Energy Secretary Federico Pena called the [Argonne and DARPA[30]] project one of 'profound importance to all Americans.' The Energy Department had funded the project in conjunction with the Human Genome Project, which had the task of mapping the entire set of human chromosomes by the year 2005. Pena said it could be the birth of a new multibillion dollar industry."

Reuters failed to report that the Human Genome Project was the name given to the DNA mapping program, largely funded by the Rockefeller and Alfred P. Sloan foundations, that provided continuity for the eugenics movement of the 1920s and 30s. As detailed previously, eugenics's offspring was the "racial hygiene" program embraced by Hitler. These political agendas each targeted certain races and populations for genocide.

Moreover, the Energy Department, especially its Atomic Energy Commission (AEC), is further implicated in the development of biological weapons for potentially genocidal applications. The AEC's director, Dr. Alfred Hellman, helped persuade an international scientific gathering, in 1968, that the Marburg virus—the mother of Ebola—was not a laboratory creation as the world's leading expert in this field, Dr. Seymour Kalter, from the Southwest Foundation's National Cancer Institute laboratories, had publicly argued.[31]

Thus, today's "biochip" program is implicated by association with the Human Genome Project, its Nazi racial hygiene program forerunners, as well as Atomic Energy Commission links to potentially genocidal biological weapons research and developments.

"With a commercial biochip to rapidly and economically perform genetic analysis [and genetic manipulations with potentially genocidal applications], within a few years we should see better pharmaceuticals developed more rapidly," said Richard McKernan, president of Packard Instrument. In agriculture, he predicted improved crop strength and breeding along with early disease detection in animals.

"The partners expect the greatest impact in the [biochip] field," Reuters relayed, to affect medical diagnostics. They wrote "researchers would be able to identify [and create] in minutes mutated genes that could lead to later medical problems such as cancer, multiple sclerosis, or Alzheimer's."[30]

All three of these illnesses, it should be recalled, have been linked to vaccine injuries, including cancers of the lung, brain, and lymph nodes.[32]

With such intense hype, all risks aside, populations will be lined up by "prevention minded" governments to be inoculated with their "biochips" by the year 2003, according to industry experts.[30]

Such "biochips" would, of course, provide far greater control over myriad human functions than a simple crystal prion might. At least many suspect this to be the case. One such petitioner for public concern was Dr. Carl W. Sanders, who received a wide audience on the internet in September, 1997. Dr. Sanders claimed to be "an electronics engineer, inventor, author and consultant to various government organizations as well as IBM, General Electric, Honeywell and Teledyne."

The Sanders alert, entitled "The Microchip and the Mark of the Beast,"[33] recalled thirty-two years of his life devoted to designing and engineering microchips for biomedical applications. Though most people would scoff at his many allegations, parts of his story at least seemed reasonable, particularly when placed in the context of well documented mind control programs as detailed in the next chapter. If only for the widespread interest it received, here's Dr. Sanders's report:

> ... In 1968 I became involved, almost by accident, in a research and development project in regard to a spinal bypass for a young lady who had severed her spine. They were looking at possibly being able to connect motor nerves etc. It was a project we were all excited about. There were 100 people involved and I was senior engineer in charge of the project. This project culminated in the microchip that we talk about now, a microchip that I believe is going to be the positive identification and "mark of the beast."

> This microchip is recharged by body temperature changes.[32] Obviously you can't go in and have your battery changed every so often, so the microchip has a recharging circuit that charges based upon the body temperature changes. Over one and a half million dollars was spent finding out that the two places in the body that the temperature changes most rapidly are in the forehead (primary position), right below the hairline, and the back of the hand (alternative position).

> Working on the microchip, we had no idea about it ever being an identification chip. We looked at it as being a very humanitarian thing to do. . . . My responsibility had to do with the design of the chip itself, not the medical side of it.

As the chip came to evolve, there came a time in the project when they said that the financial return on bypassing severed spines is not a very lucrative thing for us to be into, so we really needed to look at some other areas. We noticed that the frequency of the chip had a great effect upon behavior and so we began to branch off and look possibly at behavior modification. [See next chapter for more details.]

The project almost turned into electronic acupuncture because what they ended up with was embedding the microchip to put out a signal which affected certain areas. They were able to determine that you could cause behavior change. One of the projects was called the Phoenix [I] project which had to do with Vietnam veterans. We had a chip that was called the Rambo chip. This chip would actually cause extra adrenaline [to] flow. . . . [another stopped] estrogen flow . . . This was tested in India and other parts of the world. So here you have a birth control tool, based on a microchip.

Microchips can also be used for migraine headaches, behavior modification, uppers/downers, sexual stimulation and sexual depression. This is nothing more than electronic acupuncture . . .

As the development moved along, I left the project and came back as a consultant several times. . . . I attended one meeting wherein it was asked, "How can you control people if you can't identify them?" All of a sudden the idea came, "Let's make them aware of lost children, etc." This was discussed in meetings almost like people were cattle. The CIA came up with an idea of putting pictures of lost children on milk cartons. Since the chip is now accepted, you don't see the pictures anymore . . . It served its purpose.

As we developed this microchip, as the identification chip became the focal point, there were several things that were wanted. They wanted a name, an image (picture of your face), social security number with the international digits on it, finger print identification, physical description, family history, address, occupation, income tax information and criminal record.

I've attended seventeen "one world" meetings where this has been discussed—meetings in Brussels, Luxembourg, tying together the finances of the world.

Just recently in the newspapers they've talked about the health care program, the "Womb to Tomb" identification. . . . There are bills before congress right now that will allow them to inject a microchip into your child at the time of birth for "identification purposes." The president of the United States of America, under the "Immigration and Naturalization Control Act of 1986," Section 100, has the authority to deem whatever type of identification is necessary—whether it be an invisible tattoo or electronic media under the skin. So I think you have to look at these facts. . . .[33]

Zbigniew Brzezinski, Past Executive Director of the Trilateral Commission, the National Security Advisor to President Jimmy Carter, and advisor to four other presidents stated, "The technotronic era involves the gradual appearance of a more controlled society. Such a society would be dominated by an elite, unrestrained by traditional values." In his book, *Between Two Ages*, he wrote, "Soon it will be possible to assert almost continuous surveillance over every citizen and maintain up-to-date complete files containing even the most personal information about the citizen. These files will be subject to instantaneous retrieval by the authorities."[34]

It is unlikely that anyone making such extraordinary investments would place all of their "eggs in one basket." One control device may apparently be in the form of prion crystals. Surveillance equipment may go under the skin with biochips. The currently expanding technology called the "Health Card" or "Health Passport," discussed in greater detail in the next chapter, contains an additional tracking device.

## References

1. Thomas W. Mystery contrails: Poison from the sky. Document available on www.Islandnet.com/~wilco/. Also personal communication from Will Thomas, February 26, 1999, following his second national broadcast on "The Art Bell Show" wherein this information was also provided. See also: Staff reporters. Art Bell says everbody is sick: Watch those contrails in sky! *Contact: The Phoenix Educator*, February 16, 1999, Vol. 23, No. 13, pp. 1, 8-9. The Thomas and Bell reports were countered by independent investigator Jay Reynolds. See: "Contrail Controversy" in FTP file at www.tetrahedron.org.

According to Will Thomas (personal communication April 25, 2000), he was able to locate a patent, held by the Hughes Corporation, for the development and deployment of an aluminum oxide atmospheric spraying device. These authors theorize, and strongly suspect, this "weather modification" method might somehow serve to increase transmission of certain electromagnetic frequencies, like those produced by projects HAARP and EISCAT, for behavior modification and global population control. For more details on the Hughes patent contact Will Thomas at: wilco@islandnet.com.

In addition, see website http://www.contrailconnection.com/ for excellent color photographs of chemtrails spraying from the tail sections of aircraft whose jet engines are devoid of contrails.

Another website, http://www.earthfiles.com/earth039.html, shows chemtrails, one formed at a 90 degree angle in Three Rivers, Michigan, that according to Centers for Disease Control and Prevention, Toxicology Information Branch administrator George Prince, represents a "scary hoax." According to Prince, who admitted "extremely small quantities" of ethylene dibromide (EDB) have mysteriously been included in jet fuels, "Unless there is indeed the broad conspiracy . . . ambient air monitoring efforts conducted by the U. S. Government, state governments, and private and public research institutions would detect any widespread levels that might pose a threat to health." Mr. Prince responds to questions at 1-888-42-ATSDR, or by e-mail at ATSDRIC@cdc.gov.

2. Pettersson P and Cleaves Y. Cymatics—The Science of the Future? available only on the internet at http://www.alphaomega.se/english/cymatics.html#chladni.

3. Klein, CF. "Woven Heaven, Tangled Earth: A Weaver's Paradigm of the Mesoamerican Cosmos," in *Ethnoastronomy and Archeoastronomy in the American Tropics*, Ed. by Anthony P. Aveni and Gary Urton, *Annals of the Academy of Science*, Vol. 385, New York, 1982, p. 15.

3a. For more information on the biological and bioelectric effects of clustered water and DNA, browse the clustered water "technical background" on the internet beginning at http://www.tetrahedron.org. See also discussions in Chapter 6, references 2 and 20.

4. McClellan, R. *The Healing Forces of Music: History, Theory and Practice*, Rockport, MA: Element, Inc., 1991, p. 50.

5. Jenny, H. *Kymatik: Wellen und Schwingungen mit ihrer Struktur un Dynamik (Cymatics: The Structure and Dynamics of Waves and Vibrations)*, Basilius Press, 1967, p. 10. See also: Dr. Sir Peter Guy Manners "Healing by Sound" information at http://eclecticviewpoint.com/evmanners.html.

6. Beaulieu, J. *Music and Sound in the Healing Arts*, Station Hill Press, 1987, p. 40.

7. Guzzetta, CE. *Music Therapy: Nursing the Music of the Soul, in Music: Physician for the Times to Come*, Don Campbell, Editor, Quest Books, 1991, p. 149.

8. Gurvich AG. *Problems of Mitogenetic Radiations as an Aspect of Molecular Biology*. Moscow: Meditsina Publishing House, 1960.

9. Staff writer. Ultra-violet light and infections. *The Equinox Alternative*. Etonhall Publishing, 1998. (Available on the Internet at www.equinoxalternative.com.)

10. Kaznachayev VP, Michailova LP, et al. Apparent information transfer between two groups of cells. *Psychoenergetic Systems* 1974;1:37.

11. Kaznachayev VP and Michailova LP. *Ultra-weak Radiation from Cells as a Mechanism of Intracellular Interaction*. Novosibirsk: Nauka Publishing House, 1981.

12. Quizkenden TI and QueHee SS. Weak luminescence for the yeast Saccharomyces cerevisae and the existence of mitogenetic radiation. *Biochem Biophys Res Comm* 1974;60-2:764-769.

13. Gurvitch AA, Eremeyev VF and Karabchievsky YA. *Energy Base of the Mitogenetic Radiation and its Registration on Photoelectron Multiplier*. Moscow: Meditsina Publishing House, 1974.

14. Quizkenden TI and QueHee SS. The spectral distribution of the luminescence emitted during the growth of the yeast Saccharomyces cerevisae and its relation to mitogenetic radiation, *Photochem Photobiol* 1976;23:201-204.

15. Ruth B. Experimental investigation of low-level photon emission. In: *Electromagnetic Bio-Information*. FA Popp, G Becker, HL Konig and W Peschka, Eds. Munich: Urban and Schwarzenberg, 1979, pp. 107-122.

16. Popp FA. Being ill: when cells no longer talk to each other. *Bild Wissen* 1977;80:90-97.

17. Popp FA. Photon storage in biological systems. In: *Electromagnetic Bio-Information*. FA Popp, G Becker, HL Konig and W Peschka, Eds. Munich: Urban and Schwarzenberg, 1979, pp. 123-141.

18. Rattenmeyer M, Popp FA and Nagl W. Evidence of photon emissions from DNA in living systems. *Naturwissen* 1981;11:572-573.

19. Popp FA, Ruth B, Bahr J, et al. Emission of visible and UV radiation by active biological systems. *Collect Phenom* 1981;3:187-214.

20. Vuickenden TI and Tjlbury RN. Growth dependent luminescence from cultures of normal and respiratory deficient Saccharomyces cerevisiae. *Photochem Photobiol* 1983;37:337-344.

21. Karu TI, Kalendo VS, Letokhov VS, et al. Response of proliferating and resting tumour cells to repetitive pulsed low-intensity UV laser radiation. *Dolk Akad Nauk SSSR* 1982;262:1498-1501.

21. Contributing scientists. Ask the experts: Medicine—"What is a prion? Specifically, what is known about the molecular structure of prions and how they cause infections such as Creutzfeldt-Jakob disease? *Scientific American* on the internet. Available from file:///A/medicine14what is a prion.html.

23. Day T. UV light discovery surprises scientists. Washington State University College of Agriculture and Home Economics. Press release, November 13, 1996. (Available on the Internet from WSU file:///A/Wsu.htm) For pleomorphic theory proposed by Béchamp see: Young RO. *Sick & Tired: Reclaim Your Inner Terrain*. Unpublished manuscript. Copyright 1997 by Dr. Robert O. Young, 134 East 200 North Alpine, Utah 84004, pp. 1-3; App. D., Sect. 1, p. 2.

24. Staff writer. Zoologists identify mysterious fungus killing world's frogs and toads. Fox News Service, June 25, 1998. (Available

on the Internet from www.foxnews.com and from www.sightings.com file:///A/toadsnfrogs.htm.)

25. Case Western Reserve University. Fungus study: NIEHS, CDC fund study of fungus fatal to Cleveland infants. Announced in *Science* September, 1997. (Available on the Internet from http://jeeves. niehs.nih.gov/oc/factor/9709/fungus.htm and http://gcrc.meds.cwru. edu/stachy.htm.)

26. Orsat V and Raghavan V. Radio-frequency treatment of seed-quality wheat infected with Fusarium Graminearum. McGill University, Department of Agricultural and Biosystems Engineering, Ste-Anne de Bellevue, August 2, 1998. (Available from www.processing.com file:///A/fn96311 Wheat Fungus. htm.)

27. Calza RE and Barichievich EM. Mutagen killing and photo-reactivation in the anaerobic fungus Neocallimastix frontalis EB188. Washington State University, Pullman, WA 99164-6320. (Scientific paper available on the Internet from http://www.seqnet.dl.ac.uk/re-search/fgsc/fgn43/calza.html.)

28. Sorenson WG and Lewis DM. Organic dust toxic syndrome. In: *The Mycota*, K. Esser and P. A. Lemke, eds. Vol VII. "Animal and Human Relations." Berlin, Germany: Springer-Verlag, pp.159-172; See also Dr. Sorenson's website at http://www.hsc.wvu.edu/micro/fac-ulty/sorenson.htm.

29. Heller J, Kolbert AC, Larsen R, Ernst M, et al. Solid-state NMR studies of the prion protein H1 fragment. *Protein Science* 1996;5:1655-1661. (Also available on the Internet from http://www.cyber-dyne. com/~tom/upcoming_3D.html.)

30. Staff reporter. New "Biochips" aimed at medicine, agriculture. Reuters News Service, June 30, 1998. (Report listed on *PCWorld Today* available through the Internet from http://www.pcworld.com/pc-wtoday/article/0,1510,7313,00.html.)

The Defense Advance Research Projects Agency (DARPA) connection to Argonne Labs was brought to Dr. Horowitz's attention by Spanish journalist Roman Ribera Canet. This investigator reported for dissemination the intelligence that DARPA was born in the late 1950s to facilitate military space programs. Linked also to the Hughes Corporation, biological weapons contractors, and biowarfare research and development, in 1969, "DARPA funded ARPANET, a communications network based on phone lines, linking universities and military researchers." ARPANET became the "father" of the internet. "DARPA, along with other proprietaries and fronts for the military–industrial complex, has much to do . . . with AIDS, . . . mad cow disease, and human variant CJD. . . . According to Professor Orlin Grabbe, DARPA launders drug money on line through 'virtual' casinos" to finance itself. If you want to learn how secret DARPA is, try searching for it over the internet!

31. Horowitz LG. *Emerging Viruses: AIDS & Ebola—Nature, Accident or Intentional?* Rockport, MA: Tetrahedron Publishing Group, 1997, pp. 461-463.

32. Horowitz LG. "Horowitz 'on Vaccines'". Sandpoint, Idaho: Tetrahedron Publishing Group, 1998.

33. Dr. Sanders statement that the microchip is recharged by fluctuating body temperatures may be well founded. In fact, Joey had theorized that prion activity was likewise linked to the thermodynamics of fungal infections. Reference: Sanders CW. The microchip and the mark of the beast. *Nexus.* Posted on the web September 8, 1997, at http://www.techmgmt.com/restore/micromrk.htm.

34. McLamb J. *Operation Vampire Killer 2000.* Phoenix, AZ: Police Against The New World Order. (P. O. Box 8712, Phoenix, AZ 85066), 1996, pp. 21-22.

35. See disclaimer regarding the litigation of Tenen vs. Winter posted at: http://www.drlenhorowitz.com/news_and_articles/person. al_file/stan_tenen_correction.html

# Chapter 11.
# EISCAT and Project HAARP:
# Killing All the Birds From Iron
# Mountain With One Secret Stone

The Sun produces a wide spectrum of electromagnetic effects on planet Earth and its people. It does so by producing x-rays, ultraviolet radiation and various other light frequencies, as well as by emitting magnetic fields. This later function is a property of "solar plasma." Solar plasma is the ions and electrons from atoms blown apart at the surface of the sun by its extreme heat.

"When the solar wind plasma reaches the Earth," an international government agency reported, "these embedded magnetic fields interact with the Earth's magnetic field, distorting it to form a compression on the dayside, and a very elongated tail on the nightside, away from the Sun. The region within which the Earth's magnetic field is constrained is called the magnetosphere . . .

"The solar UV, x-rays and charged particles, also ionize the upper part of the Earth's atmosphere resulting in a region, called the ionosphere, which can be studied by radar methods."[1] (See figure 11.1.)

This report, issued by EISCAT—the European Incoherent Scatter Association that is comprised and funded by seven nations: Finland, France, Germany, Japan, Norway, Sweden and the United Kingdom—further explained the "eleven year cycle" of changing electromagnetism surrounding the earth due to changes of the solar wind and plasma.

EISCAT's authors explained that high in the Earth's atmosphere "magnetic field lines provide routes" for particles to "interact with the neutral gas to produce spectacular auroral displays . . . and additional ionization at polar and auroral latitudes. Electric fields and currents are

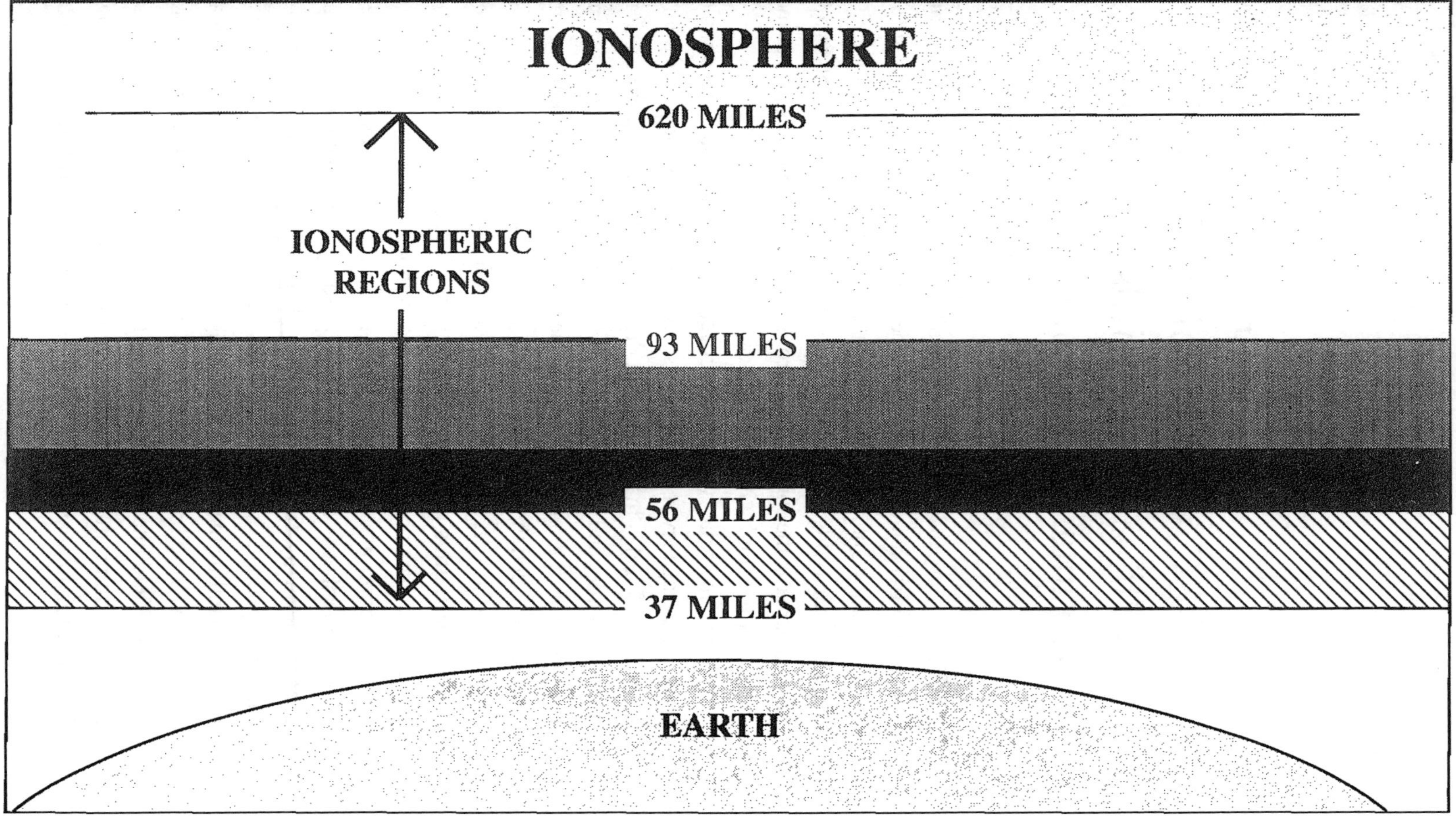

Fig. 11.1. The Ionosphere in Relation to the Earth as Reported in the HAARP Environmental Impact Statement

also transferred between the magnetosphere and the auroral zone iono-sphere."[1]

The purpose of EISCAT, its promotion stated, was to study these regions with radars "which transmit powerful radio waves into the ionosphere, where a small fraction of the energy is scattered back to the radar receiver. . . . EISCAT uses this technique" the article said, "in the study of solar-terrestrial physics. The scattered signal contains information describing the ionosphere and upper atmosphere."[1]

What EISCAT's report failed to mention was that their "scatter back" could have a profound effect on the weather and all living bioelectric systems including human beings. The authors also neglected to reveal EISCAT's connections to Cold Spring Harbor labs and the infamous "atmospheric heating project HAARP."

In other words, what EISCAT's propaganda failed to disclose was that EISCAT represented the quintessential bioelectric technology for population surveillance and control. As this chapter details, projects EISCAT and HAARP provide the bioelectric technology to kill all the Iron Mountain birds with one fell swoop from inner space.

## More Background On *The Report From Iron Mountain*[2]

Iron Mountain is located close to the town of Hudson, New York. The report by government consultants who met at this site beginning in 1963, briefly described this meeting place as "something out of [an] Ian Fleming" James Bond novel. "It is an underground nuclear hideout for hundreds of large American corporations. Most of them use it as an emergency storage vault for important documents. But a number of them maintain substitute corporate headquarters, as well, where essential personnel could presumably survive and continue to work after an attack. This latter group includes such firms as Standard Oil of New Jersey, Manufacturers Hanover Trust, and Shell."[3]

Standard Oil, of course, is owned principally by the Rockefeller family whose connections to the Committee of 300, NATO and The Club of Rome have already been detailed. Manufacturers Hanover

Trust is directed by Gabriel Hague, who is also affiliated with these largely secret organizations. Finally, according to Dr. John Coleman, Shell's controlling interests are held by Queen Elizabeth II.[4]

The Iron Mountain report,[2] "On the Possibility and Desirability of Peace," was written by anonymous authors and published in late 1967 with an introduction by Leonard C. Lewin who edited the manuscript. Its extraordinary content immediately sparked controversy and criticism of Lewin. Shortly thereafter, he reversed his position and announced that the meeting had not really happened. The report was his own satirical hoax, he retracted. By that time, the report had been so widely distributed, and believed, that its readers did not know which Lewin story to trust.

Given the relevance of *The Report From Iron Mountain* to Cecil Rhodes's century old quest to "charm young America . . . to share in a scheme to take the government of the whole world" for the "cessation of all wars" (as coordinated by a secret society under British rule), Len and Joey were left feeling the report was legitimate for at least five reasons: 1) someone with Lewin's apparent intimate knowledge of government operations and shadow governor objectives would not likely waste time, nor jeopardize his professional career, by developing and then distributing a hoax in the form of a serious work; 2) the in-depth analysis provided by the work would likely be missing in a satire; 3) a satire would likely include obviously satirical content missing in the final publication; 4) the work was published by an organization with Masonic and secret society connections—The Dial Press, Inc.; and 5) there was precedence for calling a legitimate document a satirical hoax—the old Hegelian "thesis–antithesis–synthesis" model— likewise successfully performed with *The Protocols of the Elders of Sion*. For all the above reasons, suggestions that *The Report From Iron Mountain* was a satirical hoax, were likely designed to confuse—standard counterintelligence propaganda.

Intelligent readers may judge for themselves as Figure 11.2 provides the recommendations provided by the Iron Mountain group at

**Fig. 11.2. The Report From Iron Mountain: Summary, Conclusions, Models and Substitutes for War**

SECTION 7

# SUMMARY AND CONCLUSIONS

*The Nature of War*

WAR IS NOT, as is widely assumed, primarily an instrument of policy utilized by nations to extend or defend their expressed political values or their economic interests. On the contrary, it is itself the principal basis of organization on which all modern societies are constructed. The common proximate cause of war is the apparent interference of one nation with the aspirations of another. But at the root of all ostensible differences of national interest lie the dynamic requirements of the war system itself for periodic armed conflict. Readiness for war characterizes contemporary social systems more broadly than their economic and political structures, which it subsumes.

79

373

Economic analyses of the anticipated problems of transition to peace have not recognized the broad preeminence of war in the definition of social systems. The same is true, with rare and only partial exceptions, of model disarmament "scenarios." For this reason, the value of this previous work is limited to the mechanical aspects of transition. Certain features of these models may perhaps be applicable to a real situation of conversion to peace; this will depend on their compatibility with a substantive, rather than a procedural, peace plan. Such a plan can be developed only from the premise of full understanding of the nature of the war system it proposes to abolish, which in turn presupposes detailed comprehension of the functions the war system performs for society. It will require the construction of a detailed and feasible system of substitutes for those functions that are necessary to the stability and survival of human societies.

## The Functions of War

The visible, military function of war requires no elucidation; it is not only obvious but also irrelevant to a transition to the condition of peace, in which it will by definition be superfluous. It is also subsidiary in social significance to the implied, nonmilitary functions of war; those critical to transition can be summarized in five principal groupings.

*1. Economic.* War has provided both ancient and modern societies with a dependable system for stabilizing and controlling national economies. No alternate method of control has yet been tested in a complex modern economy that has shown itself remotely comparable in scope or effectiveness.

*2. Political.* The permanent possibility of war is the foundation for stable government; it supplies the basis for general acceptance of political authority. It has enabled societies to maintain necessary class distinctions, and it has ensured the subordination of the citizen to the state, by virtue of the residual war powers inherent in the concept of nationhood. No modern political ruling group has successfully controlled its constituency after failing to sustain the continuing credibility of an external threat of war.

*3. Sociological.* War, through the medium of military institutions, has uniquely served societies, throughout the course of known history, as an indispensable controller of dangerous social dissidence and destructive antisocial tendencies. As the most formidable of threats to life itself, and as the only one susceptible to mitigation by social organization alone, it has played another equally fundamental role: the war system has provided the machinery through which the motivational forces governing human behavior have been translated into binding social allegiance. It has thus ensured the degree of social cohesion necessary to the viability of nations. No other institution, or groups of institutions, in modern societies, has successfully served these functions.

*4. Ecological.* War has been the principal evolutionary device for maintaining a satisfactory ecological balance between gross human population and supplies available for its survival. It is unique to the human species.

*5. Cultural and Scientific.* War-orientation has determined the basic standards of value in the creative arts, and has provided the fundamental motivational source of scientific and technological progress. The concepts that the arts express values independent of their own forms and that the successful pursuit of knowledge has intrinsic social value have long been accepted in modern societies; the development of the arts and sciences during this period has been corollary to the parallel development of weaponry.

### Substitutes for the Functions of War: Criteria

The foregoing functions of war are essential to the survival of the social systems we know today. With two possible exceptions they are also essential to any kind of stable social organization that might survive in a warless world. Discussion of the ways and means of transition to such a world are meaningless unless a) substitute institutions can be devised to fill these functions, or b) it can reasonably be hypothecated that the loss or partial loss of any one function need not destroy the viability of future societies.

Such substitute institutions and hypotheses must meet varying criteria. In general, they must be technically feasible, politically acceptable, and potentially credible to the members of the societies that adopt them. Specifically, they must be characterized as follows:

*1. Economic.* An acceptable economic surrogate for

the war system will require the expenditure of resources for completely nonproductive purposes at a level comparable to that of the military expenditures otherwise demanded by the size and complexity of each society. Such a substitute system of apparent "waste" must be of a nature that will permit it to remain independent of the normal supply-demand economy; it must be subject to arbitrary political control.

*2. Political.* A viable political substitute for war must posit a generalized external menace to each society of a nature and degree sufficient to require the organization and acceptance of political authority.

*3. Sociological.* First, in the permanent absence of war, new institutions must be developed that will effectively control the socially destructive segments of societies. Second, for purposes of adapting the physical and psychological dynamics of human behavior to the needs of social organization, a credible substitute for war must generate an omnipresent and readily understood fear of personal destruction. This fear must be of a nature and degree sufficient to ensure adherence to societal values to the full extent that they are acknowledged to transcend the value of individual human life.

*4. Ecological.* A substitute for war in its function as the uniquely human system of population control must ensure the survival, if not necessarily the improvement, of the species, in terms of its relation to environmental supply.

*5. Cultural and Scientific.* A surrogate for the function of war as the determinant of cultural values must

establish a basis of sociomoral conflict of equally compelling force and scope. A substitute motivational basis
for the quest for scientific knowledge must be similarly
informed by a comparable sense of internal necessity.

### Substitutes for the Functions of War: Models

The following substitute institutions, among others,
have been proposed for consideration as replacements
for the nonmilitary functions of war. That they may not
have been originally set forth for that purpose does not
preclude or invalidate their possible application here.

*1. Economic.* a) A comprehensive social-welfare
program, directed toward maximum improvement of
general conditions of human life. b) A giant open-end
space research program, aimed at unreachable targets.
c) A permanent, ritualized, ultra-elaborate disarmament
inspection system, and variants of such a system.

*2. Political.* a) An omnipresent, virtually omnipotent international police force. b) An established and
recognized extraterrestrial menace. c) Massive global environmental pollution. d) Fictitious alternate enemies.

*3. Sociological: Control function.* a) Programs generally derived from the Peace Corps model. b) A modern,
sophisticated form of slavery. *Motivational function.* a)
Intensified environmental pollution. b) New religions or
other mythologies. c) Socially oriented blood games. d)
Combination forms.

*4. Ecological.* A comprehensive program of applied
eugenics.

EISCAT and Project HAARP: Killing All The Birds

5. *Cultural.* No replacement institution offered. *Scientific.* The secondary requirements of the space research, social welfare, and/or eugenics programs.

### Substitutes for the Functions of War: Evaluation

The models listed above reflect only the beginning of the quest for substitute institutions for the functions of war, rather than a recapitulation of alternatives. It would be both premature and inappropriate, therefore, to offer final judgments on their applicability to a transition to peace and after. Furthermore, since the necessary but complex project of correlating the compatibility of proposed surrogates for different functions could be treated only in exemplary fashion at this time, we have elected to withhold such hypothetical correlations as were tested as statistically inadequate.[1]

Nevertheless, some tentative and cursory comments on these proposed functional "solutions" will indicate the scope of the difficulties involved in this area of peace planning.

*Economic.* The social-welfare model cannot be expected to remain outside the normal economy after the conclusion of its predominantly capital-investment phase; its value in this function can therefore be only temporary. The space-research substitute appears to meet both major criteria, and should be examined in greater detail, especially in respect to its probable effects on other war functions. "Elaborate inspection" schemes, although superficially attractive, are inconsistent with the basic premise

**86**

of transition to peace. The "unarmed forces" variant, logistically similar, is subject to the same functional criticism as the general social-welfare model.

*Political.* Like the inspection-scheme surrogates, proposals for plenipotentiary international police are inherently incompatible with the ending of the war system. The "unarmed forces" variant, amended to include unlimited powers of economic sanction, might conceivably be expanded to constitute a credible external menace. Development of an acceptable threat from "outer space," presumably in conjunction with a space-research surrogate for economic control, appears unpromising in terms of credibility. The environmental-pollution model does not seem sufficiently responsive to immediate social control, except through arbitrary acceleration of current pollution trends; this in turn raises questions of political acceptability. New, less regressive, approaches to the creation of fictitious global "enemies" invite further investigation.

*Sociological: Control function.* Although the various substitutes proposed for this function that are modeled roughly on the Peace Corps appear grossly inadequate in potential scope, they should not be ruled out without further study. Slavery, in a technologically modern and conceptually euphemized form, may prove a more efficient and flexible institution in this area. *Motivational function.* Although none of the proposed substitutes for war as the guarantor of social allegiance can be dismissed out of hand, each presents serious and special difficulties. Intensified environmental threats may raise ecological dangers; mythmaking dissociated from war may no longer be politically feasible; purposeful blood games and rituals can far more readily be devised than implemented. An institution combining this function with the preceding one, based on, but not necessarily imitative of, the precedent of organized ethnic repression, warrants careful consideration.

*Ecological.* The only apparent problem in the application of an adequate eugenic substitute for war is that of timing; it cannot be effectuated until the transition to peace has been completed, which involves a serious temporary risk of ecological failure.

*Cultural.* No plausible substitute for this function of war has yet been proposed. It may be, however, that a basic cultural value-determinant is not necessary to the survival of a stable society. *Scientific.* The same might be said for the function of war as the prime mover of the search for knowledge. However, adoption of either a giant space-research program, a comprehensive social-welfare program, or a master program of eugenic control would provide motivation for limited technologies.

*General Conclusions*

It is apparent, from the foregoing, that no program or combination of programs yet proposed for a transition to peace has remotely approached meeting the comprehensive functional requirements of a world without war. Although one projected system for filling the economic function of war seems promising, similar optimism cannot be expressed in the equally essential political and sociological areas. The other major nonmilitary functions of war—ecological, cultural, scientific—raise very different problems, but it is at least possible that detailed programming of substitutes in these areas is not prerequisite to transition. More important, it is not enough to develop adequate but separate surrogates for the major war functions; they must be fully compatible and in no degree self-canceling.

Until such a unified program is developed, at least hypothetically, it is impossible for this or any other group to furnish meaningful answers to the questions originally presented to us. When asked how best to prepare for the advent of peace, we must first reply, as strongly as we can, that the war system cannot responsibly be allowed to disappear until 1) we know exactly what it is we plan to put in its place, and 2) we are certain, beyond reasonable doubt, that these substitute institutions will serve their purposes in terms of the survival and stability of society. It will then be time enough to develop methods for effectuating the transition; procedural programming must follow, not precede, substantive solutions.

Such solutions, if indeed they exist, will not be arrived at without a revolutionary revision of the modes of thought heretofore considered appropriate to peace research. That we have examined the fundamental questions involved from a dispassionate, value-free point of view should not imply that we do not appreciate the intellectual and emotional difficulties that must be overcome on all decision-making levels before these questions are generally acknowledged by others for what they are.

They reflect, on an intellectual level, traditional emotional resistance to new (more lethal and thus more "shocking") forms of weaponry. The understated comment of then-Senator Hubert Humphrey on the publication of *On Thermonuclear War* is still very much to the point: "New thoughts, particularly those which appear to contradict current assumptions, are always painful for the mind to contemplate."

Nor, simply because we have not discussed them, do we minimize the massive reconciliation of conflicting interests which domestic as well as international agreement on proceeding toward genuine peace presupposes. This factor was excluded from the purview of our assignment, but we would be remiss if we failed to take it into account. Although no insuperable obstacle lies in the path of reaching such general agreements, formidable short-term private-group and general-class interest in maintaining the war system is well established and widely recognized. The resistance to peace stemming from such interest is only tangential, in the long run, to the basic functions of war, but it will not be easily overcome, in this country or elsewhere. Some observers, in fact, believe that it cannot be overcome at all in our time, that the price of peace is, simply, too high. This bears on our overall conclusions to the extent that timing in the transference to substitute institutions may often be the critical factor in their political feasibility.

It is uncertain, at this time, whether peace will ever be possible. It is far more questionable, by the objective standard of continued social survival rather than that of emotional pacifism, that it would be desirable even if it were demonstrably attainable. The war system, for all its subjective repugnance to important sections of "public opinion," has demonstrated its effectiveness since the beginning of recorded history; it has provided the basis for the development of many impressively durable civilizations, including that which is dominant today. It has consistently provided unambiguous social priorities. It is, on the whole, a known quantity. A viable system of peace, assuming that the great and complex questions of substitute institutions raised in this Report are both soluble and solved, would still constitute a venture into the unknown, with the inevitable risks attendant on the unforeseen, however small and however well hedged.

Government decision-makers tend to choose peace over war whenever a real option exists, because it usually appears to be the "safer" choice. Under most immediate circumstances they are likely to be right. But in terms of long-range social stability, the opposite is true. At our present state of knowledge and reasonable inference, it is the war system that must be identified with stability, the peace system with social speculation, however justifiable the speculation may appear, in terms of subjective moral or emotional values. A nuclear physicist once remarked, in respect to a possible disarmament agreement: "If we could change the world into a world in which no weapons could be made, that would be stabilizing. But agreements we can expect with the Soviets would be destabilizing."[2] The qualification and the bias are equally irrelevant; *any* condition of genuine total peace, however achieved, would be destabilizing until proved otherwise.

If it were necessary at this moment to opt irrevocably for the retention or for the dissolution of the war system, common prudence would dictate the former course. But it is not yet necessary, late as the hour appears. And more factors must eventually enter the war-peace equation than even the most determined search for alternative institutions for the functions of war can be expected to reveal. One group of such factors has been given only passing mention in this Report; it centers around the possible obsolescence of the war system itself. We have noted, for instance, the limitations of the war system in filling its ecological function and the declining importance of this aspect of war. It by no means stretches the imagination to visualize comparable developments which may compromise the efficacy of war as, for example, an economic controller or as an organizer of social allegiance. This kind of possibility, however remote, serves as a reminder that all calculations of contingency not only involve the weighing of one group of risks against another, but require a respectful allowance for error on both sides of the scale.

A more expedient reason for pursuing the investigation of alternate ways and means to serve the current functions of war is narrowly political. It is possible that one or more major sovereign nations may arrive, through ambiguous leadership, at a position in which a ruling administrative class may lose control of basic public opinion or of its ability to rationalize a desired war. It is not hard to imagine, in such circumstance, a situation in which such governments may feel forced to initiate serious full-scale disarmament proceedings (perhaps provoked by "accidental" nuclear explosions), and that such negotiations may lead to the actual disestablishment of military institutions. As our Report has made clear, this could be catastrophic. It seems evident that, in the event an important part of the world is suddenly plunged without sufficient warning into an inadvertent peace, even partial and inadequate preparation for the possibility may be better than none. The difference could even be critical. The models considered in the preceding chapter, both those that seem promising and those that do not, have one positive feature in common—an inherent flexibility of phasing. And despite our strictures against knowingly proceeding into peace-transition procedures without thorough substantive preparation, our government must nevertheless be ready to move in this direction with whatever limited resources of planning are on hand at the time—if circumstances so require. An arbitrary all-or-nothing approach is no more realistic in the development of contingency peace programming than it is anywhere else.

But the principal cause for concern over the continuing effectiveness of the war system, and the more important reason for hedging with peace planning, lies in the backwardness of current war-system programming. Its controls have not kept pace with the technological advances it has made possible. Despite its unarguable success to date, even in this era of unprecedented potential in mass destruction, it continues to operate largely on a laissez-faire basis. To the best of our knowledge, no serious quantified studies have ever been conducted to determine, for example:

—optimum levels of armament production, for purposes of economic control, at any given series of chronological points and under any given relationship between civilian production and consumption patterns;

—correlation factors between draft recruitment policies and mensurable social dissidence;

—minimum levels of population destruction necessary to maintain war-threat credibility under varying political conditions;

—optimum cyclical frequency of "shooting" wars under varying circumstances of historical relationship.

These and other war-function factors are fully susceptible to analysis by today's computer-based systems,[a] but they have not been so treated; modern analytical techniques have up to now been relegated to such aspects of the ostensible functions of war as procurement, personnel deployment, weapons analysis, and the like. We do not disparage these types of application, but only deplore their lack of utilization to greater capacity in attacking problems of broader scope. Our concern for efficiency in this context is not aesthetic, economic, or humanistic. It stems from the axiom that no system can long survive at either input or output levels that consistently or substantially deviate from an optimum range. As their data grow increasingly sophisticated, the war system and its functions are increasingly endangered by such deviations.

Our final conclusion, therefore, is that it will be necessary for our government to plan in depth for two general contingencies. The first, and lesser, is the possibility of a viable general peace; the second is the successful continuation of the war system. In our view, careful preparation for the possibility of peace should be extended, not because we take the position that the end of war would necessarily be desirable, if it is in fact possible, but because it may be thrust upon us in some form whether we are ready for it or not. Planning for rationalizing and quantifying the war system, on the other hand, to ensure the effectiveness of its major stabilizing functions, is not only more promising in respect to anticipated results, but is essential; we can no longer take for granted that it will continue to serve our purposes well merely because it always has. The objective of government policy in regard to war and peace, in this period of uncertainty, must be to preserve maximum options. The recommendations which follow are directed to this end.

# SECTION 8

---

# RECOMMENDATIONS

(1) WE PROPOSE THE ESTABLISHMENT, under executive order of the President, of a permanent War/Peace Research Agency, empowered and mandated to execute the programs described in (2) and (3) below. This agency (a) will be provided with nonaccountable funds sufficient to implement its responsibilities and decisions at its own discretion, and (b) will have authority to preempt and utilize, without restriction, any and all facilities of the executive branch of the government in pursuit of its objectives. It will be organized along the lines of the National Security Council, except that none of its governing, executive, or operating personnel will hold other public office or governmental responsibility. Its directorate will be drawn from the broadest practicable

95

spectrum of scientific disciplines, humanistic studies, applied creative arts, operating technologies, and otherwise unclassified professional occupations. It will be responsible solely to the President, or to other officers of government temporarily deputized by him. Its operations will be governed entirely by its own rules of procedure. Its authority will expressly include the unlimited right to withhold information on its activities and its decisions, from anyone except the President, whenever it deems such secrecy to be in the public interest.

(2) THE FIRST OF THE WAR/PEACE RESEARCH AGENCY'S two principal responsibilities will be to determine all that can be known, including what can reasonably be inferred in terms of relevant statistical probabilities, that may bear on an eventual transition to a general condition of peace. The findings in this Report may be considered to constitute the beginning of this study and to indicate its orientation; detailed records of the investigations and findings of the Special Study Group on which this Report is based, will be furnished the agency, along with whatever clarifying data the agency deems necessary. This aspect of the agency's work will hereinafter be referred to as "Peace Research."

The Agency's Peace Research activities will necessarily include, but not be limited to, the following:

(a) The creative development of possible substitute institutions for the principal nonmilitary functions of war.

(b) The careful matching of such institutions against

the criteria summarized in this Report, as refined, revised, and extended by the agency.

(c) The testing and evaluation of substitute institutions, for acceptability, feasibility, and credibility, against hypothecated transitional and postwar conditions; the testing and evaluation of the effects of the anticipated atrophy of certain unsubstituted functions.

(d) The development and testing of the correlativity of multiple substitute institutions, with the eventual objective of establishing a comprehensive program of compatible war substitutes suitable for a planned transition to peace, if and when this is found to be possible and subsequently judged desirable by appropriate political authorities.

(e) The preparation of a wide-ranging schedule of partial, uncorrelated, crash programs of adjustment suitable for reducing the dangers of an unplanned transition to peace effected by *force majeure.*

Peace Research methods will include but not be limited to, the following:

(a) The comprehensive interdisciplinary application of historical, scientific, technological, and cultural data.

(b) The full utilization of modern methods of mathematical modeling, analogical analysis, and other, more sophisticated, quantitative techniques in process of development that are compatible with computer programming.

(c) The heuristic "peace games" procedures developed during the course of its assignment by the Special

Study Group, and further extensions of this basic approach to the testing of institutional functions.

(3) THE WAR/PEACE RESEARCH AGENCY's other principal responsibility will be "War Research." Its fundamental objective will be to ensure the continuing viability of the war system to fulfill its essential nonmilitary functions for as long as the war system is judged necessary to or desirable for the survival of society. To achieve this end, the War Research groups within the agency will engage in the following activities:

(a) *Quantification of existing application of the nonmilitary functions of war.* Specific determinations will include, but not be limited to: 1) the gross amount and the net proportion of nonproductive military expenditures since World War II assignable to the need for war as an economic stabilizer; 2) the amount and proportion of military expenditures and destruction of life, property, and natural resources during this period assignable to the need for war as an instrument for political control; 3) similar figures, to the extent that they can be separately arrived at, assignable to the need for war to maintain social cohesiveness; 4) levels of recruitment and expenditures on the draft and other forms of personnel deployment attributable to the need for military institutions to control social disaffection; 5) the statistical relationship of war casualties to world food supplies; 6) the correlation of military actions and expenditures with cultural activities and scientific advances (including necessarily, the development of mensurable standards in these areas).

(b) *Establishment of a priori modern criteria for the execution of the nonmilitary functions of war.* These will include, but not be limited to: 1) calculation of minimum and optimum ranges of military expenditure required, under varying hypothetical conditions, to fulfill these several functions, separately and collectively; 2) determination of minimum and optimum levels of destruction of life, property, and natural resources prerequisite to the credibility of external threat essential to the political and motivational functions; 3) development of a negotiable formula governing the relationship between military recruitment and training policies and the exigencies of social control.

(c) *Reconciliation of these criteria with prevailing economic, political, sociological, and ecological limitations.* The ultimate object of this phase of War Research is to rationalize the heretofore informal operations of the war system. It should provide practical working procedures through which responsible governmental authority may resolve the following war-function problems, among others, under any given circumstances: 1) how to determine the optimum quantity, nature, and timing of military expenditures to ensure a desired degree of economic control; 2) how to organize the recruitment, deployment, and ostensible use of military personnel· to ensure a desired degree of acceptance of authorized social values; 3) how to compute on a short-term basis, the nature and extent of the loss of life and other resources which should be suffered and/or inflicted during any single outbreak of hostilities to achieve a desired degree of internal political authority and social allegiance; 4) how to project, over extended periods, the nature and quality of overt warfare which must be planned and budgeted to achieve a desired degree of contextual stability for the same purpose; factors to be determined must include frequency of occurrence, length of phase, intensity of physical destruction, extensiveness of geographical involvement, and optimum mean loss of life; 5) how to extrapolate accurately from the foregoing, for ecological purposes, the continuing effect of the war system, over such extended cycles, on population pressures, and to adjust the planning of casualty rates accordingly.

War Research procedures will necessarily include, but not be limited to, the following:

(a) The collation of economic, military, and other relevant data into uniform terms, permitting the reversible translation of heretofore discrete categories of information.[1]

(b) The development and application of appropriate forms of cost-effectiveness analysis suitable for adapting such new constructs to computer terminology, programming, and projection.[2]

(c) Extension of the "war games" methods of systems testing to apply, as a quasi-adversary proceeding, to the nonmilitary functions of war.[3]

(4) SINCE BOTH PROGRAMS of the War/Peace Research Agency will share the same purpose—to maintain governmental freedom of choice in respect to war and peace

until the direction of social survival is no longer in doubt —it is of the essence of this proposal that the agency be constituted without limitation of time. Its examination of existing and proposed institutions will be self-liquidating when its own function shall have been superseded by the historical developments it will have, at least in part, initiated.

the conclusion of their report.[2] Following a thorough reading of this, it may be seen that EISCAT's efforts are, in reality, and quoting directly from the report, intended to develop: 1) as part of "a giant open-end space research program, aimed at unreachable targets . . . [since] space research can be viewed as the nearest modern equivalent yet devised to the pyramid-building, and the similar ritualistic enterprises, of ancient societies;" 2) "a permanent, ritualized, ultra-elaborate disarmament inspection system, and variants of such a system" the best of which is conducted from outer space with the aid of extensive radar and surveillance technology; 3) "massive global environmental pollution" including the effect of "global warming" (generated largely by the EISCAT and HAARP atmospheric heaters), as well as the "ozone depletion" problem that has manufactured "environmental pollution" required to present an international threat that only a "one world government" can effectively handle; 4) "an acceptable threat from 'outer space'" or "an established and recognized extraterrestrial menace" that includes most of "the alien phenomena;" the cyclic solar flares described by EISCAT that are blamed for "El Nino" and related environmental damage; and the economic gain resulting from related natural disasters including hurricanes, floods, tornados, and earthquakes; 5) "a comprehensive social" control program, or "a modern sophisticated form of slavery," that, as these final chapters evidence, are likely linked to the "scatter back" of specific electromagnetic broadcasts capable of modifying, if not completely controlling human health and behavior in a program heralded for "health" and "social welfare;" and 6) a "direct eugenic management" program, or "comprehensive program of applied eugenics" for depopulation which is easily brought about by several of the above EISCAT and HAARP capabilities.[2]

Len and Joey had no idea when they began this effort that the outcome would be a complete exposé of the hitherto secret program to technologically control populations. Similarly, when they first read the *Report From Iron Mountain*,[2] they failed to recognize the full extent to which its recommendations were being implemented. After receiving from Joey the background on harmonics beginning with the vibrational frequencies hidden within the Solfeggio, later discovering the true power and meaning behind the British intelligence agency's "MI6," and DNA repair frequency "528," the collaborators were primed, but not fully prepared, to see the "big picture." The pieces fell together when Len was intuitively guided to investigate EISCAT and project HAARP in detail.

To see the big picture most clearly, and how the specifics in *The Report From Iron Mountain* are being actualized, figure 11.2 provides the summary report and conclusions from this initially secret document. Readers are urged to integrate this knowledge and then proceed to the next section describing EISCAT and HAARP's activities.

In addition, EISCAT's frequencies and their relationship to numerology is discussed in the appendix section of this book.

## EISCAT, UNFPA and Eugenics

As mentioned, EISCAT's supporting nations include "Finland, France, Germany, Japan, Norway, Sweden and the United Kingdom." Minus the United States, where HAARP is located, these nations represent the majority of NATO countries. They also just happened to be the chief funding sources for UNFPA—the United Nations Fund for Population Activities.

According to a report from the United Nations, "The U.N. Fund for Population Activities (UNFPA) is the largest multilateral source of external funding for population action programs in developing countries." Between 1969 and 1978, UNFPA "provided over $250 million in support of more than 1,200 population projects in more than 100 countries. In 1977, the Fund's annual budget, obtained from voluntary contributions, exceeded $100 million." The major donors were, once again, the principle NATO nations. "The United States in recent years has provided about 30% of total UNFPA funding."[5]

The UNFPA report continued:

Most of the projects that UNFPA supports are implemented through organizations and specialized agencies of the U.N. system, acting in their respective fields of competence. Among

# Fig. 11.3. EISCAT Links to U.S. Project HAARP and Rockefeller-Funded Cold Spring Harbor Eugenics

## 4th European Heating Seminar

**Ramfjordmoen, Tromsø, 16-19 May 1995**

*Preliminary* programme

---

General information is available.
Participants are listed separately, as are abstracts

**Events:**

- Planning of Oct/November or other Heating campaigns
- Demonstration Heating experiment of API in the lower ionosphere using Heating and Dynasonde.
  *Thursday 18 May*
- Dinner at the restaurant on "Fløya" overlooking Tromsø. Transport via Fjellheisen (cable car).
  *Wednesday 17 May*

---

**Programme:**

---

**Tuesday 16 May**

| | |
|---|---|
| 09.00 | Introductory remarks |
| | **M. Rietveld, I. Storhaug** |
| 09:15 | Welcome to EISCAT |
| | **Dr A. P. van Eyken** |

*Heating Facilities*

| | |
|---|---|
| 09.30 | EISCAT-Heating: results and future prospects |
| | **M. T. Rietveld** |
| 10.00 | US Heater plans (HAARP) |
| | **J. Rasmussen** |
| 10.45 | Remarks on the 2nd Finnish EISCAT-Heating campaign, October 1994 |
| | **T. Bösinger** |
| 11.00 | Coffee break |

*Interaction of Electromagnetic and Plasma Waves*

| | |
|---|---|
| 11.30 | Theory of electrostatic excitations in ionospheric radio Heating experiments |
| | **E. Mjølhus** |
| 12.00 | Recent Langmuir turbulence results from Tromsø Heating experiments |
| | **H. Kohl** |
| 12.30 | Lunch at Veikroa |
| 14.00 | SEE applications for studying temporal evolution of artificial ionospheric turbulence |
| | **V. L. Frolov, L. M. Kagan, and E. N. Sergeev.** |
| 14.30 | Title to be decided |
| | **B. Thidé** |
| 15.00 | Generation of broad-band artificial ELF radiation by HF heating of the |

**Welcome to the RAL EISCAT Homepage**    http://www.eiscat.ult.no/heating/sem-tlks.html    **3/9/99 1:44 AM**

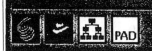

The intimate connection between Rockefeller family interests and the American, then Nazi, eugenics movement was amply documented in *The Nazi Connection: Eugenics, American Racism, and German National Socialism* by author Stefan Kühl, and later by others as reviewed in *Emerging Viruses: AIDS & Ebola—Nature, Accident or Intentional?* by Dr. Leonard Horowitz. *The Report From Iron Mountain*, and the use of EISCAT and HAARP for slavery and population management, adds another dimension to the practice of eugenics. The above documents were found on the "RAL EISCAT Homepage" on the Internet, copyrighted 1994 by Cold Spring Harbor Labs, available at http://eiscate.ag.rl.ac.uk/ and http://www.eiscat.ult.no/heating/semtlks.html

these are the U.N. Office of Technical Cooperation, the U.N. Development Program (UNDP), World Health Organization (WHO), [the] U.N. Children's Fund (UNICEF) . . . [and others].

The World Bank and its soft-loan affiliate, the International Development Association (IDA), entered the population assistance field in 1968. This reflected the Bank's conviction that rapid population growth is a major barrier to the economic and social progress of many developing countries. Supported projects have included a widening range of activities relevant to an effective population program. Assistance is provided on conventional Bank terms or, in the case of especially weak economies, on highly subsidized soft-loan terms. [Meaning repayment was not required.][5]

Bilateral assistance, the report said, came from the NATO countries and Japan. The U.S. program comprised about "two-thirds of the total over the 1965-78 period," and the entire operation was "administered by the Agency for International Development (USAID)."[5]

The "voluntary" contributors funding the lion's share of depopulation operations according to the State Department was the United States through USAID. A number of NGOs (non-governmental organizations) additionally contributed "in recognition of the need for many-sided efforts for effective overall population [control/reduction] assistance to developing countries. The Ford and Rockefeller Foundations have been major supporters of world population programs since 1965."[5]

In other words, U.S. taxpayers provided The Ford and Rockefeller Foundations, and others, with money to effectively administer eugenics. This new level of applied eugenics came in 1965 as *The Report From Iron Mountain* was being finalized. Moreover, EISCAT is linked to these same organizations and funding sources.

For instance, figure 11.3 documents the intimate links between EISCAT, America's project HAARP, and Cold Spring Harbor labs in New York—the top American eugenics laboratory, home of the "Human Genome Project." Cold Spring Harbor labs is largely funded by the Rockefeller Foundation which remains a chief benefactor of world population reduction programs, and among the earliest instigators of eugenics along with the Royal Family. This EISCAT document revealed that EISCAT's text, that is its propaganda, was issued by Cold Spring Harbor who held its copyright.[6]

The figure also shows the "Programme" from the "4th European Heating Seminar" held on May 16-19, 1995. Following a preliminary presentation entitled, "EISCAT-Heating: results and future prospects," the "U.S. Heater plans (HAARP)" program was presented by M. T. Rietveld. Thus, despite the alleged lack of U.S. funding for EISCAT, the U.S. was actively involved.

## Project HAARP and "Ionospheric Heating:" What Is It?

According to the descriptive abstract accompanying U.S. Patent number 4,686,605, HAARP's patent provides for:

> A method and apparatus for altering at least one selected region which normally exists above the earth's surface. The region is excited by electron cyclotron resonance heating to thereby increase its charged particle density. In one embodiment, circularly–polarized electromagnetic radiation is transmitted upward in a direction substantially parallel to and along a field line which extends through the region of plasma to be altered. The radiation is transmitted at a frequency which excites electron cyclotron resonance to heat and accelerate the charged particles. This increase in energy can cause ionization of neutral particles which are then absorbed as part of the region, thereby increasing the charged particle density of the region."[7]

The HAARP patent, assigned to ARCO Power Technologies, Inc., a division of the Atlantic Richfield Oil Company, entitled "Method and Apparatus for Altering a Region in the Earth's Atmosphere, Ionosphere, and/or Magnetosphere," was claimed by inventor Bernard J. Eastlund to have several uses. According to Alaskan author Eric Nashlund, who broke the HAARP story in the Australian magazine *Nexus*, these uses included:

> . . . total disruption of communications over a very large portion of the Earth . . . disrupting not only land-based communications, but also airborne communications and sea communications (both surface and subsurface) . . . missile or aircraft destruction, de-

flection or confusion. . . . Weather modification . . . by altering solar absorption . . . ozone, nitrogen etc. concentrations could be artificially increased.[7]

The patent's "prior art" section acknowledged the previous related inventions of inventor Nikola Tesla. His referenced articles had appeared during the late nineteenth and early twentieth century. In the book *Angels Don't Play This HAARP*, by authors Nick Begich and Jeane Manning, Tesla described the earliest applications of this technology in a feature story that appeared in the *New York Times* on December 8, 1915. It read:

> Nikola Tesla, the inventor, has filed patent applications on the essential parts of a machine, possibilities [of which] test a layman's imagination and promise a parallel of Thor's shooting thunderbolts from the sky to punish those who had angered the gods. . . . Suffice it to say that the invention will go through space with a speed of 300 miles a second, a manless ship without propelling engine or wings sent by electricity to any desired point on the globe on its errand of destruction, if destruction [is what] its manipulator wishes to effect.
>
> "It is not a time," said Dr. Tesla yesterday, "to go into the details of this thing. It is founded upon a principle that means great things in peace; it can be used for great things in war. But I repeat, this is no time to talk of such things."[7]

Though he obviously lacked a desire to explore details, Tesla continued:

> "It is perfectly practicable to transmit electrical energy without wires and produce destructive effects at a distance. I have already constructed a wireless transmitter which makes this possible, and have described it in my technical publications, among which I refer to my patent number 1,119,732 recently granted. With transmitters of this kind we are enabled to project electrical energy in any amount to any distance and apply it for innumerable purposes, both in war and peace. Through the universal adoption of this system, ideal conditions for the maintenance of law and order will be realized, for then the energy necessary to the enforcement of right and justice will be normally productive, yet potential, and in any moment available, for attack and defense. The power transmitted need not be necessarily destructive,

for, if [people are] made to depend upon it, its withdrawal or supply will bring about the same results as those now accomplished by force of arms."[7]

Though "heating" the atmosphere in the wake of a "global warming crisis" might seem inappropriate to everyone except Satan, the discrepancy might be reconciled with a background check on HAARP's patent assignee. Few realize that the Atlantic Richfield Oil Company is closely linked to the British Royal Family, MI6, the Committee of 300, NATO and the Illuminati's Club of Rome.[4]

## Background on ARCO

According to Dr. John Coleman, a former member of British MI6, who extensively detailed the hierarchy of the New World Order conspirators, members of the Committee of 300 include[d] Lord Hartley Shawcross and Sirs Brian Edward Mountain, Kenneth Keith, Kenneth Strong, William Stephenson, and William Wiseman. "All of the foregoing are (or were) heavily involved in key Committee 300 companies which interface with literally thousands of companies engaged in every branch of commercial activity . . . "[4] One of these companies is Atlantic Richfield. In this regard Coleman wrote:

> MI6 ran a large number of these companies through British intelligence stationed in the RCA building in New York, which was the headquarters of its chief officer, Sir William Stephenson. Radio Corporation of America (RCA) was formed by G. E., Westinghouse, Morgan Guarantee and Trust (acting for the British crown), . . . back in 1919 as a British intelligence center. . .

In addition, another affiliate of RCA was United Fruit, identified as a CIA front that was intimately linked to the assassination of President John F. Kennedy.[4,8]

Coleman continued:

> It is obvious that the communications field is tightly controlled. Going back to RCA, we find that its directorate is composed of British-American establishment figures who feature prominently in other organizations such as the CFR, NATO, the Club of Rome, the Trilateral Commission, Freemasonry, Skull and

Bones, Bilderbergers, Round Table, Milner Society and the Jesuits-Aristotle Society. Among them was David Sarnoff [RCA's president] who moved to London at the same time Sir William Stephenson moved into the RCA building in New York.

All three major television networks came as spin-offs from RCA, especially the National Broadcasting Company (NBC) which was first, closely followed by the American Broadcasting Company (ABC) in 1951. The third big television network was Columbia Broadcasting System (CBS) which, like its sister companies was, and still is, dominated by British intelligence. William Paley was trained in mass brainwashing techniques at the Tavistock Institute prior to being passed as qualified to head CBS. . . .

On RCA's board sits Thornton Bradshaw, president of Atlantic Richfield and a member of NATO, World Wildlife Fund, the Club of Rome, The Aspen Institute for Humanistic Studies, and the Council on Foreign Relations. Bradshaw is also chairman of NBC. The most important function of RCA remains its service to British intelligence.[4]

Dr. Coleman published for posterity the important organizational chart seen in figure 3.6 that summarized the Illuminati's worldwide operations.

## "The Real Problem" Regarding HAARP

"The real problem with HAARP," according to "Hugh's HAARP Info Page"—a well publicized and active "primenet.com" website—"is the news blackout."

Not so. The "real problem" is that HAARP, virtually in one fell swoop from inner space, provides the capability to fulfill the majority of population policy recommendations advanced in *The Report From Iron Mountain*. There was no mention of this critical fact on this website or any other investigation into HAARP by any author(s).

The real problem is that HAARP, given the documentation provided herein, is most likely intended to actualize the initiatives the Iron Mountain group recommended in their 1967 report. (See text in figure 11.2.) The "giant open-end space research program," of which

HAARP is a part, could easily be used as "a permanent, ritualized, ultra-elaborate disarmament inspection system." As its patent clearly indicates, HAARP's capacity to survey communications and cause "total disruption of communications over a very large portion of the Earth . . . disrupting not only land-based communications, but also airborne communications and sea communications (both surface and subsurface)" is by itself potentially lethal in unprecedented measure.

That *The Report From Iron Mountain* called for "massive global environmental pollution," while HAARP and EISCAT have demonstrated a hazardous ability to affect solar absorption, nitrogen, and ozone levels is disconcerting. Obviously the technology is far from benign as it is being used today to "heat up the earth's atmosphere" in an age when widespread climatic changes endanger virtually every living thing. This relationship alone is extraordinarily incriminating and threatening.

Additionally suspicious and troubling is the media's coverage of the "alien phenomenon" during the last part of the twentieth century. In keeping with the Iron Mountain report's recommendation to create "an established and recognized extraterrestrial menace," the HAARP and EISCAT technologies might easily come into play in the "grand finale"— Hollywood's ending to Babylonian captivity—a curtain call for the Old World of managed chaos. The profitable fright and fraud of Y2K, power outages, computer viruses, massive communications and banking failures, mortgage meltdowns, escalating "natural" disasters, terrorism and increased militarism, threatened outbreaks, and social chaos involving loss of life are all conditions demanding new forms of social control. All of this seems peculiarly similar to what the doctors from Iron Mountain prescribed.

Specifically, the atmospheric electromagnetic technologies applied by HAARP and EISCAT could acutely, or over the long term, create massive population reduction—death and destruction from natural and man-made disasters—all justifying a "flexible" military presence as proposed in the report. Further recommended on pages 99 and 100, under "the execution of the nonmilitary functions of war," the U.S. Government and its secret leaders were advised to extend "war games" methods to social and political systems. Through the creation of "quasi-adversary" proceedings,[2] such as the initiation and funding of bogus (and legitimate) terrorist organizations and events as broadcast by various news agencies,[9] and the social chaos associated with communications and energy systems failures, citizens will desire and demand more government protections, interventions, and control. In this context "threats from space," including those which are being used to justify HAARP's existence, are ideal.[2] All of this is a "real problem" with HAARP and EISCAT.

Finally, according to the report, since "excess population is war material" (p. 74), in the "peaceful" New World Order it was considered necessary to reduce excess populations in the ways cited above, as well as to develop "a comprehensive social" control program—or "slavery" in a technologically modern and acceptable manner. This topic will be discussed in the final chapter of this book. The capability to provide technological slavery is most likely to be largely provided by HAARP's and EISCAT's electromagnetic frequency generators and methodologies researched and perfected by British and American intelligence agencies since the 1940s. The "scatter back" of specific electromagnetic frequency broadcasts are capable of modifying, if not completely controlling, numerous aspects of the human condition. In this context, simple identification and surveillance programs that operate electromagnetically, including the "medical biochip," the "health passport card," and possibly even the prion crystal, may only be part of the applied science of technological slavery and "direct eugenic management" proposed in *The Report From Iron Mountain.*

### References

1. EISCAT report. The Earth's magnetosphere. Available on the Internet at http://eiscate.ag.rl.ac.uk/ (and for The EISCAT Scientific Association information see http:www.eiscat.ult.no/eiscat.html).

2. Lewin LC. et al. *Report From Iron Mountain on the Possibility and Desirability of Peace*. New York: The Dial Press, 1967, pp. 79-101.

3. Cook T. *The Mark of the New World Order*. Springdale, PA: Whitaker House, 1996, p. 125.

4. Coleman J. *Conspirators' Hierarchy: The Story of the Committee of 300*. Carson City, NV: American West Publishers, 1992, pp. 52; 159; 182-183; 187.

5. Department of State Staff. World Population: The Silent Explosion. *Department of State Bulletin*. November, 1978. pp. 1-8. The Series were available through the Correspondence Management Division, Bureau of Public Affairs, Department of State, Washington, D.C. 20520.

6. "Programme" from the "4th European Heating Seminar" held on May 16-19, 1995. Following a preliminary presentation entitled, "EISCAT-Heating: results and future prospects," the "US Heater plans (HAARP)" program was presented by M. T. Rietveld. Document available on the Internet at http://eiscate.ag.rl.ac.uk/ and http://www.eiscat.ult.no/heating/semtlks.html.

7. Manning J and Begich N. *Angels Don't Play this HAARP: Advances in Tesla Technology*. Anchorage, AK: Earthpulse Press (P. O. Box 201393, Anchorage, AK 99520), 1995, pp. 24-25.

8. Haslam ET. *Mary, Ferrie & the Monkey Virus: The Story of an Underground Medical Laboratory*. Albuquerque, NM: Wordsworth Communications (7200 Montgomery NE #280, Albuquerque, NM 87109), 1995.

9. McMahon P. FBI battles terrorism in Northwest. *USA Today*, Wednesday, December 23, 1998, p. 3A.

# Chapter 12.
# MKULTRA and the
# "Mark of the Beast"

**B**ioluminescent dinoflagellates are relatives of *Pfiesteria*. You may have seen them if you've ever walked along the ocean's shore at night. They light up, slightly blue, when energized by the crest of a wave or a splash as you moved through the water. It is the clearest example of biochemical transformation of physical matter into transmitted light energy.

Chemical stimulation by acid (10% acetic acid or vinegar) also stimulate these microorganisms to glow. So in the presence of lowered pH, they are more easily stimulated to emit electromagnetic radiation that we see as light.

A certain type of dinoflagellate—*Gymnodinium breve*—is responsible for the red tides that intoxicate shellfish and the people who eat them. It is also the red tide dinoflagellate that scientists say are to blame for the disappearance of the great Florida manatees.[1]

If someone wanted to kill off the remaining manatees, all they would need to do is seed the Florida canals with this tiny microorganism, lower the pH just right to facilitate optimal growth, and the little beasts would release their toxins and do the rest.

Similarly, if you wanted to control or even eliminate human populations, you could use very similar methods and materials.

### The CIA and Projects MKNAOMI and MKULTRA

In *Emerging Viruses: AIDS & Ebola—Nature, Accident or Intentional?* the CIA's top secret biological weapons program, MKNAOMI, was exposed as were the related efforts of scientists to produce and test numerous viruses that were descriptively and functionally identical to the AIDS virus (HIV) and Ebola. (See figure 7.1.) Later, Len learned that the entire MKNAOMI project was, in fact, a subordinate part of the CIA's "Program of Research in Behavioral Modification," that is, "PROJECT MKULTRA." In other words, as evidenced in figure 12.1, by the early 1950s the CIA administered a project to develop and test biological agents that would, "under operational conditions," precisely affect aspects of human behavior—thinking, feeling, and acting. The purpose was to render targeted populations helpless and susceptible to attack, manipulation, and even complete mind control.[2]

As defined in a memorandum from the CIA Inspector General to the Director of the agency, "MKULTRA was the principal CIA program involving the research and development of chemical and biological agents." It was "concerned with the research and development of chemical, biological, and radiological materials capable of employment in clandestine operations to control human behavior."[2]

Thus, primary emphasis of MKULTRA was on *controlling human behavior*, and the principle methods used to accomplish this included biological and radiological methods and materials. The radiological methods included the use of electromagnetic frequencies deployed to affect individuals and large populations. The biological materials included bacteria, viruses, and fungi. As documented in Chapter 8, mycoplasma, yeasts, and other fungi were researched, developed, and even transmitted to infect, affect and even kill plants, animals, and humans. This was clearly inferred when the Senate Select Committee on Intelligence reported, in addition to the CIA's interest in biological weapons for use against humans, it also asked SOD [Special Operations Division at Fort Detrick, Maryland] "to assist CIA in developing, testing, and maintaining biological agents and delivery systems," and to study the use of biological agents against crops, animals, and enemies.[2] (See figures 12.1 through 12.4.)

"MKNAOMI was [allegedly] terminated in 1970 . . ." the report stated. But we know from the documentation in *Emerging Viruses: AIDS & Ebola*, that this was clearly not the case.[3] Lawmakers and the public had only been deceived by false assurances from Henry Kissinger and President Nixon that MKNAOMI had been halted.

## PROJECT MKULTRA, THE CIA'S PROGRAM OF RESEARCH IN BEHAVIORAL MODIFICATION

# JOINT HEARING

BEFORE THE

## SELECT COMMITTEE ON INTELLIGENCE

AND THE

## SUBCOMMITTEE ON HEALTH AND SCIENTIFIC RESEARCH

OF THE

## COMMITTEE ON HUMAN RESOURCES

## UNITED STATES SENATE

NINETY-FIFTH CONGRESS

FIRST SESSION

AUGUST 3, 1977

Printed for the use of the Select Committee on Intelligence
and Committee on Human Resources

U.S. GOVERNMENT PRINTING OFFICE

96-408 O          WASHINGTON : 1977

For sale by the Superintendent of Documents, U.S. Government Printing Office
Washington, D.C., 20402
Stock No. 052-070-04357-1

that no damage was done to individuals who volunteer for the experiments."[5] Overseas interrogations utilizing a combination of sodium pentothal and hypnosis after physical and psychiatric examinations of the subjects were also part of ARTICHOKE.

The Office of Scientific Intelligence (OSI), which studied scientific advances by hostile powers, initially led BLUEBIRD/ARTICHOKE efforts. In 1952, overall responsibility for ARTICHOKE was transferred from OSI to the Inspection and Security Office (I&SO), predecessor to the present Office of Security. The CIA's Technical Services and Medical Staffs were to be called upon as needed; OSI would retain liaison function with other government agencies.[6] The change in leadership from an intelligence unit to an operating unit apparently reflected a change in emphasis; from the study of actions by hostile powers to the use, both for offensive and defensive purposes, of special interrogation techniques—primarily hypnosis and truth serums.

Representatives from each Agency unit involved in ARTICHOKE met almost monthly to discuss their progress. These discussions included the planning of overseas interrogations[8] as well as further experimentation in the U.S.

Information about project ARTICHOKE after the fall of 1953 is scarce. The CIA maintains that the project ended in 1956, but evidence suggests that Office of Security and Office of Medical Services use of "special interrogation" techniques continued for several years thereafter.

## 3. MKNAOMI

MKNAOMI was another major CIA program in this area. In 1967, the CIA summarized the purposes of MKNAOMI:

(a) To provide for a covert support base to meet clandestine operational requirements.

(b) To stockpile severely incapacitating and lethal materials for the specific use of TSD [Technical Services Division].

(c) To maintain in operational readiness special and unique items for the dissemination of biological and chemical materials.

(d) To provide for the required surveillance, testing, upgrading, and evaluation of materials and items in order to assure absence of defects and complete predictability of results to be expected under operational conditions.[9]

Under an agreement reached with the Army in 1952, the Special Operations Division (SOD) at Fort Detrick was to assist CIA in developing, testing, and maintaining biological agents and delivery

[5] Memorandum from Robert Taylor, O/DD/P to the Assistant Deputy (Inspection and Security) and Chief of the Medical Staff, 3/22/52.

[6] Memorandum from H. Marshall Chadwell, Assistant Director, Scientific Intelligence, to the Deputy Director/Plans (DDP) "Project ARTICHOKE," 8/29/52.

[8] "Progress Report, Project ARTICHOKE," 1/12/53.

[9] Memorandum from Chief, TSD/Biological Branch to Chief, TSD "MKNAOMI: Funding, Objectives, and Accomplishments," 10/18/67. p. 1. For a fuller description of MKNAOMI and the relationship between CIA and SOD. see p. 360 ff.

"In January 1973," the Senate's report continued, "MKULTRA records were destroyed by Technical Services Division personnel acting on the verbal orders of Dr. Sidney Gottlieb, Chief of TSD [Technical Services Division]." Dr. Gottlieb testified, and former Director Richard Helms confirmed, "that in ordering the records destroyed, Dr. Gottlieb was carrying out the verbal orders of then DCI [CIA Director] Helms."[2]

So if one wanted to find any remaining MKNAOMI—biological weapons research and development documents—alternative investigative channels would need to be followed. Even then, only limited evidence might be gathered.

One example of this is shown in figure 12.2—a previously classified "summary of major events and problems of the United States Army Chemical Corps: Fiscal Years 1961-1962."[3] By reading the Chemical Corps's documents certain references to top secret MKULTRA and MKNAOMI activities are implied and reasonably enlightening. The text discussed the use of "bacterial and fungal agents" that were recombined with genetic material "carrying infectivity factors . . . isolated from viruses." As seen in the document marked "CONFIDENTIAL," beginning in 1962, that is, when the "Special Virus Cancer Program" began, "new combinations of genetic factors through the mixture of infectious nucleic acids from different sources were undertaken. . . "[3] This bioweapons research was reminiscent of, and a forerunner to, the development of the "pathogenic mycoplasma" by the Armed Forces Institute of Pathology (AFIP) "Inventor" Dr. Shyh-Ching Lo[4] as discussed in Chapter 8.

By the mid-1980s, Lo and his colleagues were able to genetically engineer a lethal immune system destroying mycoplasma beginning with viral genes taken from AIDS patients. Mycoplasma associated illnesses included CFIDS, Alzheimer's, Wegener's Disease, Sarcoidosis, respiratory distress syndrome, Kiu-chi's disease, and the autoimmune diseases including collagen vascular disease, and lupus. The "*Mycoplasma fermentans* incognitas" strain Lo et al. concocted was

SECRET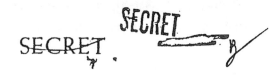

# SUMMARY OF MAJOR EVENTS
### and
# PROBLEMS

## United States Army Chemical Corps (U)

### FISCAL YEARS 1961 - 1962

PAFES 109/110

CLASSIFIED BY:

DOD DIR 5.200.IR

JUNE 1962 ON: JUNE 1992

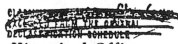

*U.S. Army Chemical Corps Historical Office*
*Army Chemical Center, Maryland*

SPECIAL HANDLING REQUIRED
NOT RELEASABLE TO FOREIGN NATIONALS
EXCEPT NONE BY AUTHORITY OF OCCMLO
12 Mar 62

THIS DOCUMENT
REGRADED UNCLASSIFIED
WHEN SEPARATED FROM
CLASSIFIED ENCLOSURES

PAGES 109 + 110

 SECRET

SECRET

COPY 6 OF 35 COPIES

CBR-S-1794-62

OCMH, SC No. 116226

(S) Research on new agents has tended to concentrate on viral and rickettsial diseases. A whole range of exotic virus diseases prevalent in tropical areas came within the screening program in FY 1961 - 62, with major effort directed at increased first-hand knowledge of these so-called arbor (i.e., arthropod-borne) viruses. The importance of epidemiological studies in connection with this area of endeavor was being emphasized. A major step forward was achieved in the development of a better known agent, the virus of psittacosis, when stabilization of the dry agent through addition of a small amount of monosodium glutamate was successfully demonstrated. This accomplishment eliminated one of the principal difficulties in the path of future development of this agent.[25]

(S) In the realm of bacterial and fungal agents, the causative organisms of histoplasmosis, leptospirosis, and cryptococcosis reached the laboratory screening stage. Work on Bacillus anthracis, an agent which has been the subject of more or less concern to the Corps for many years, went forward in the area of process research, particularly in the evaluation of drying methods. But the crucial problem of providing adequate assessment of human susceptibility to this agent remains to be solved.[26]

(U) One of the most striking lines of inquiry in the Corps program was the basic research being done by the Biological Laboratories on the genetic factors underlying the infectivity of micro-organisms. Nucleic acids carrying infectivity factors were isolated from viruses. First attempts at inducing new

---

25

Goodlow interv, 16 Feb 62.

26

(1) Ibid. (2) Technical Program Review & Analysis, Bio Labs, Jan - Mar 62, p 24.

combinations of genetic factors through the mixture of infectious nucleic acids from different sources were undertaken in FY 1962. Studies of bacterial genetics were also in progress with the aim of transferring genetic determinants from one type of organism to another.[27]

## Alarms

(C) A landmark in the long development of a practical automatic field alarm for G and V agents was reached early in the third quarter of FY 1962, when the E41R3 point detection alarm was accepted by the Army for limited production, thereby fulfilling at least a portion of the existing Qualitative Military Requirement for automatic alarms. The E41R3, which operates through a color reaction on a treated wet tape and a color-actuated audio signal, is a modified version of the E41R1 discussed in the FY 1960 Annual Summary.[28] The modifications were those suggested by deficiencies revealed during Arctic Test Board tests of the earlier model in FY 1961. Approval of the alarm for limited procurement (to satisfy an immediate operational requirement for 400 alarms) came in January of 1962.[29]

(C) An active program toward the development of a long path infra-red (LOPAIR) system for area scanning alarms reached the contracting stage before the end of FY 1962. The E49 LOPAIR system, selected for development, was the

---

[27]
    (1) Goodlow interv, 16 Feb 62. (2) Technical Program Review & Analysis, Bio Labs, Oct - Dec 61, pp 17 - 18.

[28]
    Summary of Major Events and Problems, FY 60, pp 117 - 18.

[29]
    CCTC Items 3934, 26 Dec 61, and 3950, 23 Jan 62..

414

# Fig. 12.3. Declassified U. S. Army Chemical Corps Documents Showing "Anticrop," "Antipersonnel," and "Crystalline" Biological Toxin Research in the 1950s

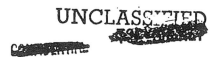

UNCLASSIFIED

Considerable progress, on the other hand, was made in the development of anticrop agents. Research resulted in improved field evaluation of potential agents, addition of 4-fluorophenoxy-. acetic acid as a standard-type agent, and demonstration of the high efficiency of the Aero 14A Airborne Spray Tank. (SECRET)

Whereas the previous chemical anticrop agents, butyl 2,4-di-chlorophenoxyacetic acid and butyl 2,4,5-trichlorophenoxyacetate were useful for curtailing the growth of broadleaf plants, the new standard-type agent, 4-fluorophenoxyacetic acid, reduces the yields of wheat and rice materially when applied in militarily feasible quantities. The agent is produced industrially by chemical companies and is available on the open market. [56]  (SECRET)

An important advance in field evaluation was the development of a miniature spraying system for disseminating liquid agents from an L-19 airplane. This system makes practicable the testing of undiluted agents on field grown crops. An effort is being made to mount the system on a truck, which can then be used at Camp Detrick.
(CONFIDENTIAL)

In conjunction with the Navy, tests were made of the Aero 14A

---

[56]
Chemical anticrop agents are discussed in:
(1) Technical Progress FY 1954, pp.56-58.
(2) Annual BW Project Report.

REGRADED UNCLASSIFIED ORDER
SEC ARMY BY TAG PER
7 9 1 3 8 4

PAGE 10 OF 11 PAGES

COPY 2 OF 25 COPIES

UNCLASSIFIED

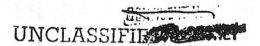

46

### Biological Warfare Research and Development

For the first time since the Chemical Corps embarked on a BW program, permission has been granted for the use of human volunteers in the evaluation of agents. A plan, drawn up at Camp Detrick, for the quantitative assessment of BW agents and vaccines has been approved by the Surgeon General and the Secretary of the Army. It is being planned to have the work carried on under contract in a medical school.[47]    (SECRET)

The funds available for BW during the fiscal year amounted to $25,440,000. By 30 June, $21,966,000 (86%) were obligated. The failure to fully obligate the funds were due to delays caused by earlier attempts to place the entire BW program under contract. Approval was obtained from higher authority to continue obligation of 1954 funds through 30 September 1954.[48]    (CONFIDENTIAL)

---

[46]
Unless otherwise noted, the section on BW is based on an interview with Dr. Charles Phillips, Camp Detrick, 28 Jul 54.
The Eighth Annual Report, Cml C Biol Labs, was not scheduled for publication until 16 Sep 54, and was therefore not available for this Summary History.
[47]
DF, DC CmlO to Hist O, OCCmlO, 3 Jun 54, sub: Summary List for Historical Report.
[48]
Review and Analysis of Chemical Corps Program, 4th Qtr FY 1954.

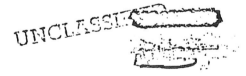

416

the M44 generator cluster respectively.[22] The Standard B classification represents the interim character of the new agent which in some respects - its prolonged time of onset of symptoms (at least two to three hours), and its dissemination in a visible cloud of smoke - falls short of optimum performance.

(C) Research was resumed during the FY 1961 - 62 period on botulinum toxin, the substance responsible for botulism. The research project on the crystalline toxin was the responsbility of CRDL, but some of the work was done by the Biological Laboratories acting as a sub-contractor. Problems in bio-assays and dissemination methods were a major concern during the period.[23]

(S) Progress toward standardizing new BW agents was slowed in 1961 - 62 by the lack of adequate extra-continental test facilities in which agent-munition combinations could be fully assayed without the limitations necessary in less remote test areas. Lack of the data such a test program could provide was responsible for the inability of the Chemical Corps to gain approval at the outset of the period for the standardization of a strain of Venezuelan equine encephalomyelitis. The requirement, new in FY 1961, that agents be type classified only in conjunction with munitions, was itself a limiting factor in consequence of the small range of formulated Army requirements for BW anti-personnel munitions.[24]

---

22

CCTC Item 3960, 26 Feb 62.

23

Quart Hist Rpt, CRDL, Jan - Mar 62 .

24

(1) Interv, Hist Off with Dr C.G. Ash, Hq EDCCM, 27 Dec 61. (2) Interv, Hist Off with Dr R.D. Housewright, Bio Labs. 16 Feb 62. (3) Interv, Hist Off with Dr R.J. Goodlow, Bio Labs. 16 Feb 62. For creation of Deseret Test Facility to expedite extra-continental test programs, see Chap I, above.

virtually identical to the strain Dr. Nicolson had found infecting fifty-percent of vets suffering with Gulf War syndrome or related CFIDS.

Also as documented in Chapter 8, Lo's application[4] referred to prion pioneer Carlton Gajdusek's work on AIDS virus-related projects akin to Robert Gallo's efforts with U.S. Army biological weapons contractor Litton Bionetics.[3a] Albeit circumstantial, these U.S. Army documents evidenced a weak link between biological weapons research on fungi, and fungal diseases, and prion research. Additionally, as seen in figures 12.2 and 12.3, this circumstantial link was strengthened by the early development of biological and chemical weapons surveillance systems, or electromagnetic technologies for use in the realm of biological and chemical warfare. As the declassified document in figure 12.2 showed, "infra-red" scanning systems were developed to quickly identify infectious agents or toxic substances in the field of military operations as early as 1962. Figure 12.3 documents that U.S. Army contractors were involved in related research and testing of "anticrop," and "antipersonnel" biological weapons including fungi.[3] Even more interesting, and related to this book's subject matter, the final page in the figure even discussed research on a "crystalline toxin" derived from another biological weapon—botulism—as early as 1961.[3a] Again, it should be recalled that this entire biological weapons program, Project MKNAOMI, was a subordinate part of the larger Project MKULTRA for mind control and population control. Infectious crystalline agents, then, were certainly considered important, even during this early period of population control research and development.[3a]

## MKULTRA for Mind and Population Control

According to the *Congressional Record*, MKULTRA began with a proposal from the Assistant Deputy Director for Plans, Richard Helms, to the DCI, outlining a special funding mechanism for highly sensitive CIA research and development projects that studied the use of biological and chemical materials in altering human behavior.

The hearings revealed that MKULTRA had been "approved by the DCI on April 13, 1953 along the lines proposed by ADDP [Assistant Deputy Director for Planning] Helms."[2]

The entire operation was kept top secret primarily because Americans themselves were to be placed at risk as targets for the research and its developments. In this regard, the Senate report stated, "Part of the rationale for the establishment of this special funding mechanism was its extreme sensitivity. The Inspector General's survey of MKULTRA in 1963 noted the following reasons for this secrecy:

> a. Research in the manipulation of human behavior is considered by many authorities in medicine and related fields to be professionally unethical, therefore the reputation of professional participants in the MKULTRA program are on occasion in jeopardy.

> b. Some MKULTRA activities raise questions of legality implicit in the original charter.

> c. A final phase of the testing of MKULTRA products places the rights and interests of U.S. citizens in jeopardy.

> d. Public disclosure of some aspects of MKULTRA activity could induce serious adverse reaction in U.S. public opinion, as well as stimulate offensive and defensive action in this field on the part of foreign intelligence services.[2]

Additional evidence that such secret experimentation on U.S. citizens continued despite Nixon's signing of the Geneva accord in 1971 is shown in figures 12.4 and 12.5. The first of these documents came from the 1976 "Foreign and Military Intelligence, Book I, Final Report of the Senate Select Committee to Study Governmental Operations with Respect to Intelligence Activities." The document discussed "Testing and Use of Chemical and Biological Agents by the Intelligence Community." It stated that "Research and development programs to find materials which could be used to alter human behavior were initiated in the late 1940s and early 1950s. These experimental programs originally included testing of drugs involving witting human subjects, and culminated in tests using unwitting, nonvolunteer human subjects . . . Few people, even within the agencies, knew of the pro-

## Fig. 12.4. U. S. Senate Select Committee's Report: Hearings on the Testing and Use of Chemical and Biological Agents By the Intelligence Community

### XVII. TESTING AND USE OF CHEMICAL AND BIOLOGICAL AGENTS BY THE INTELLIGENCE COMMUNITY[2]

Under its mandate[1] the Select Committee has studied the testing and use of chemical and biological agents by intelligence agencies. Detailed descriptions of the programs conducted by intelligence agencies involving chemical and biological agents will be included in a separately published appendix to the Senate Select Committee's report. This section of the report will discuss the rationale for the programs, their monitoring and control, and what the Committee's investigation has revealed about the relationship among the intelligence agencies and about their relations with other government agencies and private institutions and individuals.[2]

Fears that countries hostile to the United States would use chemical and biological agents against Americans or America's allies led to the development of a defensive program designed to discover techniques for American intelligence agencies to detect and counteract chemical and biological agents. The defensive orientation soon became secondary as the possible use of these agents to obtain information from, or gain control over, enemy agents became apparent.

Research and development programs to find materials which could be used to alter human behavior were initiated in the late 1940s and early 1950s. These experimental programs originally included testing of drugs involving willing human subjects, and culminated in tests using unwitting, nonvolunteer human subjects. These tests were designed to determine the potential effects of chemical or biological agents when used operationally against individuals unaware that they had received a drug.

The testing programs were considered highly sensitive by the intelligence agencies administering them. Few people, even within the agencies, knew of the programs and there is no evidence that either the executive branch or Congress were ever informed of them. The highly compartmented nature of these programs may be explained in part by an observation made by the CIA Inspector General that, "the knowledge that the Agency is engaging in unethical and illicit activities would have serious repercussions in political and diplomatic circles and would be detrimental to the accomplishment of its missions."[3]

# Fig. 12.4 cont. U. S. Senate Select Committee Report

The research and development program, and particularly the covert testing programs, resulted in massive abridgments of the rights of American citizens, sometimes with tragic consequences. The deaths of two Americans[3a] can be attributed to these programs; other participants in the testing programs may still suffer from the residual effects. While some controlled testing of these substances might be defended, the nature of the tests, their scale, and the fact that they were continued for years after the danger of surreptitious administration of LSD to unwitting individuals was known, demonstrate a fundamental disregard for the value of human life.

The Select Committee's investigation of the testing and use of chemical and biological agents also raise serious questions about the adequacy of command and control procedures within the Central Intelligence Agency and military intelligence, and about the relationships among the intelligence agencies, other governmental agencies, and private institutions and individuals. The CIA's normal administrative controls were waived for programs involving chemical and biological agents to protect their security. According to the head of the Audit Branch of the CIA these waivers produced "gross administrative failures." They prevented the CIA's internal review mechanisms (the Office of General Counsel, the Inspector General, and the Audit Staff) from adequately supervising the programs. In general, the waivers had the paradoxical effect of providing less restrictive administrative controls and less effective internal review for controversial and highly sensitive projects than those governing normal Agency activities. . . .

---

[1] Senate Resolution 21 directs the Senate Select Committee on Intelligence Activities to investigate a number of issues:

" (a) Whether agencies within the intelligence community conducted illegal domestic activities (Section 2(1) and (2));

" (b) The extent to which agencies within the intelligence community cooperate (Section 2(4) and (8));

" (c) The adequacy of executive branch and congressional oversight of intelligence activities (Section 2 (7) and (11));

" (d) The adequacy of existing laws to safeguard the rights of American citizens (Section 2 (13))."

[2] The details of these programs may never be known. The programs were highly compartmented. Few records were kept. What little documentation existed for the CIA's principal program was destroyed early in 1973.

[3] CIA Inspector General's Survey of TSD, 1957, p. 217.

[3a] On January 8, 1953, Mr. Harold Blauer died of circulatory collapse and heart failure following an intravenous injection of a synthetic mescaline derivative while a subject of tests conducted by New York State Psychiatric Institute under a contract let by the U.S. Army Chemical Corps. . . .

## Fig. 12.5. United States Annotated Title 50. War and National Defense. Chapter 32—Chemical and Biological Warfare Program. Approved 1-16-96

**§ 1520.** Use of human subjects for testing of chemical or biological agents by Department of Defense; accounting to Congressional committees with respect to experiments and studies; notification of local civilian officials

**(a)** Not later than thirty days after final approval within the Department of Defense of plans for any experiment or study to be conducted by the Department of Defense, whether directly or under contract, involving the use of human subjects for the testing of chemical or biological agents, the Secretary of Defense shall supply Representatives with a full accounting of such plans for such experiment or study, and such experiment or study may then be conducted only after the expiration of the thirty-day period beginning on the date such accounting is received by such committees.

**(b)(1)** The Secretary of Defense may not conduct any test or experiment involving the use of any chemical or biological agent on civilian populations unless local civilian officials in the area in which the test or experiment is to be conducted are notified in advance of such test or experiment, and such test or experiment may then be conducted only after the expiration of the thirty-day period beginning on the date of such notification.

**(2)** Paragraph (1) shall apply to tests and experiments conducted by Department of Defense personnel and tests and experiments conducted on behalf of the Department of Defense by contractors.

(Pub.L. 95-79, Title VIII, § 808, July 30, 1977, 91 Stat. 334; Pub.L. 97-375, Title II, § 203(a)(1), Dec. 21, 1982, 96 Stat. 1822.)

The above text has been reset verbatum from: United States Code Annotated: Title 50, War and National Defense, Chapter 32—Chemical and Biological Warfare Program, Title 50:1520 on the Use of human subjects for testing of chemical or biological agents by Department of Defense. January, 1996, pp. 510, This represents a revision from "1977 Act. House Report No. 95-194 and House Conference Report No. 95-446, see 1977 U. S. Code Cong. and Adm. News, p. 537.

grams and there is no evidence that either the executive branch or Congress were ever informed of them. The highly compartmented nature of these programs may be explained in part by an observation made by the CIA Inspector General that, 'the knowledge that the Agency is engaging in unethical and illicit activities would have serious repercussions in political and diplomatic circles and would be detrimental to the accomplishment of its missions.'

"The research and development program, and particularly the covert testing programs, resulted in massive abridgements of the rights of American citizens, sometimes with tragic consequences. . . ."[6]

The second document, figure 12.5, showed biological testing had been authorized to continue well into the 1990s. This "Title 1520" of the "United States Code Annotated Title 50, on War and National Defense" was widely circulated among U.S. patriotic, Christian, and militia groups as evidence of the government's malfeasance. This 1996 document reiterated and clarified authorizations detailed in 1977 and again in 1982. This update covered the "Use of human subjects for testing of chemical or biological agents by Department of Defense; accounting to Congressional committees with respect to experiments and studies;" [and] notification, not permission, of one unspecified local civilian official. This document stated that the only requirement for defense and intelligence agencies who wish to authorize the exposure of unwitting citizens to lethal biological or chemical agents, was the notification of one local civilian official. This was required "in the area in which the test or experiment is to be conducted . . . in advance of such test or experiment" by thirty days.[7]

The circulation of this document created such popular outrage that Senator John Glenn was obliged to sponsor a revised proposal titled: "Bill S-193 HUMAN RESEARCH SUBJECT PROTECTIONS ACT OF 1997." The bill was sent to the Senate's Labor and Human Resources Committee for final consideration and approval. It was subsequently modified to require military, medical, and intelligence contractors to fund the human experiments. No longer would taxpayers be forced to fund their own intoxication and demise.[8] Yet, according to the final "Repeal Restrictions," biological and chemical testing on U.S. citizens could continue under the guise of "medical, therapeutic, pharmaceutical, agricultural, industrial, or research activity." This allowed for alleged "protection against toxic chemicals or biological weapons," or "any law enforcement purpose, including any purpose related to riot control" providing "informed consent to the testing was obtained from each human subject in advance . . ."[8a]

Although these government investigations and documents raised a few eyebrows, they did little more than that. It appeared that government oversight committees were doing their jobs so taxpayers could rest assured. However, very little technical knowledge and too few specifics were ever discussed during these Senate intelligence committee hearings. In some cases, legislators were even given false and misleading information. As a result, the public has remained at risk.

One example of such deception is shown in figure 12.6—a declassified U.S. government memorandum discussing some intricacies of Project BLUEBIRD. Notice the deletion of critical facts. The document and project is of particular relevance to this book and chapter as it concerns the use of "sound" and the application of "ultrasonics, UHF, vibrations, monotonous sounds, concussion, etc., etc.," for hypnosis, mind control, and behavior change. The project also employed the study and use of dietary factors and foods as toxin delivery systems. In contrast to these documented facts, the 1976 Senate Select Committee's report described the CIA's Project BLUEBIRD/ARTICHOKE as simply "the earliest of the CIA's major programs involving the use of chemical and biological agents. Project BLUEBIRD was approved by the Director in 1950. Its objectives were:

> (a) discovering means of conditioning personnel to prevent unauthorized extractions of information from them by known means, (b) investigating the possibility of control of an individual by application of special interrogation techniques, (c) memory enhancement, and (d) establishing defensive means for preventing hostile control of Agency personnel."[6]

Thus, without mentioning the details, the *Congressional Records* were devoid of knowledge that the earliest BLUEBIRD experiments involved extensive use of sound and electromagnetic frequencies for

# Fig. 12.6. United States Government Office Memorandum Concerning the CIA's 1950 Top Secret Mind Control Project Bluebird

*Office Memorandum* • UNITED STATES GOVERNMENT

A/B, 4, 23/32

*A*

TO       :
Via      :
FROM     :

DATE:    3 March 1952

SUBJECT: . Attached.

> 1. The attached memorandum is an Eyes Only report for your study and consideration.

> 2. The writer has set down personal comments relative the Bluebird operation and particularly contributions or rather lack of contributions to this effort by OSI. The writer has also commented relative matters involving the medical staff in relation to the Bluebird program.

> 3. The paper is not an official document, but rather a confidential report for I & SO information only.

> 4. If you have no further use for it after reading, I will retain it in our controlled files.

 *A*

1) Sound

   What use can be made of sound for Bluebird
   application? Consider ultra-sonics, UHF,
   vibrations, monotonous sounds, concussion,
   etc., etc. (The Agency has contributed
   ▒▒▒▒▒▒cently to the "Side Tone Delay" --
   a related matter but the answers along these
   lines are a year away probably.)

   H-B/3

2) High and Low Pressures, Various Gases

   Use of gas as in the air-tight chambers and
   the effects of various gases or lack of oxygen
   on individuals should be studied. The effects
   of high and low pressures and certain gases
   are reported to be being considered b▒▒▒▒▒▒
   ▒▒▒▒▒▒▒▒▒▒▒▒▒▒), but pressure chamber
   there has not been built.

   H-B/6
   B

-3) Use of Hypnotic Techniques and Chemicals in
   Connection with the Polygraph

   Some work has been done by the writer and his
   associates in the hypnotic field with interesting results; however, insufficient work has
   been done to specifically state that individuals
   controlled by hypnotism or operating under post-
   hypnotics could

        A). beat the polygraph

        B). or take the polygraph examination
            without being detected.

   Information relative chemicals and drugs which
   could be used in beating the polygraph is very
   sketchy and inaccurate. This type of testing
   cannot easily be carried on within the Agency
   and the few tests that have been observed by
   the writer were very poorly controlled and the
   results at best were confusing.

4) Use of Bacteria, Plant Cultures, Fungi, Poisons
   of Various Types, Etc.

   Whether any of these elements would be useful
   in Bluebird techniques are unknown to the writer
   and to date, research has developed no information

that is useful along these lines. What effect
these elements would have on individuals who
are under control is unknown. However, certain
of these elements could produce bodily conditions
such as high fever, delirium, etc., but it is
doubted if these conditions could be exploited
advantageously.

5) Diet

If individuals under strict control are continuously fed food or liquid containing high quantities of salt, spices, etc. or if certain basic
food elements (such as fats, starches, proteins,
etc.) are continuously removed from the diet of
controlled individuals, will they or can they
thus be conditioned for Bluebird techniques?

There is considerable literature to indicate
that a standard Soviet and satellite technique
is the use of food containing high salt content,
which produces thirst in the subject to be in-
terrogated. The exact reasons for this are unknown, but a number of intelligent guesses can
be made.

## 20. FURTHER COMMENTS RELATIVE ELECTRO-SHOCK

As has been noted above and in conversation, there has been
a considerable amount of discussion relative possible uses of
electroshock as a weapon by Bluebird.

It has been reported to the writer that       , referred **C**
to above, believes that the electroshock or post electroshock coma **A**
can be used in obtaining information from individuals. According
to       and his associates have been able
to obtain information from subjects after the electroshock convulsion and during the coma period following the convulsion after
the initial electroshock. There is very little information on this
technique and while we are not certain that individuals who are
attempting to conceal information could be forced to give up information through this method, the idea may have some merit, but
it is apparently in experimental form only and has not been widely
tested. At least as far as the writer knows there is little, if
any, literature available relative this technique.

-14-

## Fig. 12.7. Major U. S. Military and Intelligence Agency Electromagnetic Mind-Control Projects

### Project MOONSTRUCK, 1952, CIA:

**Description—Electronic implants in brain and teeth**

Targeting—Long range; Implants introduced during surgey or surreptitiously during abduction.

Frequency range: HF–ELF transceiver implants.

Purpose: Tracking, mind and behavior control, conditioning, programming, covert operations.

Functional Basis: Electronic stimulaton of the brain, E.S.B.

### Project MK-ULTRA (BLUEBIRD/ARTICHOKE), 1953, CIA:

**Description—Electronics and electroshock**

Targeting—Short range.

Frequency range: VHF, HF, UHF, modulated at ELF. Local transmission and reception.

Purpose: Programming behavior, creation of "cyborg" mentalities.

Effects: Narcoleptic trance states, programming by suggestion.

Functional Basis: Electronic dissolution of memory, E.D.O.M.

### Project ORION (DREAMLAND), 1958, U.S.A.F.:

**Description—Drugs, hypnosis, and ESB**

Targeting—Short range, in person.

Frequency range: ELF modulation. Transmission and reception by radar and microwaves.

Purpose: Top security personnel debriefing, programming, insure security and loyalty.

Effects: Narcoleptic trance states, programming by suggestion.

Functional Basis: Electronic dissolution of memory, E.D.O.M.

## Project MK-DELTA (DEEP SLEEP), 1960, CIA:

**Description—Fine-tuned electromagnetic subliminal programming.**

Targeting—Long range.

Frequency range: VHF, HF, UHF, modulated at ELF. Transmission and reception through television and radio antennae, power lines, mattress spring coils, modulation on 60Hz wiring.

Purpose: Programming behavior and attitudes in general population.

Effects: Fatigue, mood swings, behavior dysfunction and criminality.

## Project PHOENIX II (MONTAUK), 1983, U.S.A.F., NSA:

**Description—Electronic multi-directional targeting of select population groups.**

Targeting—Medium range.

Frequency range: Radar, microwaves, EHF, UHF modulated with gigawatt through terawatt power.

Purpose: Loading of Earth grids, planetary sonombulescence to stave off geological activity, specific-point earthquake creation, population programming for sensitized individuals.

Pseudonym: "Rainbow," ZAP.

## Project TRIDENT, 1989, ONR, NSA:

**Description—Electronic directed targeting of individuals or populations**

Targeting—Large population groups assembled.

Frequency range: VHF, HF, UHF, modulated at ELF. Local transmission and reception.

Purpose: Crowd dispersion and others.

Display: Black helicopters flying in triad formation.

---

Adopted from "Major Electromagnetic Mind-Control Projects" report in *Contact: The Phoenix Educator*, July 14, 1998, p. 5.

inducing various states of mental incapacitation, persuasion, and even death.

Most revealing, the declassified document in figure 12.6 showed the initial use of "Bacteria, Plant Cultures, Fungi, [and] Poisons of Various Types" were already being considered as cofactors, or delivery systems, for mind and personnel control by the early 1950s. Though BLUEBIRD's targets were allegedly limited to individuals, BLUEBIRD evolved into ARTICHOKE and ultimately to the PHOENIX II project—also called the MONTAUK program. This activity endeavored to develop technologies and the wherewithal for "electronic multidirectional targeting of select populations." Its description and purpose was akin to those provided by project HAARP.[9]

Figure 12.7 provides a listing of the major electromagnetic mind-control projects administered by the CIA and branches of the U.S. military. The next section covers their most relevant achievements.

### Early Electromagnetics for Mind-Control

According to *Operation Mind Control*,[10] a definitive effort by investigative journalist Walter Bowart, the earliest "wireless" mind-control experiments evolved by the late 1960s. By then, the "remote control" of human cognition without the use of implanted electrodes was being pioneered by a research team at the University of California's Space and Biology Laboratory at the Los Angeles Brain Research Institute. There, Dr. W. Ross Adey developed ways of stimulating the brain using low level electomagnetic pulses. Bowart detailed the novel methods Adey used as follows:

> In one experiment, Dr. Adey analyzed the brain waves of chimpanzees who were performing tasks that involved learning. He established that there were two very distinct brain-wave patterns which accompanied correct and incorrect decisions. Building on this, Dr. Adey attempted to control the rate at which the chimps learned by applying forcefields to the outside of the head to alter behavior, moods, and attention. Dr. Adey's research indicated that his subjects were able to remember new information faster and better with stimulation.[10]

Following the assassination of John. F. Kennedy by, allegedly, Lee Harvey Oswald, an conspiracy that Bowart theorized had been accomplished using CIA mind control radio frequency technologies, Richard Helms sent a memo to Warren Commissioners. Helms, once again, was the initiator of Project MKULTRA. In his letter, Helms referred to "biological radio communication" as having something to do with the assassination. Although he failed to fully explain, he did relate his comments to electronic brain stimulation research that was underway in the United States and Russia. "Current research," Helms wrote, "indicates that the Soviets are attempting to develop a technology for control in the development of behavioral patterns among the citizenry of the USSR in accordance with politically determined requirements of the system. Furthermore, the same technology can be applied to more sophisticated approaches to the 'coding' of information for transmittal to population targets in the 'battle for the minds of men.'"[10]

Helms's comments were based on knowledge that, since 1961, Drs. W. Fry and R. Meyers at the University of Illinois had used ultrasonic waves to develop brain lesions in test subjects. Their research, according to Bowart, "demonstrated the great advantage of ultrasonics over the psychosurgical techniques which implanted electrodes in the brain. By using low-energy sound beams, Fry and Meyers stimulated or destroyed neural tissue at the point of focus of the beams without cutting or drilling into the brain."[10]

Not long after, Dr. Peter Lindstrom at the University of Pittsburgh developed "prefrontal sonic treatment" to effectively produce a lobotomy in patients with severe psychiatric disorders or untreatable pain. He used a single unfocused sound beam to kill specific nerve fiber tracts leaving adjacent cells healthy.[10]

At the same time, scientists found that monotonous rhythms could produce drowsiness and hypnotic inductions, and that specific frequency flashing strobe lights could initiate seizures in epileptics.[10]

Along with these discoveries the CIA secretly funded studies designed to test the effects of various vibrations on the brain. In one such experiment, researchers suspended a tin sheet from the ceiling connected to an electrical wave generator operating at ten cycles per second. When very large field strengths were coupled with very small volt strengths, and oscillated at the alpha frequency of brain function, human volunteers reported extremely unpleasant sensations.[10]

Similarly, at the Brain Research Institute in California, researchers examined additional effects of oscillating electromagnetic fields (EMFs) on human behavior. They exposed subjects to extremely small EMFs for only fifteen minutes and observed measurable degeneration of simple task performance.[10]

"These and other experiments," Bowart concluded, "led the cryptocracy to study the effects of very-low-frequency sound (VLF)— the opposite of ultrasonics—as an instrument of war. *Research revealed that there is a natural wave guide between the ionosphere and the earth which could be used to propagate very-low-frequency radiation, and guide it to selected locations on the earth.* Studies showed that this low-frequency sound subtly affected the electrical behavior of the brain in much the same way that Dr. Adey's studies had shown."[10] [Emphasis added due to relevance.] These were virtually the same experiments that led authorities to realize the potential use of the applications being conducted today by EISCAT and HAARP to affect behavior and even, perhaps, induce disease in large populations.

Bowart further explained, "The alpha-wave frequency of the human brain is from eight to twelve hertz (cycles per second). The ionospheric wave guide oscillates at eight hertz, making it a good harmonic carrier of low-frequency sound (LFS) waves. These are such long waves that they are virtually impossible to detect. Pentagon reports apply LFS to demobilizing the productive capacity of a civilian population in time of war."[10]

A related concern was voiced by Dr. Frank Barnaby, Director of the Stockholm International Peace Research Institute. He warned of military and intelligence agency use of this technology as follows:

"If methods could be devised to produce greater field strengths of such low-frequency oscillations, either by natural (for example, lightning) or artificial means, then it might become possible to impair the performance of a large group of people in selected regions over extended periods."[11]

Thus, early researchers found that ultrasonics, or very-low-frequency sound, harmonized with alpha rhythms might lull large populations into suggestive states wherein radio waves, as well as television, could then be used to implant suggestions. These suggestions could then affect, if not control, the behavior of millions.

As early as 1933, Soviet scientists had studied microwave irradiation to cause central nervous system changes and affect behavior. During mind control studies they observed that even low intensity microwave radiation could dangerously alter normal brain wave rhythms. Such manipulations caused drastic alterations in perception—sense of time loss included—and even hallucinations. In addition, Russian investigators learned that microwave exposures caused changes in protein metabolism and protein composition, altered white blood cell and immune system functions, and created hormonal imbalances—especially those linked to altered thyroid activity, chronic fatigue, and male sterility.[10]

Bowart also recalled the 1962 fracas between the United States and Russia over the microwave bombardment of the U.S. Embassy in Moscow. The author noted very few details regarding the issue in the news. "Perhaps," he speculated, the CIA "feared that any claim that microwave radiation could affect human behavior would bring great restrictions on the use of radar, microwave relays, and on booming microwave oven sales. But a less obvious reason suggests itself: the cryptocracy did not want to draw attention to its own use of radiation in mind control."[10]

Despite these historic facts, during the 1970s and early 1980s, most U.S. scientists remained skeptical that there was an advancing field of bioelectric mind control.[10]

Dr. Elliot S. Valenstein, the author of *Brain Control*, was one whose comments reflected a scientific naivete of this burgeoning field. He wrote, "The reports of new technical developments for brain stimulation have led to concern that it will be used as the basis of an 'electroligarchy' where people could be virtually enslaved by controlling them from within their own brains . . . there is actually little foundation for the belief that brain stimulation could be used as a political weapon. It doesn't make sense. Anyone influential enough to get an entire population to consent to having electrodes placed in its head would already have his goal without firing a single volt."[12]

Dr. Willard Gaylin concurred saying, "Electrode implantation or surgical ablation of brain sections as a direct means of political control seems unlikely—much less a threat, for example, than drugs. Such an individualized and dramatic procedure hardly seems suited to the enslavement of populations or the robotization of political leaders. Drugs, brainwashing by control of the media, exploitation of fears through forms of propaganda, and indoctrination through the sources of education, particularly if preschool education or neonatal conditioning . . . becomes an approved practice, all seem more likely methods of totalitarian control."[13]

Finally, Dr. Steven Rose, a British biochemist objected: "Unlike ancient maps marked 'here be monsters,' there will not be . . . brains transplanted into bodies or bottles, thought, memory or mind control, telepathic communication or genetic engineering, artificial intelligence or robots . . . I believe them impossible—or at least improbable; more importantly because scientific advance and its attendant technology only comes about in response to social constraints and social demands in the direction of these lurid potential developments, they do not represent, in a world beset with crises and challenges to human survival, serious contenders for our concerns."[14]

History would soon prove such nay-sayers wrong. As Bowart explained, such off base remarks by esteemed scientists could have been expected "when science is developed in a piecemeal, compartmentalized fashion, as it is under the direction of the cryptocracy. . . . Where the public is kept ignorant, and where scientists themselves are manipulated by the grant system, the balance upon which" such denials rest, heavily favors deception."[10]

For every scientist who denied that mind control existed, however, there were those who took a shining to the advancing technology for improved prospects for social control. One example was social psychologist Kenneth B. Clark, who said, "Given the urgency of the immediate survival problem, the psychological and social sciences must enable us to control the animalistic, barbaric and primitive propensities in man and subordinate these negatives to the uniquely human moral and ethical characteristics of love, kindness, and empathy . . . We can no longer afford to rely solely on the traditional prescientific attempts to contain human cruelty and destructiveness."[15]

Further advancing this thesis were Drs. Stephen Rosen, a scientist at IBM and Olaf Helmer, a founding member of the Institute for the Future. Rosen predicted a time when physical medicine would combine with the behavioral sciences to produce a new level of social control, while Olaf Helmer envisioned a state in which "slave robots" were likely to be developed from advances in mind control technologies.[10]

## Current Electromagnetic Population Control Technologies

In 1980, John Alexander, a covert operations specialist with a Vietnam war hero's background, published an article in the U.S. Army's *Military Review*, titled "The New Mental Battlefield." Alexander, a Green Berets commander who went on to complete a Ph.D. from Walden University and then became a spokesperson for Silva Mind Control, argued that offensive electronic weapons might be used to interfere with brain activity of targeted populations.

As exposed by veteran author and investigator Jim Keith, in his book *Mind Control-World Control*, "Alexander was encouraged by two senior army officials to do additional research in the field, and this led to his joining the special technologies group at Los Alamos National Laboratories." There Alexander began to collaborate with Janet Morris, another Silva Mind Control graduate and Research Director of the U.S. Global Strategy Council (USGSC) think tank. The council's chairman was Ray Cline, the former Deputy Director of the CIA. The USGSC played a major role in the creation of the Non-lethality Policy Review Group, led by Major General Chris S. Adams, USAF (retd.), former Chief of Staff, Strategic Air Command. This pioneering group, Keith explained, "encouraged the military to think in terms of 'non-lethality.'"[16]

Consistent with the recommendations made in the *Report From Iron Mountain*, in 1991, Janet Morris issued several papers promoting the concept of non-lethal warfare. She and her associates advanced certain key areas of military preparedness research. "These included technologies directed at the destruction of weapons of war, but also an increased focus on anti-personnel electomagnetics."[16]

According to Keith, Morris's recommendations for anti-personnel non-lethal warfare included very low frequency radiation weapons. These, according to her remarks in a position paper entitled, "In Search of a Non-Lethal Strategy," included, "some very low frequency sound generators." Certain frequencies generated by these devices could cause "the disruption of human organs and, at high power levels, can crumble masonry."[16]

A parallel recommendation was advanced by the U.S. Army War College's Strategic Studies Institute (SSI) in Pennsylvania. A 1994 paper originating here entitled "The Revolution in Military Affairs (RMA) and Conflict Short of War" argued that many "American strategic thinkers believe that we are in the beginning stages of a historical revolution in military affairs." The changes were destined to affect not only "the nature of warfare," but also the "global geopolitical balance." Accordingly, the RMA included, according to Keith, "a number of new avenues of warfare research that should be pursued, specifically 'behavior modification' and 'technology designed specifically for conflict short of war, especially psychological, biological, and defensive technology,'"[16] In other words, the SSI recommended "spiritual warfare" at its finest.

In this context, Gulf War Syndrome as a result of biological and/or chemical exposures might be reconciled. Why resort to bloody warfare, for instance, when "excess" military populations can be forced to consent to "nonlethal" but largely debilitating vaccinations. Here too, the "excess population" of "war material" is effectively controlled, culled, and slowly killed in an economically reliable manner.

The SSI authors lamented, however, that the use of "the new technology may . . . run counter to basic American values." Therefore, deception might be required to initiate the effort, though this too presented problems. The authors wrote, "Deception, while frequently of great military or political value, is thought of as somehow 'un-American.'"[16]

To overcome these restraints, these RMA advocates advanced the possibility of creating a "fundamental change in the United States—an ethical and political revolution [that] may be necessary to make a military revolution" possible.[16]

## New Deceptions for Implementing Surveillance Technology

The activation of project HAARP's electromagnetic radiation technologies seems particularly timely for such an insurrection. As stated above, the two contingencies—mass deception and an "ethical revolution" seem to have been conveniently incorporated into HAARP's implementation plan. Some people truly want to believe this project is for the public's good.

Likewise, in this deceptive vein, the "health passport" or "health card" introduced in the last chapter is most innovative. Herein the general use of surveillance, as with individual position locator devices, or IPLDs, have been hailed as a great social amenity versus an attack on personal freedom. Deception is the key to this successful strategy as the history of the "health card" has shown.

The RMA manifesto argued that "large numbers of Americans may find themselves in areas of instability and conflict," and that people were cautioned to be "equipped with an electronic individual position locator device (IPLD). The device, derived from the electronic bracelet used to control some criminal offenders or parolees, would continuously inform a central data bank of the individuals' locations. Eventually such a device could be permanently implanted under the skin," the SSI advanced.

In *Whatever Happened to America?*, historian Jon Christian Ryter provided a case study in a related deception. In September, 1998, he was repulsed to learn that "somehow, unbeknown to anyone, and for some as yet unexplained reason, the National ID Card that Hillary Clinton, Marc Tucker and Ira Magaziner had adroitly concealed in the failed Health Security Act of 1994 had somehow 'accidently' been passed, in a somewhat illegal and unconstitutional fashion, and was now 'the law of the land.'" The bad news eventually came from U.S. Congressional representatives Bob Barr (R-GA) and Ron Paul (L-TX) who had alerted their constituents to the sham politics.

Used in three American cities, at the time of Ryter's writing, the National Institutes of Health (NIH) introduced the card during a seminar held in Denver, Colorado, early in 1998. The word "passport," visible on the front of the card, Ryter felt, was a "tongue-in-cheek addition" since it was likely to be the precursor of a national "passport" that will largely control the public's movements within the United States.

The card, in use at the time of this writing, was said to be an effective "biometric" storage and retrieval aid. The card owner's medical history is stored on the unit as is "every conceivable piece of information about that person." Also, the card contains a "tracking device."[17]

Ryter reviewed the historic evolution of the health passport by writing that, "The plan to create and implement a National ID Card" was first made "public" in a private White House meeting November 11, 1993. It was "innocuously concealed in the Health Security Act as a 'healthcare benefits card' that the First Lady insisted had to be carried by every American—even if they refused to be covered by the plan—under penalty of law.

"The same card, in the form of a national driver's license, had just been mandated by the European Union for all of the new European States," Ryter wrote. "A brief battle was waged in Europe over this driver's license. Most Europeans had experienced national identity cards in the past and realized quickly the new universal European driver's license was an internal passport that would give their new government" an additional control device that would affect their lives. "The media immediately labeled those who resisted the EU driver's license as 'globalphobes' who were against progress, and wanted to return Europe to the days of the cold war. They were extremists.

"In the United States, the Clintons knew a National ID Card spelled problems, regardless what name was put on it. However, as a healthcare card that provided each American with thousands of dollars of free medical care, they correctly surmised that the ramblings of the right wing zealots could be easily dismissed by the mainstream liberal media. The media did its job well.

"The Health Security Act was the best thing since sliced bread and peanut butter. According to the media, the Health Security Act would provide healthcare for the millions upon millions of uninsured Americans. The media even obliged by ignoring the obviously flawed cost assessments as well."

Hillary Clinton demanded that Congress pass the Health Security Act intact. Congress balked. They read the proposal and then rejected it. It was, they declared, "the most expensive social experiment in the world."

"Buried in the National Archives, in the working papers of the Hillary Clinton healthcare plan," Ryter continued, "was a game plan in the event the Health Security Act went down in flaming defeat. The game plan? Implement another healthcare act that provided healthcare for children. No one would dare deny healthcare to children. To introduce the plan, they called on Teddy Kennedy. Kennedy failed. . . .

"Next they turned to Orrin Hatch, who teamed up with Kennedy and rammed the legislation through Congress. Healthcare for kids. Of course, everyone was in favor of it. Voting against it was a good way to lose an election. And, once the law was codified, the bureaucracy possessed the authority to simply expand it to anyone and everyone. . . ."

Introduced to members of the NIH in Denver was a card that recorded the inoculation records of children, and included everything from DNA typing to medical, psychiatric, and financial histories, as well as a tracking chip.

At a more recent NIH seminar, one of the institute's executives "proudly displayed an electronic map created by the NIH computer technicians that pinpointed every Health Passport card holder in Denver, Colorado. It was a 'living map' that" tracked each Health Passport card holder whenever and wherever they moved."[17]

## Corporal Biochips

One obvious drawback to the placement of IPLDs—individual position locator devices—in identification cards is that they may be lost or stolen. One remedy for this inconvenience is the insertion of the tracking device into the body.

In the "High-Tech Nightmare" which appeared in the July 24, 1994 issue of *The New American*, author William F. Jasper examined the future of biochip identification and tracking technology, and what the Clintons understood *before* they promoted the widespread use of their health card. Jasper wrote regarding the "smart card" as a central feature of the "health care reform" plan, "an ethical and political revolution:"

> Some "Friends of Hillary" have even grander visions. Mary Jane England, MD, a member of the executive committee of the White House Health Project and president of the Washington Business Group on Health, a national outfit comprised of some of the nation's leading corporate welfare statists, is especially

440

excited about the potential for implanting smart chips in your body. Addressing the 1994 IBM Health Care Executive Conference last March in Palm Springs, California, Dr. England said: "The smart card is a wonderful idea, but even better would be the capacity not to have a card, and I call it 'a chip in your ear,' that would actually access your medical records, so that no matter where you were . . . we would have some capacity to access that medical record. We need to go beyond the narrow conceptualization of the Smart Card and really use some of the technology that's out there. The worst thing we could do is put in place a technology that's already outdated, because all of you are in the process of building these systems. Now is the time to really think ahead. . . . I don't think that computerized, integrated medical records with a capacity to access through a chip in your ear is so far off and I think we need to think of these things."

Another article that voiced a similar interest appeared in *The Washington Times*.[18] Most interesting, the author credited the Hughes Aircraft Company with the development of the biochip technology. That is, the same Hughes company affiliated with the Howard Hughes Medical Institute, whose researchers identified the crystal-like properties of prions, as well as the *Citizen Hughes* that *The Bible Code* author of propaganda, Michael Drosnin, biographed.

Getting to the heart of the matter of radio frequency transponding biochips, here's what Martin Anderson of *The Washington Times* wrote, much of which was taken from Hughes marketing literature:

> You see, there is an identification system made by the Hughes Aircraft Company that you can't lose. It's the syringe implantable transponder. According to promotional literature it is an "ingenious, safe, inexpensive, foolproof and permanent method of . . . identification using radio waves. A tiny microchip, the size of a grain of rice, is simply placed under the skin. It is so designed as to be injected simultaneously with a vaccination or alone."

> How does it work? Well, the "chip contains a 10 character alphanumeric identification code that is never duplicated. When a scanner is passed over the chip, the scanner emits a 'beep' and your . . . number flashes in the scanner's digital display."

> Sort of like a technological tattoo. . . . Of course, most Americans will find a surgically implanted government microchip repugnant. At least for the foreseeable future, the use of this ingenious device will be confined to its current use: the tracking of dogs, cats, horses, . . . cattle [prisoners and sex offenders].

> But there is no difference in principle between being forced to carry a microchip in a plastic card in your wallet or in a little pellet in your arm. The principle that Big Brother has the right to track you is inherent in both. The only thing that differentiates the two techniques is a layer of skin.[20]

Once you denigrate the idea of privacy, all kinds of innovative government controls are possible, things that didn't even occur to Aldous Huxley when he wrote, *Brave New World*.

Terry L. Cook in his book *The Mark of the New World Order*, provided an exhaustive and enlightening review on the topic of radio frequency identification and tracking devices in modern biochip technology. Such devices use radio signals to "read" identification codes and other data stored in a "transponder." These devices provide a reliable way to "electronically detect, control, and track a variety of items, information, animals and people."[21]

Cook described the "core of the technology" as a "small, low frequency transponder attached to an object." In the typical industrial application, he explained, "a reader sends a radio signal to the passive, or battery-free, transponder. The signal charges the transponder, allowing it to return a signal carrying a unique ID code. Lasting less than one-tenth of a second, the process can take place within a "read range" of up to 15 feet. The data collected from the transponder either can be sent directly to a host computer through standard interfaces or stored in a portable reader and later uploaded to the computer for data processing. Radio frequency identification transponders are designed for long life—up to 175-250 years—according to Donald Small, of Hughes Identification Devices."[21]

Figure 12.8, provided by Terry Cook, diagrams the essential components of the injectable biochip identification and tracking system. "This type of transponder is a passive device . . . ," Cook's research

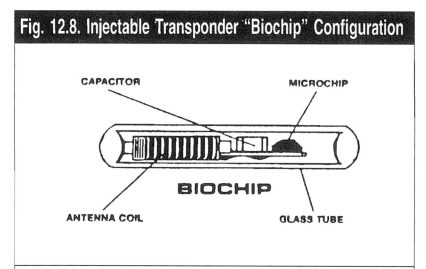

**Fig. 12.8. Injectable Transponder "Biochip" Configuration**

From: Cook, TL. *The Mark of the New World Order: 666—The Cashless Economic System of Global Electronic Enslavement.* Bend, OR: Whitaker House, 1996, p. 316

showed. "It has no batteries and never can wear out. It is energized by a low-frequency radio wave from the scanner," or from the radio emissions source such as the HAARP antennae. "Most scanners use a frequency of 125kHz, the signal used in AM medium-wave broadcasting. These low-frequency radio waves can penetrate all solid objects except those made of metal." The Electronic ID apparatus that responds to these radio signals is referred to as a RFID (Radio Frequency Identification Device). Once the scanner or radio signal is activated, "it digitally displays the decoded ID Number on a liquid biochip."[21]

Cook continued, "Texas Instruments has a brand new chip which will allow the encoding of up to nineteen digits. By combining the digits in a variety of combinations, the smallest biochip can be programmed with up to 34 billion code numbers. A spokesman from Trovan says that with the latest technology, 'the number of possible code combinations is close to one trillion.' That's a lot of identification capability!"[21]

## Considering the Capability

Figure 12.9 documents, in fact, a connecting thread, if not "smoking gun," to what otherwise might be called a baseless conspiracy theory. On February 26, 1999, the *Wall Street Journal* announced that the biochip manufacturer Hughes Corporation, linked also to *The Bible Code* propagandist Michael Drosnin, pioneering Hughes Medical Institute prion crystal research, and the Rockefeller built and funded University of Chicago, had launched a series of satellites that could easily transmit the potentially enslaving as well as pathogenic electromagnetic frequencies from space. Moreover, the Illuminati's shadow on this sobering reality is projected and documented as detailed below.[22]

The article, written by staff reporter Andy Pasztor, explained that Hughes, "the world's largest satellite maker is launching . . . a bigger and more robust generation of satellites, dubbed the 702 line, featuring nearly twice the signal strength and communications capacity of the current models. . . . The 702s [naturally, 7+2=9, or completion] also rely on a novel xenon-ion propulsion system, once the darling of science-fiction fans, which uses electric pulses instead of the combustion of chemical propellants" to slash weight, costs, and craft mortality.

According Pasztor, based on corporate announcements, just "one satellite will be able to cover a much larger chunk of the world, or ultimately beam a radio signal to a tiny antenna installed on a vehicle traveling almost anywhere on the globe." Naturally, if the antenna happened to be a prion crystal or biochip, and the vehicle human beings, recipients might cease traveling altogether depending on the frequency of the radiowave.

## Hughes and Sloan: Space Age Technology for Population Control

Hughes Electronics Corporation's parent, General Motors Corporation, was also identified in the article.[22] It might be recalled from *Emerging Viruses: AIDS & Ebola*, that Alfred P. Sloan, the former C.E.O of General Motors, created the Sloan Foundation in 1934 and

# Fig. 12.9. *Wall Street Journal* Article Linking Hughes Electronics Corporation to GM, Sloan, and Aerospace Technologies That Might Be In Use For Genocide

## CORPORATE FOCUS

# Hughes Electronics Seeks to Restore Satellite Luster

### After a Series of Performance Stumbles, Effort Is Launched to Enhance Reliability

By Andy Pasztor
Staff Reporter of The Wall Street Journal

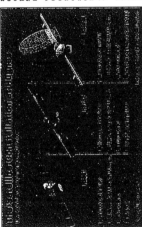

"Such initiatives are coming at a time when Hughes, a separately traded unit of **General Motors Corp.**, along with the rest of the satellite industry . . . are having to build and launch satellites faster than ever . . . .

For example, the 19 satellites Hughes plans to launch this year are nearly twice the average number it sent into orbit from 1995 to 1998. Three of the 1999 launches will involve a bigger and more robust generation of satellites, dubbed the 702 line, featuring nearly twice the signal strength and communications capacity of the current models.

One satellite will be able to cover a much larger chunk of the world, or ultimately beam a radio signal to a tiny antenna installed on a vehicle traveling almost anywhere on the globe."

later the Sloan-Kettering Institute for Cancer Research with Laurance Rockefeller at its helm.[5]

By the early 1980s, the foundation's principal scientific focus, under the neuroscience umbrella, became mass persuasion technologies. The "program in cognitive science," was a pure research program "focused on problems of understanding human mental processes." Financial aid during this program went to support "highly interdisciplinary research in psychology, linguistics, neuroscience, philosophy, anthropology, and computer science." Discoveries made during this program laid the foundation for later work that focused on "management education," or "public management."[23]

Apparently, this work was initiated as the foundation's response to Nixon administration "national security" concerns. The rising tide of racial violence and antiwar protests weighed heavy on the minds of foundation leaders. As Kissinger took control of the NSC, the CIA, the FBI, and COINTELPRO, Sloan Foundation activities reflected such adjustments. Everett Case, then the foundation's president, articulated the seriousness of the times and the need for the foundation to respond accordingly in a report published in the spring of 1968. Case wrote:

> The multiplication and growth of many of our besetting social problems seem all too reminiscent of the behavior of the cancerous cell. Who would have predicted at the beginning of this decade that racism would infect and inflame the minds of even a vocal minority of the Negroes who, in this country, have been its principal victims? Who would have foretold the rise in resort to violence not only among the swelling ranks of the criminals but also as a means of social protest and even as a weapon of dissent?[24]

Case's next paragraphs were most enlightening and relevant regarding the ideology and motivation underlying this apparent genocidal conspiracy:

> More effective techniques for the control of population growth are at hand. The genetic code has been deciphered, and the elements of DNA can now be made synthetically. So, too, the hun-

dreds of young scientists who have earned Sloan fellowships in basic research have made important contributions to our understanding of both the macrocosm and the microcosm.

It is different when one leaves the laboratory or the field experiment, and the disciplined minds they attract, for the sprawling, clamorous, and slippery problems which confront, say, the President of the United States or the Mayor of New York City. It is easy to ascribe outbreaks of urban violence to the intolerable conditions of the ghettos. It is easy to ascribe those conditions to the neglect or apathy of the landlords, to the massive immigration of unskilled and disadvantaged Negroes from the South, to the cupidity of the real estate operators and the building trades, or to the ineptitude and corruption of city officials. It is much harder to get at the *root* causes of such phenomena, and even more difficult to discover and apply effective cures.

. . . Some such observation applies as well to those who see our salvation simply in terms of a return to the "old-fashioned morality." It is not that the younger generation (and moral confusion is not limited to them) have found anything better than the golden rule or the New Testament's "Second Commandment." Indeed, many of them are seeking new ways of applying these precepts more effectively. In the canyons and ghettos of megalopolis, however, the simple injunction to "love thy neighbor as thyself" too often seems meaningless or irrelevant. Moreover, the new knowledge and new technology which we owe to science can not only change our environment in ways that bewilder and confuse, but can themselves become instruments of exploitation. By the same token, they may convert the stuff of moral and legal controversy into an academic exercise. . . .

[S]cience . . .whatever its problems, including the apprehension of a popular revulsion against its untoward consequences, . . . is an enterprise too dynamic to be "turned off" if we would, and too fundamental to our security and our economy to be abandoned if we could. Certainly the search for the causes and possible cures of cancer must be accelerated, not brought to a halt. Together with technology, engineering and management, moreover, science has an indispensable role to play in any effective assault society may launch upon the stubborn complexities of our urban problems.[24]

Thus, the Sloan Foundation implemented grant programs for "public management" as well as the Council on Foreign Relations. Fulfilling Alfred P. Sloan's published goal to take advantage of people's "ignorance of the principles of capitalism and free enterprise," the Sloan and Rockefeller influence advanced genetic engineering, cancer research, and population control agendas. The Sloan Foundation and as well Sloan's cancer center became fully entwined with the Rockefeller Foundation, Laurence Rockefeller, Cold Spring Harbor Labs, and the international blood banking industry through generous gifts to the New York City Blood Council, the New York City Blood Bank, and to world population reduction agencies including the Population Council of the City of New York assembled by Laurence Rockefeller.[5, 25]

According to numerous authors,[26-28] General Motors (GM) maintained powerful political, administrative, and financial links not only to the Rockefellers during World War II, but also to the Third Reich. I.G. Farben's president Hermann Schmitz, in fact, testified during criminal hearings that he had personally arranged a loan of RM 170 million in 1942 to the Alfred P. Sloan directed General Motors.[27] General Motors was, according to respected journalist Joseph Borkin, "married to I.G. Farben and Standard Oil under Hilter." Ethyl GmbH, the German manufacturing arm of the Standard–GM partnership, produced the tetraethyl lead I.G. Farben and the Third Reich needed for their war machine. All of this proceeded with the U.S. War Department's considered blessing.[28]

Ethylenedibromide (EDB), by the way, the human chemical carcinogen placed in JP8 jet fuel, and reportedly intoxicating chemtrails and untold populations all over North America at the time of this writing, is a close chemical relative of the deadly tetraethyl lead produced by the Standard–GM–I.G. Farben cartel.

Thus, grossly connected to the secret societies and corporations that helped fund and effect the twentieth century's greatest genocides, the General Motors Company, the Sloan Foundation, and its contemporary subsidiary the Hughes Corporation, is not only linked to the core of the Illuminati,[29] but appears to be actualizing its primary purpose—population reduction for the "rise of the Fourth Reich," that is, the New World Order.

## Final Words

Though biochip technology offers individual identification, tracking, and even "persuasion" applications that simple prion crystals can not provide, prions offer their own unique capabilities. The simple fact that prions have already been transmitted to individuals who, over the past decade consumed infected grain, beef, pork and chickens (that is, virtually everyone) has given "nonlethal warfare" administrators special disease-transmitting, population-reducing, and even mind controlling powers. Again, this is reconcilable within the context of "nonlethal warfare" and "antipersonnel" applications of very low frequency radiation weapons.

With this in mind, that is, the possible use of prions as well as biochips in military operations for "nonlethal warfare," a final word regarding the incomprehensible nature of this possibility, if not likelihood, is necessary. It might be asked, "Who in their right mind would do such a thing?" Moreover, "how could such a broad based 'conspiracy' proceed unnoticed?" Answers to these questions might be derived by scrutinizing contemporary publications in these related fields.

For instance, in a recent issue of *Aviation Week & Space Technology,* scientists and military officers broached the subject of "new peacekeeping" and "peace enforcement tactics." They were interested in weapons that could be effectively "merged with comprehensive, advanced information systems." They mentioned that space, airborne, and ground-based sensors—including unattended devices could provide the wherewithal that would "enable decisive actions in noncombat situations." From the standpoint of crowd control, or "nonlethal" military operations, information would be "processed and routed to the proper authorities in time to preclude hostile action, ideally, or to enable rapid response if firing occurs."[18]

Another military spokesperson, Gerold Yonas, stated in the same report, "that this 'system of systems' will require an up-front science-based systems engineering (SBSE) approach to ensure resources are used effectively. Sensors, information systems, communications and rules-of-engagement must be coordinated within a comprehensive architecture. 'If you don't do it all right, you won't have a symphony. And massive use of force will not work. The bad guys will win,' he said."[18]

In 1997, the U.S. Air Force increased its commitment to nonlethal mind control operations by creating a new position—Deputy Director for Information Operations. As detailed by author Jim Keith, the position established a new "offensive information warfare" division of the U.S. military. It was to be headed by Lt. Col. Jimmy Miyamoto.

The Information Operations Director's office was to coordinate with "the Joint Chiefs of Staff, the National Security Agency, Defense Intelligence Agency, the CIA, the National Reconnaissance Office, Defense Airborne Reconnaissance Office, and the National Imagery and Mapping Agency." According to *Defense Week*, the duties of the office included the coordination of non-lethality effort with the Air Force. According to the article, their psychological capacity included the projection of "persuasive messages and three dimensional pictures of clouds, smoke, rain droplets, buildings . . . The use of holograms as a persuasive message will have worldwide application."[7]

For example, even the arrival of an anti-Christ that many Christians expect will appear as an apparition to people simultaneously in different nations and continents, and in different forms depending on their religious bent, is possible today. In fact, this would be an ideal exercise for this new Information Operations–U.S. Air Force holographic imaging capability.

Returning to the incomprehensible nature of such "black ops" Keith relayed the gist of an unpublished article entitled "From PSYOP to MindWar: The Psychology of Victory," written by Colonel Michael Aquino. Failing to have the submission accepted for publication in

*Military Review*, Aquino distributed copies of the paper to his "Temple of Set" members.

Aquino's rich military background, "black magic" involvement, and biography was summarized by Keith as follows:

> Aquino received a master's degree in political science from the University of California at Santa Barbara and has reportedly qualified in Defense Attache, Strategic Intelligence, Psychological Operations, Special Forces, and the Airborne divisions in the army, supposedly reporting directly to the Joint Chiefs of Staff. Aquino reportedly served as a Tactical Psychological Operations officer in the 82nd Airborne in Vietnam, and received the Bronze Star, the Air Medal, and the Vietnamese Cross of Gallantry. In 1973 Aquino became executive officer of the 306th Psychological Operations Battalion at Fort McArthur in California. During the 1970s Aquino was a prominent member of the Church of Satan but became disillusioned with LaVey's sideshow-style antics and started his own group, the Temple of Set.[16]

The Temple of Set, according to a police intelligence report, dated July 1, 1981, "is a small group but nonetheless has several hundred members and operates on a national level. Aquino is the official head of the organization and rules the organization through a council of nine, who are in fact his chief lieutenants." Two members of the "council of nine" were also listed as Army Intel members.

Regarding Aquino's secret society or satanic cult involvement, a Pentagon spokesperson defended, "Aquino has an absolute constitutional right [to his belief]. . . . unless there is illegal behavior associated with it."[16]

"In the late 1980s," Keith continued, "Aquino and an associate, Gary Hambright, were accused by the San Francisco Police Department of being involved in a satanic child molestation ring centered around the Presidio military base where Aquino was stationed at the time. Twenty-two families filed $66 million in claims against the army. Although formal charges were never filed against Aquino, only against his associate . . .

"Apparently, there were satanic activities taking place at the Presidio at the time." This was confirmed by Bay Area reporter Linda

Goldston who "found a bunker behind the intelligence offices with ritual symbols painted on the walls. . . ."[22,30]

The Presidio, by the way, was also a west coast home for Bionetics Research labs, the biological weapons contractor that under Dr. Robert Gallo's direction, had developed countless AIDS-like and Ebola-like viruses. Additionally "coincidental" was the fact that Gallo's work and friendship intimately linked him to prion pioneer, Carlton Gadjusek who was, like Aquino, accused of child molestation.[3a] Gadjusek, unlike Aquino, was convicted of sexually abusing some of his adopted children. The Army effectively shielded Aquino from prosecution. In Gadjusek's case, the *Washington Post* reported, Gallo came to Gadjusek's aid. He posted $59,000 "of the $350,000 bond that secured his release."[31] Likewise, author David Icke effectively exposed high level public officials and secret society members who actively engage in child pornography, pedophilic molestation, and even ritualistic infant sacrificing, with legal immunity.[32]

Following the Presidio scandal, Aquino was transferred to Washington, D.C., to apply his knowledge and experience at National Defense University.

Aquino attributed the cover page of his "MindWar" article to the "HEADQUARTERS IMPERIAL STORMTROOPER FORCE/Office of the Chief of Staff/MindWar Center/Hub Four." The report discussed the applicability of psychotronic weapons including mind-altering electronic weapons based on "Lesser Black Magic." These, Aquino reported, are the sophisticated, state-of-the art, lethal and nonlethal weapons that would, from here on, serve to control humanity.[16]

## References

1. Holewa L. Scientists say red tide to blame for manatee die-off. Associated Press Wire Service, July 3, 1996 (Available through the Internet from http://www.n-jcenter.com/enviro/en703.htm); See also"Florida and Red Tide" website at http://fig.cox.miami.edu/~161hon3/temp2.htm.

2. Senate Select Committee on Intelligence. *PROJECT MKUL-TRA, The CIA's Program of Research in Behavior Modification.* Joint Hearing Before the Select Committee on Intelligence and the Subcommittee on Health and Scientific Research of the Committee on Human Resources, United States Senate, Ninety-fifth Congress, First Session, August 3, 1977. Washington, D.C.: U.S. Government Printing Office, 1977, pp. 388-390.

3. Secret Summary of Major Events and Problems, United States Army Chemical Corps, Fiscal Years 1961-1962. U.S. Army Chemical Corps Historical Office, Army Chemical Center, Maryland. Declassified document CBR-S-1794-62, OCMH, SCNo. 116226, released June, 1992; 3a. This document's reference to "crystalline toxin" reinforces the findings reported in: Scott D and Scott W. *The Brucellosis Triangle.* Sudbury, Canada: The Chelmsford Publishers, 1998 pp. 44-57.

The Scotts' investigation also determined that on January 3, 1946, George W. Merck, as U.S. biological weapons industry director, reported to the Secretary of War, Henry Stimson, on the "Production and isolation, for the first time, of a crystalline bacterial toxin, which has opened the way for the preparation of a more highly purified immunizing toxoid." In the same report, Merck noted significant advances in the biological warfare arena had been made concerning human immune mechanisms.

The remainder of this fascinating and relevant research section dealt with Carlton Gajdusek's earliest studies. As an expert in "protein chemistry" and "blood electrolyte balance," Gajdusek used Australian aboriginal and New Guinean populations to advance his career. These remote tribes, the Scotts concluded, had originally been infected with prion crystals by Japanese bioweapons researchers. Gajdusek's Australian assignment had been granted by his "biowar friend from Walter Reed Army Institute of Research, Joseph E. Smadel."

Most revealing in *The Brucellosis Triangle* is the Scotts' simple explanation of blood protein crystallization with relevance to Gajdusek's knowledge and research including his published report that the kuru epidemic was "man-made." Gajdusek was quoted by the Scotts as writing: "Continued surveillance has revealed no alteration in the unusual pattern of kuru disappearance, which indicates the *ar-*

*tificial man-made nature of the epidemic.* Kuru virus clearly has no reservoir in nature and no intermediate biological cycle for its preservation except in humans." [Emphasis added.]

The above "conclusion by Gajdusek," the Scotts reported, "fits the template of a Japanese-created infection as part of their biological warfare research."

4. Lo SC. Pathogenic Mycoplasma. United States Patent number 5,242,820, September 7, 1993. Assigned to the American Registry of Pathology, Washington, D.C. For cell cytoplasmic degenerative changes including vacuolization see p. 63; and Lo SC, Wear DJ, Green SL, Jones PG and Legier JF. Adult respiratory distress syndrome with or without systemic disease associated with infections due to *Mycoplasma fermentans. Clinical Infectious Diseases* 1993;17(Suppl 1):S259-63.

5. Horowitz LG. *Emerging Viruses: AIDS & Ebola—Nature, Accident or Intentional?* Rockport, MA: Tetrahedron Publishing Group, 1997, pp. 275-329; 401-440; for Sloan connections see pp. 476-479.

6. The entire text in figure 12.4, reset for clarity, came verbatim from: Senate Select Committee. *Foreign and Military Intelligence, Book I, Final Report of the Senate Select Committee to Study Governmental Operations with Respect to Intelligence Activities.* 94th Congress, 2nd Session. Report 94-755. Washington, D.C.: U.S. Government Printing Office, April 26 (Legislative Day, April 14),1976, pp.385-386.

7. United States Code Annotated: Title 50, War and National Defense, Chapter 32—Chemical and Biological Warfare Program, Title 50:1520 on the Use of human subjects for testing of chemical or biological agents by Department of Defense. January, 1996, p. 510.

8. Osborn K. Senator John Glenn introduces human research subject protection act of 1997. *Russian River Times*; 2;24, November 17, 1997, p. 1.; Letter to U.S. Senator John Warner's Office from political activist June S. Heyman, Tues, Nov. 18, 1997; 8a. Excerpt from 50USC Annotated, p. 138. 50 Sec. 1520 Repealed: Sec. 1520. Repealed. Pub. L. 105-85, Div. A, Title X sec. 1078 (g), Nov. 18, 1997, 111 Stat. 1916. See also Sec. 1520a. Restrictions.

9. Anonymous Internet source. "Major Electromagnetic Mind-Control Projects." *Contact: The Phoenix Educator*, July 14, 1998, p. 5.

10. Bowart W. *Operation Mind Control*. New York: Dell Publishing Co., Inc., 1978, pp. 257-271.

11. Barnaby F. *New Scientist*, June 17, 1976.

12. Valenstein E. *Brain Control*. New York: Wiley, 1973;

13. Gaylin WM, Meister JS and Neville RC. *Operating on the Mind*. New York: Basic Books, 1975;

14. Rose S. *The Conscious Brain*. New York: Knopf, 1976.

15. Clark K. *American Psychological Assoc. Monitor*, October, 1971.

16. Keith J. *Mind Control World Control: The Encyclopedia of Mind Control*. Kempton, IL: Adventures Unlimited, 1997, pp. 264; 267-269.

17. Ryter JC. The biometric National ID Card is now a reality. ScanThisNews on the Internet. http://www.networkusa.org/fingerprints.html.

18. Scott, WB. Panels' report backs nonlethal weapons. *Aviation Week & Space Technology,* October 16, 1995; and Ricks TE. Nonlethal arms: New class of weapons could incapacitate foe yet limit casualties. *The Wall Street Journal*, January 4, 1993.

19. Jasper WF. High-tech nightmare. *The New American*, July 24, 1994. In: Cook TL. *The Mark of the New World Order*. Springdale, PA: Whitaker House, 1996, pp. 304-307

20. Anderson M. High-tech national tattoo. *The Washington Times*, October 11, 1993. In: Cook TL. *The Mark of the New World Order*. Springdale, PA: Whitaker House, 1996, pp. 304-307.

21. Cook TL. *Ibid.* pp. 313-314.

22. Pasztor A. Hughes electronics seeks to restore satellite luster. *The Wall Street Journal*, Friday, February 26, 1999, p. B4.

23. Keele HM and Kiger JC. *Foundations: The Greenwood Encyclopedia of American Institutions*. London: Greenwood Press, 1982, pp. 8-9; for early history of the Sloan Foundation, see pp. 6-7.

24. Alfred P. Sloan Foundation: Report for 1967, pp. 2-6; for population control program, see p. 79.

25. For additional information cited in text see: Alfred P. Sloan Foundation: Report for 1969, pp. 70-71; for funding provided to the Council on Foreign Relations see p. 57; see also the Alfred P. Sloan Foundation: Report for 1970, pp. 36; 62-63, and the Sloan Foundation Report for 1967, p. 79. Laurance S. Rockefeller was cited in these capacities in all annual Sloan Foundation reports reviewed; see also:

*Who's Who in Finance and Industry, 17th edition, 1972-1973.* Chicago: Marquis Who's Who, Inc., 1973.; and finally, for Sloan's stock holdings in Merck & Co. and the Chase Manhattan Bank; see, The Sloan Foundation's "Schedule of Marketable Securities," listed in each annual report.

26. Coleman J. *Conspirators' Hierarchy: The Story of the Committee of 300.* Carson City, NV: American West Publishers, 1992, p. 233.

27. Manning P. *Martin Bormann: Nazi in Exile.* Secaucus, NJ: Lyle Stuart, 1981, p. 66.

28. Borkin J. *The Crime and Punishment of I. G. Farben.* Barnes & Noble Books, 1997, pp. 76-78.

29. According to Illuminati investigator and author David Icke, Howard Hughes was a descendant of Abraham Lincoln and the 1856 German monarch Leopold. Lincoln was a half brother to Leroy Springs (previously Springstein), a Rothschild relative and "chief trustee and general manager" of the Payseur conglomerate.

According to the 1854 *Congressional Record*, Daniel Payseur was the single wealthiest businessman in America. Through the Alabama Mineral Company he exercised control over the Rockefeller's Standard Oil, Alfred P. Sloan's General Motors, Boeing, Ford, Pepsi, and Coca Cola. Icke unearthed Daniel Payseur's former name—Crown Prince Louis, the son of Queen Marie Antoinette, and found he was the principle shareholder in the Virginia Company. That company, for all practical purposes, controlled the Federal Government of the United States from its inception. See Icke D. *The Biggest Secret.* Scottsdale, Arizona: Bridge of Love Publishing, 1999, pp. 191-92.

30. For a more in depth report on this case see: Goldston L. *The New Satanists.* New York: Warner Books, 1994.

31. Maass P. Colleague defends accused NIH scientist: Friend says law enforcement "setup" led to sexual abuse charges. *Washington Post,* April 8, 1996, p.1.

32. Icke D. *The Biggest Secret.* Scottsdale, Arizona: Bridge of Love Press, 1999, pp. 312-350. Lt Colonel Michael Aquino is mentioned on page 329 as having "controlled" Illuminati sex slave Cathy O'Brien. Aquino's Temple of Set, according to Icke's investigation, was inspired by "the leader of Hitler's SS, Heinrich Himmler."

# Appendix

This book is a wake-up call. The only thing that is going to save you from the increasing risk of "End Times" disease, death, and "mind-altering electronic weapons based on 'Lesser Black Magic'" is your connection to God. This is the prophetic understanding and teaching of virtually every prophet and reputable seer throughout history.

The mathematical encryptions in the King James Bible as revealed herein pave the way for additional studies in this regard. The release of this book will undoubtedly prompt other investigators to further advance knowledge in this field for the evolution of "Godkind."

Due to limitations in these authors' knowledge of music, cryptography, ancient astrology, astral-physics, and mathematics, the following decoded segments, Pythagorean patterns, and numerical formulations, in addition to those considered earlier in this book, provide only a perfunctory beginning for investigators to pursue more in depth studies.

## Conclusions and Directions

This book raises far more questions than it answers while foreshadowing a new beginning for humanity. Research into these questions offers the hope that people will advance free versus enslaved, healthy versus diseased, and divinely inspired versus spiritually deprived.

Since quality of life for a person, or society in general, depends mainly on the quality of the questions being asked at any given time— higher quality questions determining higher quality outcomes—this summary and conclusion section advances several critical questions in an effort to guide future research efforts of readers and investigators from various disciplines.

Clearly, the questions raised by the revelations contained in this book are multidisciplinary. The first few chapters raised questions concerning physics, music, and mathematics. Chapters three through five advanced questions for historians and religious scholars. The latter chapters raised urgent challenges to various fields of biomedicine and bioethics. The final chapters prescribed sobering reflections for social and political scientists regarding the nature of our psychosocial evolution—from whence we, the masses, came, largely engineered, and where mankind is headed in the coming decades.

## The Solfeggio Frequencies

To begin, perhaps the most startling issue that demands interpretation are the mathematical electromagnetic frequency codes revealed in the Torah, the King James Bible, and other Bibles that followed. Questions concerning these revelations are most appropriate for physicists and religious scholars alike. Were these frequencies placed in the scriptures by God as many religious fundamentalists will be inclined to argue? Or were they among the most important arcana—the "treasure" hidden by the Jewish scholars in Alexandria who issued the Septuagint (LXX) that was later recovered by the Templars and refashioned by King James and Francis Bacon in the Authorized Bible for convenience and likely artifice?

These authors believe the codes were not hidden by God, but by manipulative men. Though it might be validly argued that the Bible contains legitimate divine encryptions, and God may have withheld important knowledge from people, like loving parents often do with immature children, it is challenging to assume this is the case with the verse numbers in Numbers 7:12-84. The inane repeating quality of this text further differentiates it from other Biblical writings that articulate God's ways and laws. The purpose of the Bible, after all, was to document God's omnipotent word, laws, and dealings. It attests to God's desire that his will and ways be known, and his laws be followed for the benefit of all. One would have to argue that Moses, this section's author, must have been inspired by God to repeat largely inane verses to shield future Levi priest incryptions.

One could argue this, and further, given the urgent "End Times" issues facing humanity, that these authors were divinely inspired to receive and transmit this truth.

However, one would still need to reconcile the Templar connection to King James and the mass of incriminating evidence, including Francis Bacon's connection to the secret societies that had furthered the esoteric sciences, if not genocides, since at least the time the Anunnaki are believed to have created the Brotherhood of the Snake. (Read William Bramley's *Gods of Eden* [Avon, 1993].) Given this evidence, these authors feel justified in concluding these codes were more likely incorporated by entities inclined to mystify, deceive, and control humanity.

## Sound Research: Implications for Spiritual Evolution

Another important question, now theoretically plausible, is were these specific codes used by God for creation and destruction? Were the Solfeggio tones used to generate the cosmos? If so, what was the role played by each of the six harmonic tones? Did each one degree higher frequency follow *Webster's* definitions? Which frequency contributed most to the "big bang;" the creation of Adam and Eve, to angels, and aliens (if aliens existed before earthlings as some evidence suggests and many investigators argue)? Finally, what role might each frequency play in reestablishing peace on Earth?

Regarding this latter question, one physicist and musician who the authors contacted to perform a cursory examination of these special codes reported some fascinating findings. Joseph DeBrouse, a developer of advanced music therapy equipment, first found that the series of six tones were harmonically related. For instance the first three tones—frequencies 396, 417, and 528—shown in figure A1 produce a tonal disparity of six and three respectively. This disparity added equaled nine (9) which, as Joey noted earlier, suggests completion. Furthermore, adding each of the three-digit frequency codes by themselves, and then together, produced eighteen (18), twelve (12), and fifteen (15), which yielded forty-five (45). This is a perfect harmonic fourth of half an octave, as four times 45 equals 180, which is half of 360; and which in terms of degrees represents a full circle.

## Figure A1. Harmonic Relationships and Disparity of the Solfeggio Tones

396—3+9+6=18
417—4+1+7=12
528—5+2+8=15

Disparity of 6
Disparity of 3

9

**45**x4th Harmonic=180=1/2 circle
**45**x8th Harmonic=360=full circle

G=396÷9=44=F
G#= 417÷3=139=C#
C= 528÷6=88=F

2nd Harmonic
Equals Octave

C to F is a Natural 4th Harmonic
G# to C# is a Natural 4th Harmonic

Wedding
March Interval

D#/E=639÷9=71=C#
F#= 741÷3=247=B
G#/A=852÷6=142=C#

2nd Harmonic
Equals Octave

F# to B is a Natural 4th Harmonic
G# to C# is a Natural 4th Harmonic

Wedding
March Interval

A similar disparity occurs in the case of the tones "Ut" and "Fa" when divided by 6 and 9 to produce the 2nd harmonic.

An analysis of the six Solfeggio frequencies provided by physicist and musician Joseph DeBrouse. The figure details extraordinary harmonic relationships between the tones produced by the frequencies encoded in the King James Bible, in the Book of Numbers 7:12-83, including an association with Revelation's 144,000 and the "wedding march."

## Figure A2. Harmonic Relationships and Errata Concerning the Solfeggio Tones

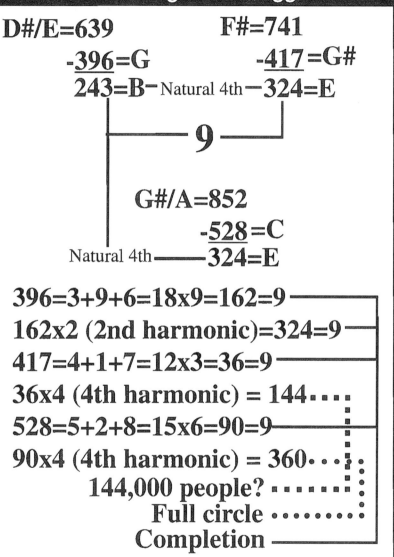

D#/E=639       F#=741

  -396=G         -417=G#

  243=B— Natural 4th —324=E

————— 9 —————

G#/A=852

  -528=C

Natural 4th ——— 324=E

396=3+9+6=18x9=162=9

162x2 (2nd harmonic)=324=9

417=4+1+7=12x3=36=9

36x4 (4th harmonic) = 144....

528=5+2+8=15x6=90=9

90x4 (4th harmonic) = 360...

144,000 people? .......

Full circle .........

Completion

The interval from "Mi" to "So" is known in music as the "devils tone" because of its offensive quality. It may be the principle harmonic, augmented 4th, for wielding destructive power.

Also shown in Figure A2, the first three tones of the Solfeggio scale are G, G#, and C. Their frequencies divided by their Pythagorean sums produce 44, 139, and 88, or the tones F, C# and F respectively—the last being an octave harmonic of the first. Moreover, G# to C#, and C to F are the common "natural 4th" tones associated with the "wedding march interval." This is likewise seen with the intervals F# to B, and G# to C# in the highest two tones derived from frequencies 741 and 852.

This knowledge breeds more excitment considering the analyses shown in Figure A2. Here, subtracting the first three Bible tone frequencies from the last three frequencies of the Solfeggio scale, the frequency tones 243 or B, 324 or E, and 324 or E are generated. All three of these frequencies reduced to their Pythagorean single digit produce 9—completion—and 999 laterally.

Much cataclysmic speculation surrounded the year of this book's first edition; the final year of the twentieth century, 1999. Many computers were allegedly programmed to cease operations, or "complete their program" in lieu of their hyped Y2K glitch in 1999. As discussed in the previous two chapters, regardless of fear profiteering, projects EISCAT and HAARP hold the capacity to interfere with earth's power grids to effect global chaos.

Additionally relevant to this great tribulation and greater healing, by multiplying the code 936 times the double digit sums of the first three Solfeggio frequencies, this yields 162, 36 and 90. These are a 2nd, 4th, and 4th harmonic respectively. By multiplying the numbers 162, 36, and 90 times 2, 4, and 4 respectively, the outcomes are: 324, 144, and 360. As shown in Figure A2, each of these reduced to their single Pythagorean digit equal 9—completion. The vital number 144,000, again, was predicted in the final book of the Bible—Revelation—as God's "*bride;*" the people empowered to lead the wedding march into the Messianic Age. (More on the 144,000 follows.)

Also, the number 144,000 (as seen in Figure A2) is associated with the 4th harmonic of the notes G, G# and C. Multiplying this number then times 4 equals 576. Recalling that the Jewish calander year for 1999, the year of this book's first printing, was 5760, and like the original number of 144,000, reducing this to the Pythagorean single digit by adding 5+7+6 = 18, or once again 9—completion, the year 5760, as well as the initial revelation of these tones, may be important to the 144,000 crusaders for God discussed in the Bible. In this case, completion of the Old World of chaos and beginning of the New World Order, in the best sense, that is, the Messianic Age, may depend on this musical knowledge and harmonic activity.

Likewise, multiplying the number 90 times 4 (associated with the 4th harmonic) equals 360—full circle which is completion, or once again, 9.

Finally, DeBrouse noted that the interval from Mi to So, also known as the "devils tone," is an augmented 4th. It is a highly disruptive and disturbing tone combination, and may be associated with destructive effects.

Given the above intriguing, albeit superficial analysis, the frequency codes within the King James Bible urges additional research in the use of the six Solfeggio tones and the hymn to St. John the Baptist. It may be that by assembling merely 144,000 people in an arena to simultaneously summons, through this song, the New Messianic Age—the "MI-ra gestorum," or miracle of all miracles—will be produced.

## Characteristics of the 144,000

Figure 13.5 presents 144 characteristics of the 144,000 members of God's valiant "End Times" crusaders, educators, and prophets. The following paragraphs summarize, from scripture, the unique characteristics of this divinely inspired group:

Revelation (7:2,3; 14:4) predicted that the 144,000 will be gathered, like the first fruit of the final harvest, and "sealed" just prior to

## Figure A3. Characteristics of the 144,000 New Messianic Age Crusader

1. Abiding in Him—1John 3:6
2. Ability—1Peter 4:11 I; Cor 10:13; Phil. 3:21; Titus 1:9
3. Affectionate—Romans 12:12:10
4. Appreciative—1Chron. 16:8-10,34
5. Attentive—Luke 19:48
6. Blameless—Phil. 3:6; I Cor. 1:7,8; 1Thess. 5:23; 2 Peter 3:14
7. Bold—Prov. 28:1; Phil. 1:14; 1Thess. 2:2; Eph. 6:20
8. Brave—1Sam. 17:32-37; 30:all; Judges 7:19, 22.
9. Caring—Luke 10:34; 1Cor. 12:25.
10. Charitable—1Cor. 13; 1Tim. 1:5.
11. Cheerful—Prov. 15:13; Matt. 9:2, 14:27; John 16:22.
12. Clean—Isa. 1:16; Ps 19:9; 24:4; 51:10.
13. Compassionate—Rom. 9:15.
14. Confident—Job 4:6; 2Cor. 7:16; 1John 2:28.
15. Conscientious—2Cor. 4:2; Heb. 13:18.
16. Considerate—Gol. 6:1.
17. Consistent—Col. 1:17 in Him; Luke 12:15.
18. Constructive—Eph. 2:20, 21; 4:16.
19. Contented—Phil. 4:11; ITim. 8:6; Heb. 13:5.
20. Contrite—Ps 34:18; 51:17; Isa. 66:2.
21. Courageous—Deut. 31:6; Joshua 1:7; Ps. 27:14.
22. Courteous—I Peter 3:8.
23. Decisive—Joel 3:14.
24. Dedicated—IKings 8:63; Heb. 9:18-28 (covenant ~with blood).
25. Desirable—Deut. 18:6.
26. Determined—ICor. 2:2.
27. Devout—Luke 2:25; Acts 2:5.
28. Diligent—2 Cor. 8:22; 2Peter 3:14.
29. Earnest—Rom. 8:19; Luke 22:44; 2Cor 1:22; 5:2.
30. Energetic—Isa. 40:29-31.
31. Exemplary—ITitus 2:7.
32. Expecting (Advent)—Titus 2:13; 2Peter 3:12.
33. Expressive—2 Tim. 2:2, 7, 14-15, 23-26.
34. Faithful—IThess. 5:24; Gal. 5:22; 2Peter 1:5.
35. Fastidious—Ps. 51:10; 2 Cor 5:17; Jude 24.
36. Faultless—Jude 21-25.
37. Fervent—Rom.12:11.
38. Friendly—Prov. 18:24; James 2:23,24.
39. Gallant—Eph 1:3; 6:11-19.
40. Generous—Luke 11:13; Matt. 2:8.
41. Gentle—Gal. 5:22; James 3:17.
42. Glad—1Chron. 16:31; Ps. 35:27; 68:3,4.

43. Glorified—Isa. 26:15; Ps. 16:9; John 17:10; Rom 8:21-28.
44. Godly—I Peter 3:15-18.
45. Good—Gal. 5:22.
46. Gracious—Ps. 45:2; John 1:16; Rom 1:5, 16:20; 2 Thess. 2:16; James 4:6; 2 Peter 3:18.
47. Grateful—Ps. 107:15; 145:2,3.
48. Happy—Deut. 33:29; IPeter 3:14.
49. Harmless—Matt. 10:16; Phil. 2:15.
50. Healthy—3John 2; (vegetarian— Gen. 1:29).
51. Helpful—Ps. 20:1,2; 63:7; Hosea 13:9; Acts 26:22; Heb 4:16; Isa. 41:10.
52. Holy—Lev. 20:7; Deut. 7:6-9; Rom. 12:1,2; ICor 3:17; 7:34; Col. 1:22; Eph. 1:4; IPeter 1:15,16.
53. Honest—Isa. 33:15; Rom. 12:17; 1Cor 8:21.
54. Honorable—1Chron. 28:28; 1Sam. 2:30; Ps. 96:6; Prov. 15:33; Rom 2:10; 12:10.
55. Hopeful—I Peter 1:13; Rom. 5:5; 12;12.
56. Hospitable—Rom 12:13.
57. Humble—2Chron. 7:14; 2Cor. 10:5; James 4:10.
58. Industrious—Rom. 12:11.
59. Innocent—Job 4:17; Deut. 21:8.
60. Jubilant—IChron. 29:10-16.
61. Joyful—Ps. 65:19; Isa. 49:13; 52:6-10.
62. Just—Lev. 19:35, 36; Isa. 16:7; Heb. 2:4.
63. Kind—ICor. 13:4; Eph. 4:32.
64. Kingly—Rev. 1:6; 3:21.
65. Knowledgeable—2 Chron. 1:10; Isa. 11:9.
66. Law-abiding—Rom. 8:1,2; 1John 2:5.
67. Longsuffering—Gal. 5:22; Eph 4:2.
68. Loveliness of disposition— John I:29; Isa. 53:7.
69. Loving—Eph. 4:2; Phil. 2:2; 1John 4:16-19.
70. Lowly—Ps. 138:6; Prov. 3:34; 11:2; 16:19; Matt. 11:29.
71. Loyal—I Am. 15:22,23; Danl. 3:16-28; 6:20-27.
72. Mannerly—ICor. 15:33.
73. Meek—Matt. 5:5; I Peter 3:4; James I 21-27.
74. Merciful—Matt. 5:7.
75. Moderate (Temperence)—Gal. 5:23; 2Peter 1:6; I Cor. 9:25; Titus 1:8; 2:2.

# Fig. A3. (Cont.) Characteristics of the 144,000 New Messianic Age Crusader

76. Moral (obey law)—Deut. 7.
    Matt. 7:12; 5:17-20; Rom. 13:10.
77. Neatness—1Cor. 14:40.
78. New Creative—2Cor. 5:17; Eph. 4:24.
79. Noble—Jer. 2:21; Acts 17:11.
80. Nourished—Isa.1:2; 1Tim. 4:6.
81. Obedient—2 Cor. 10:5,6;
    1Peter 1:14,22.
82. Open—Ps. 98:2; 146:8.
83. Optimistic—2 Cor. 6:10.
84. Ordained—Eph. 2:10; Rev. 1:6.
85. Orderly—Ps. 119:133; 1Cor. 14:40.
86. Partaker—Eph. 3:6; Heb. 3:14; 6:4;
    1Peter 4:13; Jos. 1:4.
87. Patient—Rev. 14:12; Rom. 5:3; 12:12;
    Col. 1:11; 2Thess 3:5.
88. Peacable—Rom. 12:18; James 3:18.
89. Peacemaker—Matt. 5:9.
90. Perfect—Eph. 4:11; 2Cor. 13:9.
91. Persevering—Eph. 6:8; James 3:18.
92. Persistent—1Kings 18:43, 44;
    Ps. 90:2; 119:142; 145:13.
93. Pious—1Tim 5:4.
94. Positive—Ps. 17:1,2; 40:8.
95. Praising—Ps. 138;11; 148:5;
    Isa. 15:1; Rev. 14:3; 15:3,4; 19:6-8.
96. Prayerful—Rom. 12:12.
97. Prompt—Ps. 119:60.
98. Pure—Matt. 5:8; Rom. 14:20;
    2Tim. 2:22; 5:22.
99. Quiet—1Cor. 14:33; 1Peter 3:4.
100. Quick (haste to obey)—
    Ps. 70:1; 119:88,149.
101. Radiant (light)—Matt. 5:14.
102. Ready (wedding is ready)—
    Matt. 22:8; 25:6; Isa. 58:12.
103. Rejoicing—Matt. 5:12; Rom. 12:12.
104. Repentant—Matt. 9:13;
    2Cor. 7:9,10.
105. Reverent—lev. 19:30; Heb. 12:28.
106. Righteous—Ps. 33:1; 97:12;
    lJohn 3:7.
107. Reasonable—Isa. 1:18; 1Sam. 12:7.
108. Responsible—Ps. 31:23,24;
    1Tim. 1:12.
109. Responsive—2Sam. 1:7; Isa. 6:8.
110. Sanctified—Ezek.20:12-20;
    1Peter 3:15.
111. Secure—Judges 18:10; Job 11:18;
    Prov. 3:29.
112. Serene—Psalm 17:7.
113. Sincere—Eph. 6:24; Phil. 1:10;
    2Cor. 8:8.
114. Spiritual (Holy Spirit indwells)—
    Rom. 8:4-14.

115. Stable—Ps. 119:38; Rom. 16:25;
    2Thess. 2:17.
116. Steadfast—Ps. 14:7; 16:8.
117. Strong—Prov. 21:14; Haggai 2:4.
118. Studious—2Tim 2:15.
119. Sure—Ps. 19:7; 2Peter 1:10.
120. Sympathetic—Jer. 31:25;
    John II:36; 16:22.
121. Symmetrical—John 17:23.
122. Tactful—James 3:13.
123. Teachable—Job 34:32; Ps. 25:5.
124. Tender—Eph. 4:32.
125. Thankful—Ps. 100:4; Col. 3:15.
126. Thrifty—John 6:12.
127. Truthful—2Chron. 18:15; Ps. 15:2.
128. Trusting—2Sam. 22:3; Ps. 4:5; 71:5;
    Isa. 26:2,3.
129. Understanding—2Tim. 2:7.
130. Undivided (Unity)—Eph. 4:12-13;
    Phil. 1:27.
131. Unwavering—1Peter 1:5,13.
132. Unwearied—Isa40:31; Gal. 6:9.
133. Valiant—Heb. 11:34.
134. Victorious—1Cor.15:57; 1John 5:4.
135. Vigilant—1Peter 4:7; 5:8-11;
    2Tim. 4:5.
136. Virtous—Phil. 4:8; 2Peter1:5;
    Prov. 12:4.
137. Watchful-Matt. 24:42; Kar. 16:13;
    1These. 5:6; Rev. 16:15.
138. Well-balanced-James 1:8.
139. Wise—Jer. 9:23,24; Micah 6:8;
    2Tim. 3:15; James1:5.
140. Worshipful—1Chron. 16:29; Ps. 96:6;
    Matt. 4:10.
141. eXcellent—Phil. 1:10; 2Cor. 4:7;
    (majesty) Heb. 1:1-8.
142. Yahsua's mind—Eph. 3:17; 4:23;
    Phil 2:5.
143. Yielding—Phil. 2:5; Heb. 12:11.
144. Zealous—Acts 21:20; Titus 2:14.

the final plagues. The concept of "sealed" implies that this unique "famuli tuorum"—the "particularly chosen group" of scholarly and magical servants—will be so loyal, so desirous to know truth and God, that they will be unable to go backwards. They will have virtually gained entrance into heaven. So much truth and power will come to these 144,000 inspired souls that they will be "sealed" to advance God's will and enjoy His everlasting love.

The 144,000 will become the largest assembly of souls ever saved in one short time. They will formulate from both race and grace, and develop from twelve increments of 12,000, each of these representing the original lineages of the twelve tribes of Israel as promised to Abraham and the world. According to Joel 2:2 and 8; and Revelation 7, they will develop into the greatest spiritual army ever empowered on the planet, not to be killed or destroyed while battling for humanity's salvation—the spiritual renaissance. Like God's "bride," according to Revelation 14:12, they will come together to complete the final harvest of His work on earth.

This "sealing" will also signify God's final judgement made at the end of the last seven years. The 144,000 will be judged much earlier than the masses because of their precise biblical understanding and/or their intimate relationship with God. According to Revelation 14:10-12, this judgement will also signify and declare their power to walk victoriously over sin in its totality, much like Job had done.

Revelation 14:10-12 also predicted that the world, at this time, will also be receiving a destructive type of "sealing" related to the "Mark of the Beast." Different from the prions and biochips described in the previous chapter, this mark, more than anything else, issues from a false form of worship.

Unlike the vast majority who become infected and afflicted by the "defiled women" that the Bible teaches is a metaphor for the "harlot churches"—churches that teach false doctrines—the 144,000 will be like a pure virgin that goes forth to teach true redemption. Unlike the masses then, the 144,000 will be guiltless and without fault. They will be spared the "Mark of the Beast," or refuse it. (Rev 14:3-5.)

The 144,000 will learn and teach how to trust Him, communicate with Him, and be led by Him in an unprecidented measure. They will proclaim the accuracy of the scriptures and his commandments in the final days. That is, in the midst of a massive tribulation that occurs as a result of failing to acknowledge clear truth and righteousness, the 144,000 will lead others to the gates of heaven on earth. (Rev. 7:9-11.)

The 144,000's commission will be much like the disciples at Pentecost—to be divinely empowered with extraordinary faith, knowledge, and ability. As described in Joel 2:2-18, the appointment of the distinctive "sealing" will primarily result for those chosen as a result of: stern faithfulness, sincere refined biblical knowledge, tremendous transformation in their whole personages, and a willingnes to be used continuously and unconditionally by God. They will forever follow in the "Lamb's" footsteps to share their experiences that no other creation has ever encountered.

These blessings, provided these chosen few, according to Revelation 8:15-17, will be tremendous both on earth and in eternity.The group will have extraordinary powers to rise to every occasion where faith and spiritual understanding are seriously questioned for its absolute light. (Joel 2:5-7.)

Based on Joel 2:27-28, and Revelation 7:12 and 19:10, it is presumed the 144,000 will be the most intelligent people in the world regarding all truth. They will also be the most discerning, loving, wise, and prophetically educated.

Their purposes will include that of destroying the New World Order's beastly power. This spiritually chosen "famuli tuorum" will prove to everyone everywhere that regardless of severe frailties, and a cursed nature for the last 6,000 years, humanity can choose total submission to the Holy Spirit, even in the midst of the Great Tribulation. (Rev. 14:10.)

### The Meaning of "Atonement"

The first appendicial pattern of relevance to this book concerns the term "atonement." The word is most heavily cited in the Bible in Leviticus—the third book of Moses. Traditionally, the word implies becoming one with God, turning from "sin," and returning to the Godly practices as defined by the Ten Commandments.

Leviticus's references to atonement, in particular, are required to develop a more complete understanding of the six numerical "tone" frequencies encrypted in the fourth Book of Moses—Numbers, beginning in Chapter 7, verse 12.

This link between these two Bible books involves the description of the lamb and bullock sacrifices made starting in Leviticus 23:26 when "the Lord spake unto Moses . . ." As seen below, the numerical sequence of 4, 5, 6, and 7 is gained using Pythagorean analyses of the chapter and verse numbers in which the word atonement was cited. For instance, in Lev. 23:26=5+8=13=4. (See appendix Fig. A4.)

Likewise, in Numbers, beginning with the first day's offering, the repeating sequence begins with verse 13, or 1+3=4.

Apparently the first four digits of this sequence are significant. When they are added, that is, 4+5+6+7, they yield 22.

Again, there are 22 letters in the Hebrew Alphabet, and 22 degree differences between musical note vibrations in the musical scale.

In addition, the numbers referred to in the verses containing the word "atonement" are significant in a similar musical sense. For instance in Leviticus 25:9 the King James Bible records "Then shalt thou cause the trumpet of the jubilee to sound on the tenth day of the seventh month, in the day of atonement shall ye make the trumpet sound throughout all your land." The tenth day (10) of the seventh month (7) added yields 17, or 1+7=8. It is apparently no "coincidence" there are 8 octaves in the full musical scale, and 8 is the number for God.

Moreover, if we were to add the number twenty-two (22) obtained from the pattern in Leviticus and twenty-two (22) obtained in the first four repeating sequences in Numbers, that equals 44 or, once again, 8. The number eight (8), as stated early in this book, is also associated with the words "GOD," "FAITH," and "TRUST." Again, in PSALM 119, it was no accident the Hebrew alphabet was placed eight (8) verses apart, which led Joey to the code in "A Song of Degrees."

## Figure A4. Numerical Correlates to "Atonement"*

(Lev 23:26 = 5+8=13=**4**) And the Lord spake unto Moses, saying,

(Lev23:27 = 5+9=14=**5**) Also on the tenth *day* of this seventh month *there shall be* a dy of atonement: it shall be an holy convocation unto you; and ye shall afflict your souls, and offer an offering made by fire unto the Lord.

(Lev 23:28 = 5+10=15=**6**) And ye shall do no work in that same day: for it *is* a day of atonement, to make an atonement for you before the Lord your God.

(Lev 25:9 = 7+9=16=**7**) Then shalt thou cause the trumpet of the jubile to sound on the tenth *day* of the seventh month, in the day of atonement shall ye make the trumpet sound throughout all your land.

* All verses are from the Authorized King James Bible

Finally, these investigators have repeatedly felt that the frequent italicizing of certain words in the Bible, for no apparent reason, represented some additional encryption. As in the example shown in figure A4, the italicized words *day*, *there shall be*, *is*, and *day* in Leviticus verses 23:26 through 25:9, that dealt with atonement, provided a numerical code of 7, 1, 3 = 11, or half of 22—that is, a half tone in music. Moreover, the numerical code for "day" is 4, 1, 7—identical to the frequency of the tone "Re."

An additional code of potential significance was found in the very next Leviticus verses that totaled 4, 5, 6, and 7, that is, verses 23:35—23:38. (See appendix figure A5.) Here the italicized words are: *shall*, *be*, *therein*; *is*, *and*, *therein*; and *are*, *to*, *be* in verses 35, 36, and 37 respectively. These words deciphered total 6 derived from the Pythagorean sequence 3,9,3, where the final 3 occurs in verse 23:37—a verse that by itself totals 6 as well. As seen earlier in figure 5.6 these

| Figure A5. Subsequent Numerical Correlates in LEVITI-CUS Suggesting Links to Musical Mathematics |
| --- |

(Lev 23:35 = 5+8=13=**4**) On the first day *shall be* an holy convocation: ye shall do no servile work *therein*..

(Lev 23:36 = 5+9=14=**5**) Seven days ye shall offer an offering made by fire unto the Lord: on the eighth day shall be an holy convocation unto you; and ye shall offer an offering made by fire unto the Lord: it *is* a solemn assembly; *and* ye shall do no servile work *therein*.

(Lev 23:37 = 5+10=15=**6**) These *are* the feasts of the Lord, which ye shall proclaim *to be* holy convocations, to offer an offering made by fire unto the Lord, a burnt offering, and a meat offering, a sacrifice, and drink offerings, every thing upon his day:

(Lev 23:38 = 5+11=16=**7**) Besides the sabbaths of the Lord, and beside your gifts, and beside all your vows, and beside all your freewill offerings, which ye give unto the Lord.

* All verses are from the Authorized King James Bible

3,9,6; 9,3,6; and 6,3,9 repeating patterns are associated with the frequency tones of the Solfeggio, especially the tones "Ut" and "Fa."

Though obviously not definitive, these possible and apparent relationships between encrypted Bible sequences and musical mathematics provide ample food for thought and further study.

### Genesis in the King James Bible

The word "genesis" does not appear in the King James Bible except in the title of Moses' first book called GENESIS. According to *Webster's Dictionary*, the term and its relatives are defined as:

**gen-e-sis** . . . [L, fr. Gk, fr. *gignesthai* to be born — more at KIN] (ca. 1604) : the origin or coming into being of something.

**Genesis** *n* [Gk] : the mainly narrative first book of canonical Jewish and Christian Scriptures — see BIBLE table

**gene-splicing** . . . *n* (ca. 1978) : any of various techniques by which recombinant DNA is produced and made to function in an organism

The above partially being derived from "gen-" which *Webster's* records as:

**gen** . . . [perh. fr. general information] (1940) *chiefly Brit* : information 2a

¹**gen-** *or* **geno-** *comb from* [Gk *genos* birth, race, king — more at KIN] 1 : race <*geno*cide. 2: genus : king <*geno*type>

²**gen-** *or* **geno-** *comb from* : gene <*gen*ome>

**-gen** *also* **gene** *n comb from* [F -*gène,* fr. Gk -genes born; akin to Gk genos birth] 1 : producer <androgen> 2 : one that is (so) produced <culti*gen*>

It is interesting to note, given the connections between British royalty, MI6, Freemasonry, the depopulation of "dysgenic" races, and the third tone "MI"—528—the frequency associated with repairing DNA (whereas MI—5+2+8=15=1+5=6, or MI6) that the use of the term "genesis" began in England around the time of King James's rule and the start of his authorized Bible project. Moreover, that Webster even cites "gen" as *"chiefly Brit"*ish is disconcerting as are the related references to "genocide," "gene-splicing," and the human "genome" project. As this book documents, bloodline purity, as well as current world depopulation efforts, are ongoing preoccupations for Royal Family and secret society members.

It should also be noted that the word "genesis" does not appear in *Strong's Concordance.* However the associated word—genealogies— is found eight (8) times in eight (8) verses as shown in appendix A6. As detailed earlier, the number eight is a sacred number associated with "God," and its square, eight times eight, or sixty-four (64), is also mathematically and spiritually significant. (See Chapter 2 for more details.)

Finally, when the word "KIN" is cross-referenced as Webster recommends while investigating "genesis," "gene," and "genocide," the

## Figure A6. Eight (8) References to "Genealogies" in Eight (8) King James Bible Verses

(1 Chr 5:17 KJV) All these were reckoned by genealogies in the days of Jotham king of Judah, and in the days of Jeroboam king of Israel.

(1 Chr 7:5 KJV) And their brethren among all the families of Issachar were valiant men of might, reckoned in all by their genealogies fourscore and seven thousand.

(1 Chr 7:7 KJV) And the sons of Bela; Ezbon, and Uzzi, and Uzziel, and Jerimoth, and Iri, five; heads of the house of their fathers, mighty men of valour; and were reckoned by their genealogies twenty and two thousand and thirty and four.

(1 Chr 9:1 KJV) So all Israel were reckoned by genealogies; and, behold, they were written in the book of the kings of Israel and Judah, who were carried away to Babylon for their transgression.

(2 Chr 12:15 KJV) Now the acts of Rehoboam, first and last, are they not written in the book of Shemaiah the prophet, and of Iddo the seer concerning genealogies? And there were wars between Rehoboam and Jeroboam continually.

(2 Chr 31:19 KJV) Also of the sons of Aaron the priests, which were in the fields of the suburbs of their cities, in every several city, the men that were expressed by name, to give portions to all the males among the priests, and to all that were reckoned by genealogies among the Levites.

(1 Tim 1:4 KJV) Neither give heed to fables and endless genealogies, which minister questions, rather than godly edifying which is in faith: so do.

(Titus 3:9 KJV) But avoid foolish questions, and genealogies, and contentions, and strivings about the law; for they are unprofitable and vain.

* All verses are from the Authorized King James Bible

following definitions present, and are interrelated as well by their twelfth century (12c) period code:

¹**kin** . . . [ME, fr. OE *cynn*; akin to OHG *chunni* race, L genus birth, race, kind, Gk *genos*, L *gignere* to beget, Gk *gignesthai* to be born] (bef. 12c) 1 : a group of persons of common ancestry : CLAN 2 a: one's relatives : KINDRED b : KINSMAN <he wasn't any ~ to you — Jean Stafford> 3 *archaic* : KINSHIP

**kindly** . . . *n* [ME, fr. OE cyndelic, fr. cynd] (bef 12c) 1 a obs: NATURAL b archaic : lawful 2 : of an agreeable or beneficial nature : PLEASANT <~climate> 3 : of a sympathetic or generous nature

472

**kin-dred** . . . *n* [ME, fr. kin + OE *raede*n condition, fr. *raedan* to advise, read] (12c) 1 a : a group of related individuals b : one's relatives 2: family relationship : KINSHIP

**king** . . . *n* [ME, fr. OE cyning; akin to OHG kuning king. OE *cyan* : one whose position is hereditary and who rules for life b : a paramount chief 2 *cap* : GOD, CHRIST 3 : one that holds a pre-eminent position; *esp* : a chief among competitors 4 : the principal piece of each color in chess having the power to move ordinary one square in any direction and to capture opposing pieces but being obliged never to enter or remain in check . . .

The relationship of the latter definition to "genesis," "gene," and "genocide," or even "eugenics" is remarkable.

By searching *Webster's* word columns for the "bef. 12c" or "12c" period reference prior to "kin," "kindly," "kindred," and "king," the first such entry can be found in the first entry of the K words. This definition, as seen below, also provides a connection to numerology. It cites the important halftone number eleven (11). Also there is a "coincidental" reference to 64k in computer memory—that is, the all important square of eight (8), which is eight times itself or sixty-four (64):

**k** . . . *n, pl* **k's** or **ks** . . . *often cap, often attrib* (bef. 12c) 1 a : the 11th letter of the English alphabet b : a graphic representation of this letter c : a speech counterpart of orthographic k 2 : a graphic device for reproducing the letter k 3 : one designated *k* esp. as the 11th in order or class 4 : something shaped like the letter K 5 : a unit vector parallel to the z-axis 6 [*kilo*] : THOUSAND <a salary of $24K> 7 [kilo]: a unit of computer storage capacity equal to 1024 bytes <a computer memory of 64K> 8 *cap* : STRIKEOUT

## The Words Eight (8) and Nine (9)

The word "eight" appears eighty times in eighty Bible verses, appropriate for a number ascribed to God's infinite perfection. The word "nine" appears 50 times in 49 verses (5+4+9=18=9). Again, could these be "coincidences?" Appendix figure A7 cites the passages that contain the word eight.

## Figure A7. Eighty (80) Verses in Which the Word "Eight" (8) is Cited in the King James Bible

(Gen 5:4 KJV) And the days of Adam after he had begotten Seth were eight hundred years: and he begat sons and daughters:

(Gen 5:7 KJV) And Seth lived after he begat Enos eight hundred and seven years, and begat sons and daughters:

(Gen 5:10 KJV) And Enos lived after he begat Cainan eight hundred and fifteen years, and begat sons and daughters:

(Gen 5:13 KJV) And Cainan lived after he begat Mahalaleel eight hundred and forty years, and begat sons and daughters:

(Gen 5:16 KJV) And Mahalaleel lived after he begat Jared eight hundred and thirty years, and begat sons and daughters:(Gen 5:17 KJV) And all the days of Mahalaleel were eight hundred ninety and five years: and he died.

(Gen 5:19 KJV) And Jared lived after he begat Enoch eight hundred years, and begat sons and daughters:

(Gen 17:12 KJV) And he that is eight days old shall be circumcised among you, every man child in your generations, he that is born in the house, or bought with money of any stranger, which is not of thy seed.

(Gen 21:4 KJV) And Abraham circumcised his son Isaac being eight days old, as God had commanded him.

(Gen 22:23 KJV) And Bethuel begat Rebekah: these eight Milcah did bear to Nahor, Abraham's brother.

(Exo 26:2 KJV) The length of one curtain shall be eight and twenty cubits, and the breadth of one curtain four cubits: and every one of the curtains shall have one measure.

(Exo 26:25 KJV) And they shall be eight boards, and their sockets of silver, sixteen sockets; two sockets under one board, and two sockets under another board.

(Exo 36:9 KJV) The length of one curtain was twenty and eight cubits, and the breadth of one curtain four cubits: the curtains were all of one size.

(Exo 36:30 KJV) And there were eight boards; and their sockets were sixteen sockets of silver, under every board two sockets.

(Num 2:24 KJV) All that were numbered of the camp of Ephraim were an hundred thousand and eight thousand and an hundred, throughout their armies. And they shall go forward in the third rank.

(Num 3:28 KJV) In the number of all the males, from a month old and upward, were eight thousand and six hundred, keeping the charge of the sanctuary.

(Num 4:48 KJV) Even those that were numbered of them, were eight thousand and five hundred and fourscore.

(Num 7:8 KJV) And four wagons and eight oxen he gave unto the sons of Merari, according unto their service, under the hand of Ithamar the son of Aaron the priest.

(Num 29:29 KJV) And on the sixth day eight bullocks, two rams, and fourteen lambs of the first year without blemish:

(Num 35:7 KJV) So all the cities which ye shall give to the Levites shall be forty and eight cities: them shall ye give with their suburbs.

(Deu 2:14 KJV) And the space in which we came from Kadeshbarnea, until we were come over the brook Zered, was thirty and eight years; until all the generation of the men of war were wasted out from among the host, as the LORD sware unto them.

(Josh 21:41 KJV) All the cities of the Levites within the possession of the children of Israel were forty and eight cities with their suburbs.

* All verses are from the Authorized King James Bible

(Judg 3:8 KJV) Therefore the anger of the LORD was hot against Israel, and he sold them into the hand of Chushanrishathaim king of Mesopotamia: and the children of Israel served Chushanrishathaim eight years.

(Judg 12:14 KJV) And he had forty sons and thirty nephews, that rode on threescore and ten ass colts: and he judged Israel eight years.

(1 Sam 4:15 KJV) Now Eli was ninety and eight years old; and his eyes were dim, that he could not see.

(1 Sam 17:12 KJV) Now David was the son of that Ephrathite of Bethlehemjudah, whose name was Jesse; and he had eight sons: and the man went among men for an old man in the days of Saul.

(2 Sam 23:8 KJV) These be the names of the mighty men whom David had: The Tachmonite that sat in the seat, chief among the captains; the same was Adino the Eznite: he lift up his spear against eight hundred, whom he slew at one time.

(2 Sam 24:9 KJV) And Joab gave up the sum of the number of the people unto the king: and there were in Israel eight hundred thousand valiant men that drew the sword; and the men of Judah were five hundred thousand men.

(1 Ki 7:10 KJV) And the foundation was of costly stones, even great stones, stones of ten cubits, and stones of eight cubits.

(2 Ki 8:17 KJV) Thirty and two years old was he when he began to reign; and he reigned eight years in Jerusalem.

(2 Ki 10:36 KJV) And the time that Jehu reigned over Israel in Samaria was twenty and eight years.

(2 Ki 22:1 KJV) Josiah was eight years old when he began to reign, and he reigned thirty and one years in Jerusalem. And his mother's name was Jedidah, the daughter of Adaiah of Boscath.

(1 Chr 12:24 KJV) The children of Judah that bare shield and spear were six thousand and eight hundred, ready armed to the war.

(1 Chr 12:30 KJV) And of the children of Ephraim twenty thousand and eight hundred, mighty men of valour, famous throughout the house of their fathers.

(1 Chr 12:35 KJV) And of the Danites expert in war twenty and eight thousand and six hundred.

(1 Chr 16:38 KJV) And Obededom with their brethren, threescore and eight; Obededom also the son of Jeduthun and Hosah to be porters:

(1 Chr 23:3 KJV) Now the Levites were numbered from the age of thirty years and upward: and their number by their polls, man by man, was thirty and eight thousand.

(1 Chr 24:4 KJV) And there were more chief men found of the sons of Eleazar than of the sons of Ithamar; and thus were they divided. Among the sons of Eleazar there were sixteen chief men of the house of their fathers, and eight among the sons of Ithamar according to the house of their fathers.

(1 Chr 25:7 KJV) So the number of them, with their brethren that were instructed in the songs of the LORD, even all that were cunning, was two hundred fourscore and eight.

(2 Chr 11:21 KJV) And Rehoboam loved Maachah the daughter of Absalom above all his wives and his concubines: (for he took eighteen wives, and threescore concubines; and begat twenty and eight sons, and threescore daughters.)

(2 Chr 13:3 KJV) And Abijah set the battle in array with an army of valiant men of war, even four hundred thousand chosen men: Jeroboam also set the battle in array against him with eight hundred thousand chosen men, being mighty men of valour.

(2 Chr 21:5 KJV) Jehoram was thirty and two years old when he began to reign, and he reigned eight years in Jerusalem.

(2 Chr 21:20 KJV) Thirty and two years old was he when he began to reign, and he reigned in Jerusalem eight years, and departed without being desired. Howbeit they buried him in the city of David, but not in the sepulchres of the kings.

(2 Chr 29:17 KJV)  Now they began on the first day of the first month to sanctify, and on the eighth day of the month came they to the porch of the LORD: so they sanctified the house of the LORD in eight days; and in the sixteenth day of the first month they made an end.

(2 Chr 34:1 KJV)  Josiah was eight years old when he began to reign, and he reigned in Jerusalem one and thirty years.

(2 Chr 36:9 KJV)  Jehoiachin was eight years old when he began to reign, and he reigned three months and ten days in Jerusalem: and he did that which was evil in the sight of the LORD.

(Ezra 2:6 KJV)  The children of Pahathmoab, of the children of Jeshua and Joab, two thousand eight hundred and twelve.

(Ezra 2:16 KJV)  The children of Ater of Hezekiah, ninety and eight.

(Ezra 2:23 KJV)  The men of Anathoth, an hundred twenty and eight.

(Ezra 2:41 KJV)  The singers: the children of Asaph, an hundred twenty and eight.

(Ezra 8:11 KJV)  And of the sons of Bebai; Zechariah the son of Bebai, and with him twenty and eight males.

(Neh 7:11 KJV)  The children of Pahathmoab, of the children of Jeshua and Joab, two thousand and eight hundred and eighteen.

(Neh 7:13 KJV)  The children of Zattu, eight hundred forty and five.

(Neh 7:15 KJV)  The children of Binnui, six hundred forty and eight.

(Neh 7:16 KJV)  The children of Bebai, six hundred twenty and eight.

(Neh 7:21 KJV)  The children of Ater of Hezekiah, ninety and eight.

(Neh 7:22 KJV)  The children of Hashum, three hundred twenty and eight.

(Neh 7:26 KJV)  The men of Bethlehem and Netophah, an hundred fourscore and eight.

(Neh 7:27 KJV)  The men of Anathoth, an hundred twenty and eight.

(Neh 7:44 KJV)  The singers: the children of Asaph, an hundred forty and eight.

(Neh 7:45 KJV)  The porters: the children of Shallum, the children of Ater, the children of Talmon, the children of Akkub, the children of Hatita, the children of Shobai, an hundred thirty and eight.

(Neh 11:6 KJV)  All the sons of Perez that dwelt at Jerusalem were four hundred threescore and eight valiant men.

(Neh 11:8 KJV)  And after him Gabbai, Sallai, nine hundred twenty and eight.

(Neh 11:12 KJV)  And their brethren that did the work of the house were eight hundred twenty and two: and Adaiah the son of Jeroham, the son of Pelaliah, the son of Amzi, the son of Zechariah, the son of Pashur, the son of Malchiah,

(Neh 11:14 KJV)  And their brethren, mighty men of valour, an hundred twenty and eight: and their overseer was Zabdiel, the son of one of the great men.

(Eccl 11:2 KJV)  Give a portion to seven, and also to eight; for thou knowest not what evil shall be upon the earth.

(Jer 41:15 KJV)  But Ishmael the son of Nethaniah escaped from Johanan with eight men, and went to the Ammonites.

(Jer 52:29 KJV)  In the eighteenth year of Nebuchadrezzar he carried away captive from Jerusalem eight hundred thirty and two persons:

(Ezek 40:9 KJV)  Then measured he the porch of the gate, eight cubits; and the posts thereof, two cubits; and the porch of the gate was inward.

(Ezek 40:31 KJV)  And the arches thereof were toward the utter court; and palm trees were upon the posts thereof: and the going up to it had eight steps.

(Ezek 40:34 KJV)  And the arches thereof were toward the outward court; and palm trees were upon the posts thereof, on this side, and on that side: and the going up to it had eight steps.

(Ezek 40:37 KJV)  And the posts thereof were toward the utter court; and palm trees were upon the posts thereof, on this side, and on that side: and the going up to it had eight steps.

(Ezek 40:41 KJV)  Four tables were on this side, and four tables on that side, by the side of the gate; eight tables, whereupon they slew their sacrifices.

(Micah 5:5 KJV) And this man shall be the peace, when the Assyrian shall come into our land: and when he shall tread in our palaces, then shall we raise against him seven shepherds, and eight principal men.

(Luke 2:21 KJV) And when eight days were accomplished for the circumcising of the child, his name was called JESUS, which was so named of the angel before he was conceived in the womb.

(Luke 9:28 KJV) And it came to pass about an eight days after these sayings, he took Peter and John and James, and went up into a mountain to pray.

(John 5:5 KJV) And a certain man was there, which had an infirmity thirty and eight years.

(John 20:26 KJV) And after eight days again his disciples were within, and Thomas with them: then came Jesus, the doors being shut, and stood in the midst, and said, Peace be unto you.

(Acts 9:33 KJV) And there he found a certain man named Aeneas, which had kept his bed eight years, and was sick of the palsy.

(1 Pet 3:20 KJV) Which sometime were disobedient, when once the longsuffering of God waited in the days of Noah, while the ark was a preparing, wherein few, that is, eight souls were saved by water.

* All verses are from the Authorized King James Bible

## Lunar "Points of Reference"

In addition to the above biblical references to numbers, including the important number eight (8), there are numerous numerological references in the Bible in conjunction to solar and lunar cycles, and the movement of these influential spheres. Music and vibrational frequencies are intimately linked to mathematics and spirituality as additionally documented in the Bible. Examples include the following:

The word Moon appears 51 times in 51 Bible verses—5 + 1 = 6. God vibrationally spoke the world into existence in six days. He rested on the seventh, when, like those who witnessed the six day miracle at Jeracho, all celebrated the results of the vibrational labor on the seventh day.

Furthermore, there are six musical notes in the ancient Solfeggio, and 6 + 6 = 12 with twelve signs of the Zodiac and twelve months in the ancient and accurate Biblical calendar (whereas 1 + 2 = 3) and every third year was a leap year whereby the twelfth month is repeated. This worked out perfectly with three year cycles of 156 weeks (where 1 + 5 + 6 = 12 or 1 + 2 = 3) in the Pythagorean skein. Such lunar cycles were the key to musical mathematics with quarter, half, and full notes etc. in music derived from quarter, half and full moon phases.

Thus, lunar cycles were vital to the development of the ancient Jewish calendar that had twelve (and every three years thirteen) months, and was based on four lunar phases that took twenty-eight days to complete as seen in appendix figure A8. This calender was far more spiritually functional and practically accurate than the Roman calendar used today.

Indeed, there has been a vile attack on mathematical and temporal accuracy, impacting spiritual evolution. For instance, people are taught "there are three hundred and sixty five days in a year." With seven (7) days a week and fifty-two (52) weeks a year, the mathematics show that seven times fifty-two equals 364 not 365!

If we revert back to the ancient calendar, the mathematical accuracy returns with the use of the twenty-eight day cycle and thirteen month year as 13 x 28 = 364.

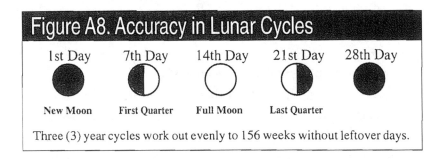

### Figure A8. Accuracy in Lunar Cycles

| 1st Day | 7th Day | 14th Day | 21st Day | 28th Day |
|---------|---------|----------|----------|----------|
| New Moon | First Quarter | Full Moon | Last Quarter | |

Three (3) year cycles work out evenly to 156 weeks without leftover days.

## Christ's Accurate Birth and Ascension Dates

With the Roman calendar and time deceptions continuing, along with many other falsehoods, one important hoax that Jeshua asked Joey to rectify herein was perpetrated by Lawrence Gardner. Recall that Gardner said he was "the appointed historian and sovereign gene-alogist to *thirty-three* royal families," emphasis added, and "Britain's Grand Prior of the Sacred Kindred of St. Columba–the Royal Ecclesiastical Seat of the Celtic Church," and that he had "access to Celtic Church records dating back to 37 A.D." As explained in Chapter 3 of this book, Mr. Gardner, like other disinformation specialists, is likely a historian who mixes deception with historic facts to mislead the public in support of covert agendas. These investigators, using Joey's original research, caught Gardner in a solid ruse regarding Jesus' alleged birthdate.

Gardner claimed in his works that Jesus, *not* a legitimate messiah, had been born in March rather than in September, the customary time for royalty to be born.[1] He explained this switching of birthdates occurred as a convenience perpetrated by the Jewish leaders, including Jesus's parents. This "miraculous" birth, then, Gardner suggested, is just another hoax designed to make something ordinary appear special.

In fact, as evidenced in appendix figures A9 and A10, Jesus' birthdate, place, and time *was* extraordinary. These graphs were generated by a computer program designed to accurately account for the historic data, both temporal and astronomical. The program was developed by a NASA contractor who had successfully tested the software at the national space agency. As shown, looking East from Bethlehem, at a 51.2 degree angle (5+1+2=8) from the horizon, on the morning of September 15, 5 B.C., "one very large star" was seen that was only seen once more in that location viewing from Jerusalem almost 33 years later. That is, on March 28, 28 A.D. the stars Venus and Regulus directly aligned to produce the illusion of a single "Star of Bethlehem." This computer study was repeated for verification searching 5,000 years before to 5,000 years after **September 15, 5 BC.** The phenomenon did not recur in all that time. In other words, *in 10,000 years checked, September 15, 5 B.C., Christ's apparent true birthday, and March 28, 28 A.D., the apparent date of his ascension, were the only times in which two major celestial bodies—Venus and Regulus—perfectly aligned, along with the rest of the Zodiac, to create the illusion of a single Star of Bethlehem.*

---

[1] Gardner L. "Bloodlines of the Holy Grail." A lecture presentation recorded at Yale University in 1994; and Gardner L. *Bloodline of the Holy Grail: The Hidden Lineage of Jesus Revealed.* Rockport, MA: Element Books, 1996.)

# Figure A9. The View From Bethlehem on September 15, 5 B.C.

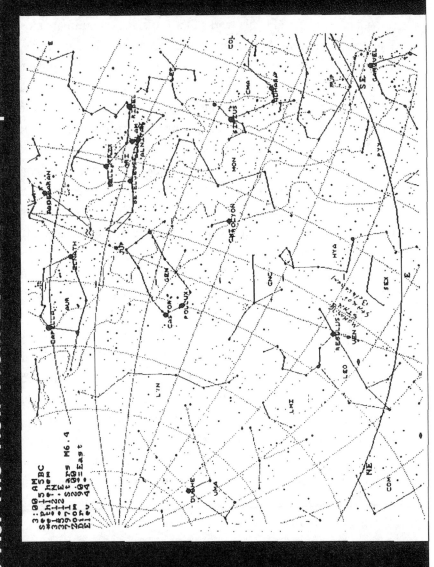

# Figure A10. The View From Jerusalem on March 28, 28 A.D.

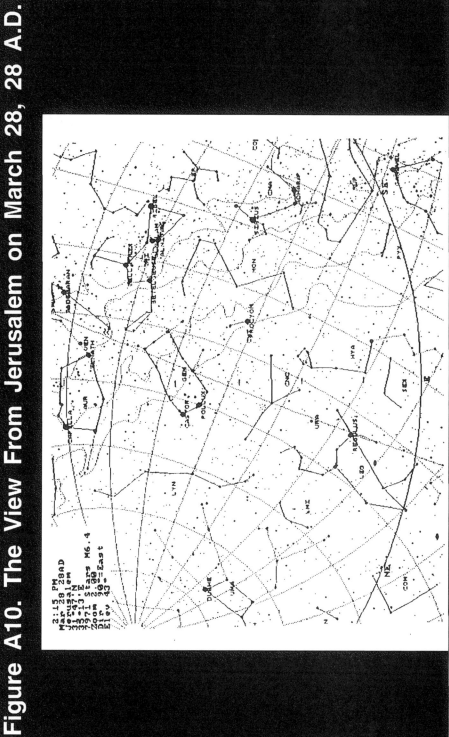

Additionally fascinating was the fact that when the computer printed the birthdate graphic shown in figure A9, it automatically substituted an asterik—a "star"—in place of the "B" in Bethlehem. It made this unique "error" repeatedly and, according to the program's users, it never did it before or after when analyzing any other date and place.

Finally, from *Webster's Dictionary*, the definition of Regulus, the star that combined with loving Venus to produce the "Star of Bethlehem," is shown below:

> **regulus** . . . *n* [NL, fr. L, petty king, fr. *reg-*, rex king — more at ROYAL] 1 *cap* : a first-magnitude star in the constellation Leo 2 [ML, metallic antimony, fr. L] : the more or less impure mass of metal formed beneath the slag in smelting and reducing ores. B. an impure intermediate product obtained in smelting ores. [1550-60: <regulus little king (diminutive of rex); formerly applied to antimony because it readily combines with gold the king of metals); see ULE] regulus: Marcus Atilus died 250? B.C. Roman General.

Indeed, Jesus was "the little King" with a big loving job to perform for the impure "slag" for which he took the heat. He was figuratively the gold sent to amalgamate the less pure masses.

### Freemasonry Past History and Present Deceptions

Given the above, the authors believe it unlikely a "coincidence" that the ancient craft of Freemasonry applies "Seven liberall Sciences" that include the "sixth science . . . called Musicke [with 6 essential notes of the Solfeggio]; that teacheth a man of songe and voice, of tongue and orgaine, harpe and trompe.

"And the seaventh science is called Astronomye; and that teacheth a man the course of the sunn, moone and starrs.

"These be . . . all founded by one Science, that is to say Geometrie." This was written in *The History of Freemasonry: Its Legendary Origins*, and "Geometrie" is itself the in depth field of study called the fifth "liberall Science" among the seven taught.[2]

---

[2] Mackey AG. *The History of Freemasonry: Its Legendary Origins*. New York: Gramercy Books & Random House, 1996, pp. 18, 19, 51 and 62.)

The second science taught the Freemasons "is Rhethoricke" that "teacheth a man to speake faire in subtill termes." The "third is Dialectyke" that "teacheth a man for to discern or know truth from false."

Joey had learned from studying the Aprocrapha about the tricks of language from the "wisdom of Solomon." King Solomon understood how language, voice, tones and vibrations could be used constructively and destructively as the Freemasons also learned and kept secret from at least the time they made off with King Solomon's treasure and arcana.

Their sciences, according to Freemasonry, as well as modern language, is believed to have evolved from the sons of Genesis's Lameche, who had two wives—Ada and Sella. The King James Bible (Gen 4:19 and 4:23) provided the names "Adah and Zillah, Hear my voice: ye wives of Lamech, hearken unto my speech . . ." This was the apparent beginning of the English alphabet letters "A to Z."

Lamech appears twelve times in eleven verses of the King James Bible. These numbers added produce the number five using the Pythagorean skein. The number five was assigned to the most important science of Freemasonry, the science of geometry which was used by Nimrod who built Babylon and the Tower of Babel.

Nimrod, the son of Cush (Gen 10:8) founded Freemasonry, not King Solomon as many Freemasons are led to believe. Interestingly, Nimrod is cited four (4) times in the King James Bible in four (4) verses (Gen 10:8, 10:9; 1Chr 1:10; Micah 5:6). Four plus four equals eight (8)—the mighty number applied to God—the symbol for infinity.

Finally, many Masons themselves were deceived by the teaching that Babel or Babylon was a city of intellectual darkness, and supposedly there the "light of Masonry was for a time extinguished, to be re-illumined only" after the Temple of Solomon was built. In fact, Babylonia "was undoubtedly the fountain of all Semitic science and architecture, as also the birthplace of Operative Masonry."[1]

## EISCAT's Frequencies

According to EISCAT's home page on the Internet, produced and directed by the Rutherford Appleton Laboratory in Rutherford England, the EISCAT Scientific Association is "an international research organization operating two incoherent scatter radar systems, at UHF [ultra high frequency] (931) and VHF [very high frequency] (224), in Northern Scandinavia." (See Chapter 11's reference 1.)

You may recall that the frequencies of the Solfeggio encoded in the King James Bible were:

1. Ut = 396 = 9
2. Re = 417 = 3
3. Mi = 528 = 6
4. Fa = 639 = 9
5. Sol = 741 = 3
6. La = 852 = 6

First notice the perfectly patterned order in the 100s, 10s, and 1s columns above.

Notice the two EISCAT frequencies 931 and 224 are close to one degree above and below the sacred frequencies of the Solfeggio scale, metaphorically "framing," or "containing" these holy tones.

Notice also that the repeating Pythagorean integers are 9, 3, 6 total 18 or 9 which, according to the major arcana implies completion, and according to the "Tarot Divinatory Meanings,"[5] as seen in figure A11, implies "deception" from "hidden enemies" and "caution" during "spiritual advancement." The number 3 in the figure represents "fruitfulness, action and creativity; the number 6 means "LOVERS—a test which you will pass, a new love." So all of God's Solfeggio codes seem humanly challenging though positive.

In contrast, EISCAT's frequencies are 9 + 3 + 1 = 13 the sign of "DEATH." 13 reduced further equals 1 + 3 = 4. The number 4 denotes the "EMPEROR: power, effectiveness, and reason.

Any way you add them, EISCAT's two frequencies combined equal 12—"Hanged Man, wisdom from self-sacrifice," or 21—"UNI-

## Figure A11. The Major Arcana—Tarot Divinatory Meanings

0   FOOL: Folly, foolishness, extravagance.

1   MAGICIAN: Skills, will power, self confidence.

2   HIGH PRIESTESS: Science, education, knowledge.

3   EMPRESS: Fruitfulness, action, creativity.

4   EMPOROR: Power, effectiveness, reason.

5   HIEROPHANT: Mercy and goodness.

6   LOVERS:  A test which you will pass, a new love.

7   CHARIOT: Triumph, overcoming obstacles.

8   STRENGTH: Spiritual power.

9   HERMIT: Caution or spiritual advancement.

10  WHEEL OF FORTUNE: Good fortune, success, luck.

11  JUSTICE: Balance, justice, equilibrium.

12  HANGED MAN: Wisdom as a result of self-sacrifice.

13  DEATH: An evolutionary change or transformation.

14  TEMPERANCE: Combine or unite seemingly unlike things, moderation.

15  DEVIL: Something must happen, but in the long run it is for the good.

16  TOWER: Ruin, catastrophe, disruption.

17  STAR: Hope and a bright future.

18  MOON: Deception, hidden enemies.

19  SUN: Happiness and contentment.

20  JUDGEMENT: Renewal, rebirths.

21  UNIVERSE: Assured success, completion.

Religious fundamentalists believe the Tarot represents an avoidable evil. This assessment is based on several Bible verses, most importantly Deuteronomy 18.9-14. Here occult practices including "soothsaying," or consulting with spirits, are referred to as "abominable." Such practices have, however, been consistently used by secret society leaders who continued to deceive the masses, violate God's laws, and commit genocide. Figure adapted from: Kraig DM. *Modern Magick: Eleven Lessons in the High Magickal Arts*. St. Paul, MN: Llewellyn Publications, 1992, pp. 14-15.

VERSE, assured success, completion." Both reduce to 3 meaning "EMPRESS"—fruitfulness, action, creativity.

In essence, EISCAT's frequencies denote completion by the "EMPEROR" and "EMPRESS" who powerfully rule to reap the creative fruits of their actions.

## Judeo-Christian Warnings

Many religious fundamentalists believe the Tarot represents an avoidable evil. For instance, several authors wrote for inclusion in this book, that Isaiah 47.9-14 and Deuteronomy 18.9-14 clearly tells why the kingdom of spiritual Babylon, whose devotees practice such occult methods, will be destroyed. They suggested reading these verses "prayerfully." Isaiah 47:13-14, specifically warns, "Thou art wearied in the multitude of thy counsels. Let now the astrologers, the stargazers, the monthly prognosticators, stand up, and save thee from these things that shall come upon thee. Behold, they shall be as stubble; the fire shall burn them; they shall not deliver themselves from the power of the flame. . . ."

Other passages in the Bible, including Daniel 2:10 and Kings II 21:6, similarly caution against practices guided by spiritism.

In the *Complete Jewish Bible*, Deuteronomy 18.9-14 likewise counsels the high Levi priests:

> When you enter the land ADONAI your God is giving you, you are not to learn how to follow the abominable practices of those nations.[10] There must not be found among you anyone who makes his son or daughter pass through fire, a diviner, a soothsayer, an enchanter, a sorcerer,[11] a spell-caster, a consulter of ghosts or spirits, or a necromancer.[12] For whoever does these things is detestable to ADONAI, and because of these abominations ADONAI your God is driving them out ahead of you.[13] You must be wholehearted with ADONAI your God.[14] For these nations, which you are about to dispossess, listen to soothsayers and diviners; but you, ADONAI your God does not allow you to do this.

Thus, it might be quite rationally argued that those who practice occult methods, or spiritism, may not only learn to rely on these practices more, and on almighty God less, but to this measure they will know God less. In so doing, they will reduce, or even lose, their potential for a full relationship with God and the truly divine and miraculous power that accompanies this intimate and optimal association with the King of the Universe.

It is these authors' contention that God gave us these laws for a reason. In this case, so that we might not be deceived into thinking that we can use these things, rather than relying on Him, to illuminate our paths or empower our lives. Unfortunately, many people lack this discretion. As Isaiah 47:8 and 10 twice states, they "dwellest carelessly," and their esoteric ". . . knowledge, it hath perverted thee; and thou hast said in thine heart, I *am*, and none else beside me." This is the egocentric trap that God's word counsels us to avoid.

Like modern science and technology, it might be argued, occult practices might be used for good *or* evil. However, in any and every case its fruits are inferior to, and most often undermine, God's creations. It is sobering, for instance, to recognize that the cryptocracy that funded Hitler's occultist rise to power, and dramatically benefited by waging incessant wars, developed the nuclear, and more recently as evidenced in this book, the bioelectric and biogenetic technologies empowering these same shadow governors to manipulate and kill even larger populations of God's children more effectively and efficiently.

## Herbs in the Bible

The word "herb" is found in the King James Bible nineteen (19) times in 19 verses, and the plural of it, "herbs," is found eighteen (18) times in 18 verses.

"All you have to do is read it from the beginning," recommended Reverend Matthew Dougherty, a Bible scholar. "GENESIS 1:29 says 'I have given you every plant yielding seed which is upon the face of all the Earth, and every tree with seed in its fruit; you shall have them for food.'

"What that passage means," Rev. Dougherty preached, "is every-thing we could ever need to keep our bodies fit and healthy is here in nature as a gift from God. The Bible tells us Methuselah and others lived for more than 900 years. The Israelites endured grueling slavery in Egypt and a tortuous trek through the desert, and yet there's no evidence of disease, stress or exhaustion. How can this be?

"Their knowledge of natural cures kept them in prime physical condition!"

Magnus Harrison, a well known herbalist expanded on Rev. Dougherty's enthusiasm: "In the Book of Isaiah, the leaf of the willow tree is mentioned as a remedy for fevers. And now we realize willow leaves contain salicin, the chemical which led to the creation of aspirin in the early 1900s.

"Other Bible cures are being proved equally effective. The more we look, the more we discover these remedies really are gifts from God."

For example, artichokes are really edible thistles, appreciated for their delicious heart and fleshy leaves. But did you know that the Bible authorized people to eat them for medicinal reasons?

"Modern studies have proven that artichokes help digestion, and have vital minerals like potassium, phosphorus, and iron," Rev. Dougherty advised. "Artichokes work well against blood-clotting cholesterol. A chemical called cyanin was taken from artichokes and used to make a cholesterol-lowering drug."

Another example is aloe. Proverbs 7:17 states, "I have perfumed my bed with myrrh, aloes, and cinnamon." According to the Book of John, Jesus was embalmed with aloe. It is well known that aloe is good for the skin, speeds wound healing, and also works as a laxative.[3]

Figure A12 provides an extensive alphabetical listing of herbs, their biblical references, and their therapeutic uses where indicated. This list was provided courtesy of the University of Maryland and is freely downloadable from its website.

# Figure A12. Biblical Herbs and Their Known Uses

| Herb Name(s)/Family | Biblical Reference | Uses/Indications |
|---|---|---|
| **FERULA GUMMOSA** Boiss. "Galbanum" (CELERY FAMILY) | "I grew tall ... like cassia and camel's thorn I gave forth the aroma of spices, and like choice myrrh I spread a pleasant odor, like galbanum, onycha and stacte, and like the fragrance of frankincense in the tabernacle." Ecclesiasticus 24: 14-5. | |
| **FICUS CARICA L.** "Fig Tree" (MULBERRY FAMILY) | And Isaiah said, take a lump of figs. And they took and laid it on the boil and he recovered..." II Kings 20. | CANCER; LEUCODERMA; RINGWORM; Thrush; Wounds. |
| **FICUS SYCOMORUS L.** "Mulberry Fig", "Sycamore Fig", "Sycomore" (MULBERRY FAMILY) | "...I was an herdman, and a gatherer of sycomore fruit..." Amos 7. | Burns; Cancer; Cirrhosis; Dermatosis; Dyslactea; Scrofula; Sore Throat. |
| **FRAXINUS ORNUS L.** Manna Ash (OLIVE FAMILY) | "...Behold, we have sent you money to buy burnt offerings, and sin offerings, and incense, and prepare ye manna..." Baruch 1. | CONSTIPATION; Fever; Gonorrhea; Malaria. |
| **GOSSYPIUM HERBACEUM L.** "Cotton" (MALLOW FAMILY) | There were white cotton curtains and blue hangings caught up with cords of fine linen..." Ester 1. | CANCER; CONTRACEPTIVE; Dermatitis; Dyslactea; Gout; Malaria. |
| **GUNDELIA TOURNEFORTII L.** "Tournefort's Gundelia" "Tumbleweed" (ASTER FAMILY) | "O my God, make them like *whirling* dust, like chaff before the wind." | |
| **\*HALOXYLON PERSICUM** Bge. "White Saxaul" "Adah" (Biblical) "Ada (Arabic) | "Lamech said to his wives 'Adah and Zilla, hear my voice" Genesis 4: 23. | |
| **HAMMADA SALICORNICA** (Moq.) Iljin "Hammada" "Lye"(Biblical) "Rimth" (Arabic) (LAMBSQUARTER FAMILY) | "Though you wash youself with lye and use much soap, the stain of your guilt is still before me...." Jeremiah 2:22. | |
| **HEDERA HELIX L.** "Ivy" (ARALIA FAMILY) | "...they were compelled to go in procession to Baccus carrying ivy..." II Maccabees 6. | Cancer; Corns; Impotence; Malaria; Rheumatism; Toothache. |
| **HORDEUM VULGARE L.** "Barley" (GRASS FAMILY) | "...Let thistles grow instead of wheat and cockle instead of barley..." | DYSPEPSIA; Fractures; Orchitis; Parotitis; Sunstroke; Tuberculosis. |
| **HYACINTHUS ORIENTALIS L.** "Hyacinth", "Lily of the Valley (Biblical)" (LILY FAMILY) | "...I am the rose of Sharon, and the lily of the valleys..." Song of Solomon 2. | Dysuria; Jaundice; Leucorrhea. |

# Figure A12. Cont. Biblical Herbs and Their Known Uses

| Herb Name(s)/Family | Biblical Reference | Uses/Indications |
|---|---|---|
| **HYOSCYAMUS AUREUS L.** "GoldenHenbane" "Shikkeron"(Biblical) (POTATO FAMILY) | "The bundary goes out to the shoulder of the hill north of Ekron, then the boundary bends round to Shikkeron, and passes along to Mount Baalah, and goes out to Jabneel." Joshua 15: 11. | NARCOTIC. |
| **HYOSCYAMUS MUTICUS L.** "Henbane" "Shikkeron"(Biblical) (POTATO FAMILY) | "The bundary goes out to the shoulder of the hill north of Ekron, then the boundary bends round to Shikkeron, and passes along to Mount Baalah, and goes out to Jabneel." Joshua 15: 11. | NARCOTIC. |
| **IRIS PSEUDACORUS L.** "Yellow Flag", "Lily" (Biblical)" (IRIS FAMILY) | "...he shall grow as the lily, and cast forth his roots as Lebanon..." Hosea 14. | Bruises; Cholera; CONSTIPATION; Hepatosis; Rheumatism; Sciatica. |
| **JUGLANS REGIA L.** "Carpathian or Persian Walnut," "English Walnut," "Nuts" (WALNUT FAMILY) | "...I went down into the garden of nuts to see the fruits of the valley, and to see whether the vine flourished, and the pomegranates budded..." Song of Solomon 6. | Alopecia; Cancer; Flu; Gingivitis; Halitosis; Headache. |
| **JUNCUS EFFUSUS L.** "Bog Rush", " Soft Rush", " Flag (Biblical)" (RUSH FAMILY) | "...The seeds and the flags shall wither..." Isaiah 19. | Anuria; Cough; Dropsy; Insomnia; Sore Throat; Stones. |
| **JUNIPERUS EXCELSA Bieb.** "Grecian Juniper", "Algum (Biblical)" (JUNIPER FAMILY) | "...Send me also cedar trees, fir trees, and algum trees, out of Lebanon...." II Chronicles 2. | Cough; Dyspepsia; Hepatosis; Rheumatism; Wounds. |
| **JUNIPERUS OXYCEDRUS L.** "Brown Juniper", "Cade", "Heath (Biblical)" "Prickly Juniper", "Cedar" (JUNIPER FAMILY) | "...For he shall be like the heath in the desert..." Jeremiah 17. | Alopecia; Cancer; Dermatitis; Eczema; Leprosy; Pruritis; Psoriasis. |
| **JUNIPERUS PHOENICIA L.** "Phoenician Juniper" "Aroer" (Biblical); Arar"(Arabic) | "From Aroer, which is on the edge of the valley of the Arnon." Deuteronomy 2:36. | |
| **LACTUCA SATIVA L.** "Lettuce" (ASTER FAMILY) | "...eat it with unleavened bread and bitter herbs... " Numbers 9. | Burns' Cough; Cancer; Impotence; INSOMNIA; Nymphomania. |
| **LAURUS NOBILIS L.** "Bayleaf", "Sweet Bay", "Grecian Laurel", "Green Bay (Biblical)" (LAUREL FAMILY) | "...I have seen the wicked in great power, and spreading himself like a green bay tree...." Psalm 37 | DIABETES; Dyspepsia; Earache; Insomnia; MIGRAINE; PAIN. |
| **LAWSONIA INERMIS L.** "Henna", "Egyptian Privet", "Mignonette" "Camphire (Biblical)" (LOOSESTRIFE FAMILY) | "...My beloved is unto me as a cluster of camphire in the vineyards..." Song of Solomon 1. | CANCER; Dermatitis; Inflammation; SUNBURN; URTICARIA; Rheumatism. |

490

# Figure A12. Cont. Biblical Herbs and Their Known Uses

| Herb Name(s)/Family | Biblical Reference | Uses/Indications |
|---|---|---|
| **LENS CULINARIS Medik.** "Lentil" (LEGUME FAMILY) | "....Then Jacob gave Esau bread and pottage of lentiles; and he did eat...." Genesis 25. | FETAL ALCOHOL SYNDROME; SPINAL BIFIDA. |
| **LILIUM CANDIDUM L.** "Madonna Lily" (LILY FAMILY) | "...to feed in the gardens, and to gather lillies..." Song of Solomon 6. | CANCER; Corns; Dermatitis; Dropsy; Epilepsy. |
| **LINUM USITATISSIMUM L.** "Flax", "Linen (Biblical)" (FLAX FAMILY) | "...And he took it down, and wrapped it in Linen... "Luke 23. Arthritis; Bronchitis; | CANCER; CARDIOPATHY; Cold; DERMATITIS; INFLAMMATION; Rheumatism. |
| **LIQUIDAMBAR ORIENTALIS Miller** "Storax" "Sweet Gum" "Balm" (Biblical) (STORAX FAMILY) | "...Ishmaelites coming from Gilead, with their camels bearing gum, balm, and myrrh, on their way to carry it down to Egypt. " Genesis 37: 25. | |
| **LOLIUM TEMULENTUM L.** "Darnel" , "Tares (Biblical)" (GRASS FAMILY) | "...But while men slept, his enemy came and sowed tares among the wheat...." Matthew 13. | Colic; Leprosy; MIGRAINE; Rheumatism; Toothache. |
| **LYCIUM EUROPAEUM Linn.** "European Box Thorn", " Desert Thorn", "Bramble (Biblical)" (POTATO FAMILY) | "...who cut up by mallows by the bushes..." Job 30. | COLD, COUGH, Gravel; IN-FLAMMATION; Jaundice; SORE THROAT. |
| **MALUS SYLVESTRIS Mill.** "Apple" (ROSE FAMILY) | "Sustain me with raisins, refresh me with apples; for I am sick with love." Song of Solomon2:5. | CONSTIPATION. |
| **MALVA SYLVESTRIS L.** "Blue Mallow" (MAL-LOW FAMILY) | "...who cut up by mallows by the bushes..." Job 30. | COLD, COUGH, Gravel; INFLAM-MATION; Jaundice; SORE THROAT. |
| **MANDRAGORA OFFICINARUM L.** "Loveapple", "Mandrake" (POTATO FAMILY) | " ....The mandrakes gave a smell..." Song of Solomon 7. | ASTHMA; INSOMNIA; COUGH; HAYFEVER; RHEUMATISM; VERTIGO. |
| **MATRICARIA AUREA (Loefl.)** Sch. Bip (Syn.ANTHEMIS SP sensu Zohary. "Dog Chamomile" (ASTER FAMILY) | "All flesh is grass, and all its glory like the flower of the grass.The grass withers, and the flower falls; but the word of the Lord abides forever." I Peter 1:24. | Cold; Conjunctivitis; Cough; Debility; Diabetes; ENTERAL-GIA; Fever; Gingivosis;Headache; Myalgia; Neuralgia; Neurosis; Toothache; Wounds. |

# Figure A12. Cont. Biblical Herbs and Their Known Uses

| Herb Name(s)/Family | Biblical Reference | Uses/Indications |
|---|---|---|
| MENTHA LONGIFOLIA (L.) Huds. "Biblical Mint" "Horsemint" "Mint" (MINT FAMILY) | "Biblical Mint" "Horsemint" "Mint" (MINT FAMILY) "...for ye tithe mint and rue and all manner of herbs...." Luke 11. | COLD Dermatitis; DYSPEPSIA; HEADACHE; Impotence; PAIN; RHEUMATISM. |
| MORUS NIGRA L. "Black Mulberry", "Purple Mulberry", "Sycamine (Biblical)" (MULBERRY FAMILY) | "...And to the end they might provoke the elephants to fight, they shewed them the blood of grapes and mulberries..." 1 Maccabees 6. | Conjunctivitis; Dysmenorrhea; Fever; Sorethroat. |
| MYRTUS COMMUNIS L. "Myrtle" (MYRTLE FAMILY) | "...I will plant in the wilderness the cedar, the shittah tree, and the myrtle, and the oil tree...." Isaiah 41 | Asthma; bronchitis; Cancer; Hemorrhoids; Polyps; Smallpox; TUBERCULOSIS. |
| NARCISSUS TAZETTA L. "Narcissus", "Buttercup", "Rose (Biblical)" (AMARYLLIS FAMILY) | "...The wilderness and the solitary place shall be glad for them; and the desert shall rejoice, and blossom as the rose...." Isaiah 35. | CANCER; Epilepsy; Fever; Mastitis; Ophthalmia. |
| NARDOSTACHYS JATAMANSI DC. "Spikenard" (VALERIAN FAMILY) | "...Thy plants are an orchard of pomegranates, with pleasant fruits: camphire with spikenard..." Song of Solomon 4. | ARRHYTHMIA; CARDIOPATHY: Chorea; CRAMPS; DYSMENORRHEA; Epilepsy; Headache; INSOMNIA; Leprosy. |
| NASTURTIUM OFFICINALE R. Br. "Watercress" (MUSTARD FAMILY) | "...Eat it with unleavened bread and bitter herbs..." Numbers 9. | Asthma; CANCER; COLD; Dermatitis; Nephrosis; Tuberculosis. |
| NERIUM OLEANDER L. "Rose (Biblical)" (DOGBANE FAMILY) | "...Hearken unto me, ye holy children, and bud forth as a rose growing by the brook of the field." Ecclesiasticus 39. | POISONOUS: Cancer; Cardiopathy; Dermatitis; Edema; Hypertension; Leprosy; Ringworm. |
| NIGELLA SATIVA L. "Black Cumin", "Fitch (Biblical)" (BUTTERCUP FAMILY) | "...For the fitches are not thrashed with a threshing instrument. ..but the fitches are beaten out with a staff...." Isaiah 28. | ARTHRITS:ASTHMA, BRONCHITIS; Colic; Cough; Dermatitis; DYSMENORRHEA; Orchitis; RHEUMATISM. |
| NOTOBASIS SYRIACA (L.) Coss. "Syrian Thistle" "Thorn" (ASTER FAMILY) | "I will flail your flesh with the thorns of the wilderness and with briers" Judges 8:7. | |
| NYMPHAEA ALBA L. "Waterlily", "Lotus", "Lily (Biblical)" (WATERLILY FAMILY) | "...And upon the top of the pillars was lily work...." 1 Kings 7. | Cancer; Cramps; Diarrhea; Fever; INSOMNIA. |
| OLEA EUROPEA L. "Olive (Biblical)" (OLIVE FAMILY) | "...His branches shall spread, and his beauty shall be as the olive tree..." Hosea 14. | CANCER; CARDIOPATHY; Dermatitis; HYPERTENSION; Sore Throat; Sunburn. |

# Figure A12. Cont. Biblical Herbs and Their Known Uses

| Herb Name(s)/Family | Biblical Reference | Uses/Indications |
|---|---|---|
| **ORIGANUM MARU L.** "Egyptian Marjoram," " Hyssop (Biblical)" (MINT FAMILY) | "...He spoke of trees, from the cedar that is in Lebanon to the hyssop that grows out of the wall. 1 Kings 4:33." | COLD; COLIC; Polyps; RHEU-MATISM; Sprain; Swelling. |
| **ORIGANUM SYRIACUM L.** "Syrian HYssop" "Hyssop (Biblical)" (MINT FAMILY) | " ....Purge me with hyssop and I shall be clean..." Psalms 51 | COLD; COLIC; Polyps; RHEUMATISM; Sprain; Swelling. |
| **ORIGANUM SYRIACUM L.** "Syrian HYssop"" Hyssop (Biblical)" (MINT FAMILY) | "...Purge me with hyssop and I shall be clean..." Psalms 51 | COLD; COLIC; Polyps; RHEU-MATISM; Sprain; Swelling. |
| **ORNITHOGALUM UMBELLATUM L.** "Star of Bethlehem", "Dove's Dung (Biblical)" (LILY FAMILY) | "...and the fourth part of a cab of dove's dung for five pieces of silver..." II Kings 6. | POISONOUS Adenopathy; Cachexia; Debility; Infections; Parotitis |
| **PALIURUS SPINA-CHRISTI** Mill "Crown of Thorns (Biblical)" (BUCKTHORN FAMILY) | "...And when they had platted a crown of thorns..." Matthew 27. | Diarrhea; Dystonia; Dysuria. |
| **PANCRATIUM MARITIMUM L.** "Sea Daffodil" "Sea-Shore Lily" (AMARYLLIS FAMILY) | "I will be as the dew to Israel; he shall blossom as the lily, he shall strike root as the poplar" Hosea 14: 5. | |
| **PANICUM MILIACEUM L.** "Proso Millet", "Millet (Biblical)", "Pannag (Biblical)" (GRASS FAMILY) | "...Take thou also unto thee wheat, and barley, and beans, and lentiles, and millet and fitches, and put them in one vessel, and make thee bread thereof..." Ezekiel 4. | Abscesses; Cancer; Gonorrhea; Infection; Momordicism. |
| **PAPAVER RHOEAS L.** "Common Poppy", "Flanders Poppy", (POPPY FAMILY) | "All flesh is grass, and all its beauty is like the flower of the field...The grass withers, the flower fades; but the word of our God will stand for ever." Isaiah 40: 6-8. | |
| **PAPAVER SOMNIFERUM L.** "Opium Poppy", "Poppyseed Poppy", "Gall" (POPPY FAMILY) | "...they gave him vinegar to drink mingled with gall: and when he had tasted thereof he would not drink..." Matthew 27. | CANCER; COUGH; Dysentery; INSOMNIA;Impotence;PAIN; TOOTHACHE. |
| **PHOENIX DACTYLIFERA L.** "Date Palm" (PALM FAMILY) | "...and brought them to Jericho, the city of palm trees..." II Chronicles 28. | Asthma; Cough; Fever; Gonorrhea; Toothache; Tuberculosis. |

# Figure A12. Cont. Biblical Herbs and Their Known Uses

| Herb Name(s)/Family | Biblical Reference | Uses/Indications |
|---|---|---|
| PHRAGMITES AUSTRALIS (Cav.) Triri. ex Steud. "Common Reed" "Pen (Biblical)" (GRASS FAMILY) | "...I will not with ink and pen write unto thee..." III John 13. | Burns; Bronchitis; Cholera; Diabetes; Jaundice' Leukemia. |
| PINUS BRUTIA Tenore "Brutian Pine", "Thick Tree (Biblical)" (PINE FAMILY) | "...Go forth unto the Mount, andfrtch olive branches, and pine branches...and myrtle branches, and palm branches, and branches of thick trees to make booths..." Nehemiah 8. | Catarrh; Cough; Gonorrhea; Hepatosis; Nephrosis; Rheumatism. |
| PINUS HALEPENSIS Mill. "Aleppo Pine", "Fir (Biblical)" (PINE FAMILY) | "...as for the stork, the fir trees are her house..." Psalms 104. | Catarrh; Cough; Gonorrhea; Hepatosis; Nephrosis; Rheumatism. |
| PINUS PINEA L. "Stone Pine" "Holm" (Biblical) | "He cuts down cedars; of he chooses a holm tree or an oak and lets it grow strong amonbg the trees of the forest; he plants a cedar and the rain nourishes it." Isaiah 44:14. | |
| PISTACIA LENTISCUS L. "Mastic", "Mastick Tree (Biblical)" (CASHEW FAMILY) | "...who answered, Under a mastick tree..." Susanna 51. | Cancer; Cholecocystosis; Cough; Diarrhea; Hepatosis; Itch; Rheumatism. |
| PISTACIA TEREBINTHUS L. "Cyprus Turpentine", "Teil Tree", "Turpentine Tree (Biblical)" (CASHEW FAMILY) | "...As the turpentine tree I stretched out by branches..." Ecclesiasticus 24. | Cancer; Cough; Diarrhea; Fever; Inflammation. |
| PISTACIA VERA L. "Pistacio-nut", "Nuts (Biblical)" (CASHEW FAMILY) | "...carry down the man a present, a little balm, and a little honey, spices, and myrrh, nuts and almonds..." Genesis 43. | Amenorrhea; Bruises;Cough; Dysentery; Impotence; Pruritus; Rheumatism. |
| PLATANUS ORIENTALIS L. "Plane Tree", " Chestnut (Biblical)" (SYCAMORE FAMILY) | "...And Jacob took him rods of green poplar, and of the hazel and chestnut tree..." Genesis 30. | Cancer; Diarrhea; Dysentery; Inflammation; Ophthalmia; Rheumatism. |
| POPULUS ALBA L. "Poplar (Biblical)" (WILLOW FAMILY) | "...and Jacob took him rods of green poplar..." Genesis 30. | ARTHRITIS; Dermatitis; FEVER; Rheumatism; Snakebite; TOOTHACHE. |
| POPULUS EUPHRATICA Oliv. "Euphrates Aspen", " Willow (Biblical)" (WILLOW FAMILY) | "...We hanged our harps upon the willows in the midst thereof..." Psalms 137. | ARTHRITIS; Dermatitis; FEVER; Rheumatism; Snakebite; TOOTHACHE. |
| PRUNUS ARMENIACA L. "Apricot" , "Chinese Almond", "Apple (Biblical)" (ROSE FAMILY) | "...A word fitly spoken is like apples of gold in pictures of silver..." Proverbs 25 | Asthma; CANCER; Cough; Laryngitis; Ophthalmia; Rheumatism. |

# Figure A12. Cont. Biblical Herbs and Their Known Uses

| Herb Name(s)/Family | Biblical Reference | Uses/Indications |
|---|---|---|
| **PRUNUS DULCIS** (Mill.) D.A. Webb "Almond" (ROSE FAMILY) | "...and carry down the man a present, a little balm, a little honey, spices, and myrrh, nuts, and almonds..." Genesis 43. | Acne; Asthma; CANCER; Cough; Dermatitis; Laryngitis; Neuralgia. |
| **PTEROCARPUS SANTALINUS L.** "Red Saunders", "Almug (Biblical)" (LEGUME FAMILY) | "...brought in from Ophir great plenty of almug trees..." I Kings 10. | Dermatosis; DYSENTERY; Fever; Headache; Inflammation; Malaria; Toothache. |
| **PUNICA GRANATUM L.** "Pomegranate", "Grenada" (POMEGRANATE FAMILY) | "...I would cause thee to drink of spiced wine of the juice of my pomegranate..." Song of Solomon 8. | Bronchitis; CANCER: Conjunctivitis; DYSENTERY: DYSMENORRHEA; ESTROGENIC; HEMOR- RHOIDS; INFERTILITY; SORE THROAT; STOMATITIS; WORMS. |
| **QUERCUS AEGILOPS L.** "Valonia Oak", "Dyer's Oak", "Oak (Biblical)" (OAK FAMILY) | "...And as an oak, whose substance is in them, when the cast their leaves..." Isaiah 6. | Burns; Cancer. |
| **QUERCUS COCCIFERA L.** "Kermes Oak"," Scarlet (Biblical)" (OAK FAMILY) | "...And he shall take to cleanse the house two birds, and cedar wood, and scarlet, and hyssop..." Leviticus 14. | Cancer; Fever; Sores; Wounds. |
| **QUERCUS ILEX L.** "Holly Oak", " Oak (Biblical)" (OAK FAMILY) | "...and she was buried beneath Bethel under an oak..." Genesis 35. | Cancer; Fever; Liver problems; Tumors. |
| **REICHARDIA TINGITANA** (L.) Roth. "Poppy-leaved Reichardia" "Bitter Herb" (Biblical) (ASTER FAMILY) | "...with unleavened bread and bitter herbs they shall eat it." Exodus 12:8. | |
| **RETAMA RAETAM** (Forsk.) Webb. & Berth. "White Broom", "Juniper (Biblical)" (LEGUME FAMILY) | "...went a day's journey into the wilderness, and came and sat down under a juniper tree..." I Kings 19. | Arthritis; Diarrhea; Fever; Ophthalmia; Pain; Sore. |
| **RHAMNUS PALAESTINA Boiss** "Palestine Buckthorn", "Hedge (Biblical)" (BUCKTHRON FAMILY) | "...whoso breaketh an hedge, a serpent shall bite him..." Ecclesiastes 10. | Cancer; Constipation. |
| **RICINUS COMMUNIS L.** "Castorbean", " Palma Christ", " Gourd (Biblical)" (SPURGE FAMILY) | "...And the Lord God prepared a gourd, and made it to come up over Jonah, that it might be a shadow over his head...Jonah 4. | Abscess; Bunion; CANCER; Conjunctivitis; DERMATITIS; Gout; Headache; Lumbago; Rheumatism; Sciatica. |
| **ROSA PHONECIA Boiss.** "Phoenician Rose" (ROSE FAMILY) | "...whereup they grew roses and lilies..." 11 Esdras 2. | SCURVY. |

# Figure A12. Cont. Biblical Herbs and Their Known Uses

| Herb Name(s)/Family | Biblical Reference | Uses/Indications |
|---|---|---|
| **RUBIA TINCTORUM L.** "Dyer's Madder" "Puah" (Biblical) (COFFEE FAMILY) | "...There arose to deliver Israel Tola, the son of Puah, son of Dodo...." Judges 10: 1. | |
| **RUBUS SANGUINEUS** Friv. "Bramble" "Thorn"(Biblical) (ROSE FAMILY) | "Thorns and snares are in the way of the perverse; he who guards himself will keep far from them. Proverbs 22:5. | |
| **RUBUS SANCTUS** Schreb. "Blackberry" , "Bramble (Biblical)" (ROSE FAMILY) | "...nor of a bramble bush gather thy grapes..." Luke 6. | |
| **RUMEX ACETOSELLA** Linn. "Sheep Sorrel" (BUCKWHEAT FAMILY) | "...eat it with unleavened bread and bitter herbs..." Numbers 9. | Cancer; Dyspepsia; Epithelioma; Fever; Jaundice. |
| **RUSCUS ACULEATUS L.** "Butchers Broom", "Knee Holly", "Brier (Biblical)" (BUTCHER'S BROOM FAMILY) | "...And there shall be no more a pricking brier unto the house of Israel..." Ezekiel 28. | Chilblains; Dyspnea; Dysuria; FEVER; Jaundice; Nephrosis. |
| **RUTA GRAVEOLENS L.** "Rue" ,"Garden Rue" , "German Rue", "Herbygrass" , "Herbe of Grace" (CITRUS FAMILY) | "...But woe unto you, Pharisees! for ye tithe mint and rue and all manner of herbs..." Luke II. | POISONOUS; Colic; CRAMPS; Dyspepsia; Epilepsy; Hysteria; Rheumatism; VITILIGO. |
| **SACCHARUM OFFICINARUM L.** "Sugarcane" , " Sweet Cane (Biblical)" (GRASS FAMILY) | "...Thou has bought me no sweet cane with money..."Isaiah 43. | Cancer; Cold; Cough; Dysentery; Hemorrhoids; Laryngitis; Pertussis; Sore Throat. |
| **SALICORNIA EUROPEA L.** "Glasswort", " Sope (Biblical)" (LAMBSQUARTER FAMILY) | "...for he is like a refiner's fire, and like fuller's sope..." Malachi 3. | Cancer; Tumors. |
| **SALIX ALBA L.** "Willow" (WILLOW FAMILY) | "...And they shall spring up as among the grass, as willows by the water course..." Isaiah 44. | ARTHRITIS; COLD: FEVER: FLU: RHEUMATISM; TOOTHACHE. |
| **SALIX BABYLONICA L.** "Weeping Willow", " Willow (Biblical)" (WILLOW FAMILY) | "...We hanged our harps upon the willows in the midst thereof..."Psalms 137 | ARTHRITIS; COLD; FEVER; FLU; RHEUMATISM; TOOTHACHE. |
| **SALIX FRAGILIS** Linn. "Crack Willow", "Red-Wood Willow ", "Kashmir Willow" (WILLOW FAMILY) | "...the willows of the brook compass him about..." Job 40. | ARTHRITIS; COLD: FEVER; FLU; RHEUMATISM; TOOTHACHE. |
| **SALSOLA KALI L.** "Glasswort", "Saltwort" (LAMBSQUARTER FAMILY) | "...for though thou wash thee with nitre, and take thee much sope..." Jeremiah 2. | Cancer; Dropsy; Dysmenorrhea; Infections; Worms. |

496

# Figure A12. Cont. Biblical Herbs and Their Known Uses

| Herb Name(s)/Family | Biblical Reference | Uses/Indications |
|---|---|---|
| **SALVIA JUDAICA Boiss.** "Judean Sage", "Candle-stick (Biblical)" (MINT FAMILY) | "...And he made the candlestick of pure gold...." Exodus 37. | |
| **SARCOPOTERIUM SPINOSUM** (L.) Spach. "Thorny Burnet" "Thorn" (Biblical) (ROSE FAMILY) | "Therefore I will hedge up her way with thorns. . ." Hosea 2: 6. | |
| **SAUSSUREA LAPPA** (Decaisne) C.B. Clarke "Indian Orris", "Kuth", "Costus Oil" "Cassia (Biblical)" (ASTER FAMILY) | "...All thy garments smell of myrrh, and aloes, and cassia..." Psalms 45. | ASTHMA; BRONCHITIS; CHOLERA; COUGH;Dermatosis; Dyspepsia; Smallpox; Stomachache; Tuberculosis. |
| **SCOLYMUS HISPANICUS L.** "Golden Thistle", "Thistles" (ASTERACEAE) | "...Thorns shall grow over its strongholds, nettles and thistles in its fortresses." Isaiah 34: 13. | |
| **SCOLYMUS MACULATUS L.** "Golden Thistle", "Brambles" (ASTERACEAE) | "...As a lily among brambles, so is my love among maidens." Song of Solomon 2: 2. | |
| **SENNA ALEXANDRINA** Miller (Syn. CASSIA SENNA L). "Alexandrian Senna" "Indian Senna" "Senna" "Burning Bush (Biblical) (LEGUME FAMILY) | "And the angel of the Lord appeared to him in a flame of fire out of the midst of a bush; and he looked, and lo, the bush was burning. . ." Exodus 3:2. | CONSTIPATION; Cramps; Gastrosis. |
| **SILYBUM MARIANUM** Gaertn. "Thistles", "Milk Thistle" (ASTERACEAE) | "...Thorns also and thistles shall it bring forth to thee; and thou shalt eat the herb of the field..." Genesis 3. | Asthma; Calculus; CIRRHOSIS; Fever; HEPATITIS; JAUNDICE; Pluerisy; PSORIASIS; Splenitis. |
| **SINAPIS ARVENSIS L.** "Charlock", "Field Mustard" " Nettle (Biblical)" (MUSTARD FAMILY) | "...it was all grown over with thorns and nettles had covered the face...." Proverbs 24. | Arthritis; BRONCHITIS; CANCER; COLDS; Pluerisy; Pneumonia; Rheumatism. |
| **SOLANUM INCANUM L.** "Sodom Apple", "Palestine Nightshade", "Brier (Biblical)" "Jericho Potato" (POTATO FAMILY) | "...and it shall burn and devour his thorns and briers in one day..." Isaiah 10. | POISONOUS: CANCER; Dermatitis; MELANOMA; Pleurisy; Sore Throat; Toothache. |
| **SOLANUM SODOMEUM L.** "Vine of Sodom" (POTATO FAMILY) | "...For their vine is of the vine of Sodom, and of the fields of Gomorrah..." Deuteronomy 32. | POISONOUS: CANCER; Cystitis; Dermatitis; MELANOMA;Pleurisy; RINGWORM; Sore Throat; Toothache. |

# Figure A12. Cont. Biblical Herbs and Their Known Uses

| Herb Name(s)/Family | Biblical Reference | Uses/Indications |
|---|---|---|
| SORGHUM BICOLOR (L.) Moeiich "Sorghum", "Milo", "Broomcorn", "Hyssop (Biblical)" (GRASS FAMILY) | "...they filled a spunge with vinegar, and put it upon hyssop, and put it to his mouth..." John 19. | Burns; Cancer; Dysuria; Epilepsy; Flu; Measles; Nephrosis; Stomach-ache. |
| STYRAX BENZOIN Dryand "Onycha (Biblical)" (STORAX FAMILY) | "...Take unto thee sweet spices, stacte and onycha..." Exodus 30. | BRONCHITIS; Cancer; LARYNGI-TIS; Mastitis; Ringworm; Shingles. |
| STYRAX OFFICINALIS L "Stacte (storax)" (STORAX FAMILY) | "...Take unto thee sweet spices, stacte, and onycha, and gal-banum; these sweet spices with pure frankincense: of each shall there be a like weight: And thou shalt make it a perfume...." Exodus 30. | Arthritis; BRONCHITIS; Cancer; Cold; Hysteria; Sores; Spermator-rhea. |
| SUEDA SPP "Sea Blite" "Shahor"=Black (Hebrew)" "Ashhur" (Biblical) | "Ashhur" (Biblical) " Ashhur, the father of Tekoa, had two wives." I Chronicles 4:5. | |
| TAMARIX APHYLLA (L.) Karst "Tamarisk", "Grove (Biblical)" (TAMARISK FAMILY) | "...And Abraham planted a grove in Beer-sheba. .." Genesis 21. | Eczema; Infertility; Impotence; Ophthalmia; Psoriasis; Splenitis; Syphilis. |
| TARAXACUM OFFICINALE Weber ex Wigg. "Dandelion" (ASTER FAMILY) | "...eat it with unleavened bread and bitter herbs..." Numbers 9. | CANCER; DIABETES; HEPATI-TIS; Rheumatism; Sciatica. |
| TETRACLINIS ARTICULATA (Vahl) Masters " Sandarac", " Thyine (Biblical)" (CYPRESS FAMILY) | "...and all thyine wood, and all manner vessels of ivory..." Revelation 18. | Dermatitis; Migraine; Neckache. |
| TRIGONELLA FOENUM-GRAECUM L. "Fenugreek" "Leek (Biblical)" (LEGUME FAMILY) | "... We remember the fish...and the leeks..." Numbers 11. | Alopecia; DIABETES; DYSLACTEA; Dyspepsia; HYPERCHOLESTER-OLEMIA; Leukorrhea; MICROMAS-TIA; Pain; RHEUMATISM; Swelling. |
| TRITICUM AESTIVUM L. "Wheat" "Corn (Biblical)" (GRASS FAMILY) | "...And he slept and dreamed the second time: and, behold, seven ears of corn came up upon one stalk, rank and good..." Genesis 41. | Diarrhea; Leprosy; Menorrhagia; Neuras-thenia; Sunstroke; Syphilis; Tuberculosis. |
| TRITICUM SPELTA L. "Spelt" " Rie (Biblical)" (GRASS FAMILY) | "...But the wheat and the rie were not smitten...." Exodus 9. Aegilops. | |
| TULIPA MONTANA Lindl. "Mountain Tulip" (LILY FAMILY) | "The flowers appear on the earth, the time of singing has come, and the voice of the turtledove is heard in our land." Song of Solomon 2: 12. | |

# Figure A12. Cont. Biblical Herbs and Their Known Uses

| Herb Name(s)/Family | Biblical Reference | Uses/Indications |
|---|---|---|
| **TYPHA AUSTRALIS** Schum & Thonn. "Cattail", "Reed (Biblical)" (CATTAIL FAMILY) | "...and they smote him on the head with a reed... " Mark 15. | Epilepsy; Insanity; Tumors; Wounds. |
| URTICA DIOICA L. "Stinging Nettle", "Common Nettle", "Greater Nettle" (NETTLE FAMILY) | "...and thorns shall come up in her palaces, nettles and brambles in the fortresses thereof..." Isaiah 34. | ALLERGY; ARTHRITIS; HAY FE-VER; PROSTATITIS; RHEUMATISM. |

Courtesy of the University of Maryland Botany Department. Freely downloadable file available at http://www.inform.umd.edu/UMS+State/MD_Resources/DBFP/pictures/mdheader.gif">; See also: http://www.inform.umd.edu/PBIO/MEDICAL_BOTANY/module12c.html"><b><u>Next

### *TIME*ly Propaganda in the Herb Industry

Following millenniums of successful unregulated use of Godly herbal provisions, herbs have suddenly come under fire by governing officials worldwide. At the same time more and more regulations threaten consumer access to previously available beneficial herbs, as well as other nutritional supplements including vitamins and minerals, the entire herb industry is targeted for a worldwide pharmaceutical industry takeover. Could these occurrences be part of the larger conspiracy unearthed in this book?

Apparently so. In fact, this herbal matter provides an ideal multidisciplinary case study in the interrelated fields of mind control, mass mediated propaganda, and the eugenics agenda including population control and population reduction.

*TIME* magazine in a cover story entitled "The Herbal Medicine Boom" (November 23, 1998) provided a particularly deadly form of persuasive prose. Months before the report, Food and Drug Administration (FDA) and the World Health Organization (WHO) officials met behind closed doors to plan and actualize a German proposal to "standardize" herbs, vitamins, minerals and the like. The *TIME* article, along with similar features on CNN (September 1, 1998), and in *USA Today* (October 14, 1998), provided insidious cover for these mostly secret dealings. Instead of learning the truth, North Americans were inundated with messages designed to persuade them, and the nutritional supplement industry at large, that they would be far safer if leading pharmaceutical firms, most of them German, continued their international herb industry takeover.

The German proposal advanced what had been officially, and traditionally, called "Codex Alimentarious"—a fancy Latin phrase meaning the "standardization of nutritional supplements." The proposal, supportive to the monopolization practices of the Rockefellers, Rothshilds, and the British, was likewise supported by FDA chiefs. According to consumer activists, including John Hammel who represented the interests of the National Health Federation (NHF) and the Life Extension Foundation at the European meetings, the FDA fully intended to "harmonize" with the German-advanced WHO standards. Of course it was all promulgated in the names of "science" and "public health." Hammel returned from the Codex session, however, warning consumers to beware that these individuals and institutions had far less noble histories and motives. The "high-minded" efforts were rooted in a half-century-old plan to monopolize the world's drug and chemical cartels for direct control over large populations as discussed in earlier chapters.

*TIME*'s feature began by heralding the "flower power" of American baby boomers. The yuppies had created an herbal industry, staff writers said, selling more than $12 billion worth of nutritional supplements annually in the 1990s. Industry investors had witnessed a return on their investments of more than 15 percent. The gold rush had been buffeted by Americans who "today make more visits to nontraditional physicians, including naturopaths who *claim* [emphasis added] expertise in herbs and other natural therapies, than to their family doctors. And they spend almost as much out of pocket (not reimbursed by health insurance) on alternative medicine ($27 billion) as on all unreimbursed physician services ($29 billion)." Thus, *TIME* reported, major pharmaceutical companies were wise to enter the rapidly growing herb market.

The emphasis above was added to display the subtle use of language to deceive and persuade. Naturopaths only *claim* expertise whereas physicians *are* experts, or so *TIME* subtly implied. Perhaps its editors were ignorant of the fact that certified naturopaths *are experts in herbal healing*. Still, the slip displayed a bias that, at least, was subliminally deceptive. Are there no shysters or quacks among the medical deity—the M.D.s? And that's just the beginning.

"The frantic expansion of the market," *TIME* continued, came ". . . at some risk to consumers. These products are not regulated in the U.S. nearly as strictly as over-the-counter drugs or even foods—in sharp contrast to countries like Germany." *TIME*'s "experts" claimed that parts of the industry resembled "a Wild West boomtown, where some 800 lightly regulated U.S. companies" competed ferociously with "fly-by-night hucksters."

"Frantic expansion?" People routinely used and prescribed herbs for thousands of years. As shown in figure A12, dozens of botanicals had been successfully used throughout biblical history to treat a variety of maladies.

But *TIME* warned that "experts" were rightfully concerned. "'When you open a bottle of nutritional supplements, you don't know what's inside,' said Jeffrey Delafuente, a pharmacy professor at Virginia Commonwealth University in Richmond. 'There may be some ingredients not listed. You do not know how much active ingredient is in each tablet. They can make all kinds of claims that may not be accurate.'"

Was this not the case for pharmaceuticals as well? *TIME* made no mention of the fact that, despite public safety assurances, toxic ingredients contaminated many highly touted and trusted FDA approved vaccines. For example, since the 1960s to the time of this writing, the FDA had turned a blind eye to as many as 100 cancer-causing monkey viruses per dose of licensed oral polio vaccines (OPV)—a vaccine said to be "required" despite the availability of religious exemptions in forty-eight states.

Most people would be shocked to learn the contents of, and inconsistencies in, virtually all vaccines. Take for instance the chicken pox vaccine produced by Merck, Sharp & Dohme that was heavily marketed in 1998. Baby boomers' memories of chicken pox were missing a week or two of school, staying home, and watching cartoons. Beginning in 1998, with the licensing of the risky chicken pox vaccine, people were repeatedly told how dangerous chicken pox was, and how Merck's vaccine was highly recommended if not urgently needed by children. Parents remained clueless regarding the contents of this vaccine: monosodium glutamate, mercury, aluminum, and formaldehyde derivatives for "stability" and "sterility;" herpes viruses that may have included, besides the chicken pox virus,

502

other strains, as well as "foreign RNA and DNA"—a pleasant way of saying "carcinogens or mutagens whose origins are not entirely known."

And what about the costly and highly toxic cancer and AIDS drugs that were routinely placed on the "fast track" for testing and approval? Had consumers been made aware of the ingredients and risks in these routinely prescribed and severely toxic pharmaceuticals?

Herb consumers were mostly moved, said *TIME*, by their desire to "seize control of their medical destinies. The perceived coldness and remoteness of conventional medicine and red-tape-tangled managed care." *TIME* failed to mention the more than one million north Americans who are killed, or irreversibly maimed, each year by pharmaceutical side effects or mistaken prescriptions.

Still, "some unwary consumers, though, have been getting hurt" by herbs, *TIME* revealed. One woman experienced a "painful burning" in her skin triggered by St. John's wort taken to combat her depression. "The woman's distress points up the danger of taking herbs without considering the side effects or gauging other risks," the authors warned. "Last year a tea made from the Chinese kombucha mushroom that was promoted as a remedy for cancer caused four people to be hospitalized for conditions ranging from jaundice to headaches and nausea." Overwhelming reason to have the FDA regulate the entire herb industry?

"Placebo effect" is really at the root of symptom relief in many herbally deceived yuppies, *TIME* reported. "Last week the *Archives of Family Medicine*, a sister publication of *JAMA*, reported a study suggesting that echinacea was no better at preventing colds than a placebo (a pill with no active ingredients). But the researchers conceded that their sample size, 302 volunteers, may have been too small to detect modest differences and concluded that more study was needed."

Deceptive propaganda! The vast majority of people who take echinacea for sinus congestion experience substantial relief for hours without the toxic side effects commonly associated with prescribed and over-the-counter antihistamines. *TIME* failed to mention this but admitted, "The researchers didn't test whether echinacea alleviates colds already in progress."

"The history of diet supplements is rife with fads that fizzled or proved dangerous to health," *TIME* recalled. That's part of the reason why "physicians have legitimate concerns about the safety, efficacy and potential misuse of the herbal products that their patients are snapping up. . . .doctors tend to be more demanding of proof. Or as Dr. Yank Coble of the American Medical Association puts it, 'In God we trust.' All others must have data."

Right on! Thank God for the wary nature of the AMA. The organization whose doctors routinely recommended cigarette smoking, thalidomide, silicone breast implants, and today ritalin and aspartame.

As in the related *USA Today* herbal expose, *TIME* placed their "precautions" adjacent beautiful colored photographs of the "natural" substances in question. "Don't assume that 'natural' means safe," they said, "unless you want to risk ending up like Socrates, who committed suicide by drinking hemlock. More recently," they added, "folks have suffered liver damage from sipping teas brewed from comfrey, an herb that is used in poultices and ointments to treat sprains and bruises and should never be taken internally."

Special warnings were distributed throughout these pieces of yellow press. Hypertensives were cautioned against using ginseng. Men with enlarged prostates were warned against using saw palmetto due to the occurrence of "rare stomach problems." Several notices were placed for pregnant and nursing women. Even garlic should "not be used while nursing," *TIME* reported. Had these authors known this previously they would have alerted nursing mothers to avoid eating at Italian restaurants!

All of this effort, however, served a higher purpose—to inform us of the great disservice leaders of the nutritional supplement industry had done. How they dared defend consumers unfettered access to vitamins, minerals, herbs, and health foods. "Since Republican Senator

Orrin Hatch of Utah rammed through the 1994 Dietary Supplement Act—with the enthusiastic support of a supplement industry largely based in his state—herbs and other supplements have been all but exempt from federal oversight," *TIME* chided begrudgingly, then said it was time to put a stop to such reprehensible special interest group behavior.

## The German Herbal Alternative

The German model for standardizing the nutritional supplement industry, surprise, surprise, heavily favored the WHO's developing Codex Alimentarious legislation, much to the glee of the Rockefeller and German-led pharmaceutical barons. Quite matter of factly, *TIME* revealed that, "This week the U.S. Pharmacopeia, a nonprofit organization, published the first American standards for the potency of nine herbs, including chamomile, feverfew, St. John's wort and saw palmetto. Manufacturers that adhere to those standards can add the letters NF, for national formulary, to their labels."

And who was most apt to conduct research and standardize their herbs according to *TIME*? Why of course, only the "trusted brands like Bayer . . . and well known companies such as Warner-Lambert [makers of] (Sudafed, Benadryl and Listerine) . . . [and] SmithKline Beecham (Tagamet HB, Contac, NicoDerm CQ) . . . The entry of these brands," *TIME* assured, "and the growing body of serious research on herbal remedies are lifting some of the stigma attached to these products—and cutting through some of the claptrap one can still hear about mystical recoveries in many a juice bar or organic grocery."

Bayer? A "trusted" company? As a parent to the infamous IG Faben company—partnered with the Rockefeller Standard Oil Company and Hitler's Third Reich, Bayer's highest officials were also top commanding officers in the Nazi SS. Such men were entrusted with the knowledge that concentration camp showers rained Zyclone B gas over millions of unwitting holocaust victims. The German mega-corporation held the patent on this genocidal product and made fortunes

# Figure A13. CFR Members in the Media

*Air Force Times/Army Times/ Defense News/Federal Times/Navy Times* (Marine Corps Edition)/ *Military Market/ Space Times*
    Vice President and Executive Editor James S. Doyle

**American Journal** (Radio)
    Senion Supervising Producer Dennis O' Brian

*American Journalism Review*
    Contributing Editor Hodding Carter III
    Contributing Editor Henry Catto

*American Purpose*
    Editor George Weigel

*American Specatator*
    Editor-n-Chief R. Emmett Tyrrell Jr.
    Board Member Midge Decter
    Board Member Jeane J. Kirkpatrick

*The Anniston Star*
    Editor, Publisher Henry Brandt Ayers

**Associated Press**
    Vice President Claude Erbsen

*The Atlantic Monthly*
    President and Chairman of the Board Mortimer B. Zuckerman
    Contributing Editor Thomas Powers

*Business and Society Review*
    Editor and Publisher Theodore Cross

*Business Week*
    Editor-in-Chief Stephen B. Shepard
    Editorial Pge Editor Bruce Nussbaum

*The Capital*
    Publisher Phillip Merrill

**Capital Cities/ABC Inc.**
    (Corporate Member)Chairman and CEO Thomas S. Murphy
    Directors:
      • Robert P. Bauman
      • Nicholas F. Brady
    ABC-TV President Roone Ariedge
    *This Week* Host David Brinkley
    ABC-TV Anchor Diane Sawyer
    ABC-TV Anchor Barbara Walters

*Chicago Tribune*
    NY Bureau Chief Lisa Anderson

*Christian Science Monitor*
    Columnist (Robert) John Hughes

*Commentary*
    Editor-at-Large Norman Podhoretz

**Corportion for Public Broadcasting**
    *NewsHour* Executive Editor, Anchor James C. Lehrer
    *NewsHour* Program Director Susan Mills
    *NewsHour* Senior Producer for Foreign Affairs Michael David Moesettig
    *NewsHour* National Correspondent Charlayne Hunter-Gault
    *Firing Line* Host William F. Buckley Jr.
    *The McLaughlin Group* Panelist Morton Kondracke
    *Washington Week in Review* Panelists:
      • Thomas L. Friedman
      • Georgie Anne Geyer
      • Jack Nelson
    Maryland Public Television *To the Contrary* Panelists:
      • Lynn Martin
      • Eleanor Holmes Norton
      • *Frontline Station* WGBH-TV Producer June Victoria Cross
    Children's Television Workshop Chairman David Van Buren Britt

*Culturefront*
    Edtorial Advisory Board Members:
      • Linda Chavez
      • Nathan Glazer
      • Ronald Steel

*Dallas Morning News*
    International Affairs Correspondent James Landers
    Editorial Page Editor Rena Pederson

**Dow Jones And Co. (Corporate Member)**
    President of Dow Jones International Group Karen Elliott House
    *Wall Street Journal*
      Chairman and CEO Peter R. Kann
      Managing Editor Paul E. Steiger
      Editorial Page Editor Robert L. Bartley
      Foreign Editor John Bussey
      Staff Reporter Robert S. Greenberger
      Deputy Editor Daiel Henninger (cont.)
    *Wall Street Journal* (cont.)
      Weekend Editor Lee Lescaze
      Deputy Editor George Mellcan
      Staff Reporter Carla Robbins
      Political Coordinator Gerald F. Selb
      Editorial Board Amity Shales
      Contributing Editor Mark Helprin

Adapted from: "Shadows across the land: Current CFR dominance over government, foundations, media, and industry." In: *Conspiracy for Global Control—Special Report. The New American.* Gary Benoit, ed., 1997, pp. 15-16.

*Wall Street Journal* - Europe, Managing
Editor Fredrick Schumann Kempe

**The Farm Journal**
Washington Editor Sonja Hillgren

*Forbes*
Chairman Casper W. Wenberger
Reporter Justin Doebele

*Foreign Affairs*
Editor James F. Hoge Jr.
Publications Director David Kellogg

*Foreign Policy*
Editor Charles William Maynes
Associate Editor Thomas Omestad

**Freedom Review**
Publisher Adrian Karatnycky

**Gannett Company Inc.**
Board Member Andrew F. Brimmer
Gannett News Service Washington
Correspondent Wendy Margaret Koch

*Global Oil Stocks & Balances/*
*Petroleum Intelligence Weekly*
Publisher Edward L. Morse

*Harper's Magazine*
Editor Lews H. Lapham
Contributing Editor David Rieff

*Harvard Business Review*
Senior Editor Nancy Nichols

**Hearst Book Group**
President and CEO Howard Kaminsky

*Hispanic* (magazine)
Editor and Publisher Alfredo J. Estrada

**National Empowerment Television**
Freedom's Challenge Host
Paula Jon Dobrinasky

*Industry Week*
Contributing Editor Richard Osborne

*Institutional Investor*
Founder and Chairman Emeritus
Gilbert E. Kaplan

*The Nation*
Editor Katrina vanden Heuvel
Music Editor Edward Said

*The National Interest*
Publisher Irving Kristol

*National Journal*
Contributing Editor William Schneider
Contributing Editor Bruce Stokes

*National Review*
Editor-at-Large William F. Buckley
President Thomas L. Rhodes
Senior Editor Peter W. Rodman
Contributing Editor Eliot Abrams
Contributing Editor Eliot A. Cohen
Contributing Editor Vin Weber

**NBC TV**
Anchor and Managing Editor Tom Brokaw
Chief Economics Correspondent
Irving R. Levine

**New Media Time Inc.**
Editor Walter Seff Isaacson

*The New Republic*
Senior Editor Michael Lind
Contributing Editor Eliot A. Cohen
Contributing Editor Jacob Hellbrunn
Contributing Editor Charles Krauthammer
Contributing Editor Ronald Steel
Literary Editor Leon Wieseltier

*Newsday*
Editorial Page Editor James M. Klurfeld

*New York Daily News*
Chairman and Co-Publisher
Mortimer B. Zuckerman

*New York Review of Books*
Editor Robert B. Silvers
Contributor Joan Didion

**The New York Times Company**
Board Members:
• Richard L. Gelb
• George B. Munroe
• Donald M. Stewart
• Cyrus R. Vance
*New York Times*:
Executive Editor Joseph Lelyveld
Asst. Managing Editor Warren Hoge
Asst. Managing Editor Jack Rosenthal
Editorial Board David Unger
Editorial Board Karl E. Meyer
Editorial Board Michael Weinstein
Editorial Board Steven R. Weisman
Editorial Page Board James L. Greenfield
Associate Editorial Page Editor
Robert B. Semple, Jr.
Opinion Page Columnist
Thomas L. Friedman
Columnist Anthony Lewis
Columnist Flora Lewis
Columnist A.M. Rosenthal
UN Bureau Chief Barbara Crossettte
Police Bureau Chief Clifford Krauss
*Boston Globe* Editorial Page Editor
H.D.S. Greenway

**News America Publishing Inc.**
Chairman Rupert Murdock
*New York Post* Editorial Page Editor
Eric Breindel

507

from its use in "showers" taken allegedly, like vaccines are today, for "public health" and "disinfection."

More recently, Bayer was entrusted to supply American hemophiliacs with freeze dried blood clotting factor VIII. Unfortunately they knew it had become contaminated with the AIDS virus (HIV). They distributed it anyway. The known contamination led to the expected deaths of several hundred hemophiliacs. The rest of the 10,000 hemophiliacs were premeditatively killed by the Rockefeller controlled blood bankers who knew that between 1980 and 1986 their HIV contaminated blood supplies would deliver AIDS to unwitting thousands.

As mentioned earlier in this book, according to CBS News correspondent Paul Manning in *Martin Bormann: Nazi in Exile* (Lyle Stuart Inc., 1981) the Rockefeller Standard Oil company and its partner, I.G. Farben, invested huge sums of money from the Nazi war chest to help actualize Hitler's proclaimed "vision of a thousand-year Third Reich [and] world empire. Remember this next time you swallow Bayer aspirin or such*TIME*ly propaganda.

*TIME* also mentioned SmithKline Beecham as another "trusted" company. Its editors, we suppose, hadn't received word of the class action lawsuit filed in 1998 against the company on behalf of multiple sclerosis victims—people immunologically and neurologically impaired by SmithKline's hepatitis B vaccine. As a result of the evidence compiled during the litigation, French public health officials suspended all hepatitis B inoculations of children in that country. That, however, didn't stop U.S. government "requirements" of the vaccine for infants.

Sure, you can trust Warner-Lambert too said *TIME*, whose parent company, Time Warner, Inc., is just coincidentally related, and whose president, Richard D. Parsons, and Gerald M. Levin—the Chairman, President and CEO of Time Warner Entertainment Company, and Norman Pearlstine—*TIME*'s Editor-in Chief, and Henry Miller—*TIME*'s Editorial Director, and many more *TIME* relatives are esteemed members of the Council on Foreign Relations (CFR). (See figure A13.)

Indeed the *TIME* is right to trust German, British, and other shadow governors who are far stricter regulators than the United States and Canadian governments regarding public access to herbs. Perhaps North Americans should all move to Europe as well to be spared the risk of exposure to unstandardized herbs; to safely retreat from the nutritional "hucksters." Maybe *TIME* magazine directors should move there as well. But then again, maybe they already have.

## Advancing Research in Herbology and Naturopathy

Chapter 6 provided the Pythagorean skein number equivalents for common herbs and diseases. Based on the mathematical and spiritual revelations contained in this book's earlier chapters, this practice, though potentially sound in theory, raises important questions for research and challenges in clinical practice.

This system, for instance, while providing a generic guide for diagnosis and treatment, a basis for further research, and additional justification for naturopathic approaches to healing, is not definitive. Traditionally, naturopathic diagnostic and therapeutic applications have demanded practitioners' knowledge, skills, and intuitive sensitivities. Intuition, of course, is largely a spiritual function. This will become increasingly, not decreasingly, more important in light of these findings.

When the authors, for example, attempted to assign number values to the array of essential oils, that, like herbs, carry unique electromagnetic frequencies, difficulties arose. They realized that oils may be referred to by more than one name, including Latin and English versions. When their number equivalents were deciphered, different names provided dissimilar values. This necessitated applying kinesiology and/or radionic techniques in an effort to determine the correct numbers. As with the use of divining rods to locate water wells, radionics relies heavily on electromagnetic, intuitive, and/or spiritual forces to correctly identify the numerical equivalent. Even then, empirical research was required to assess the validity of each oil in the treatment of similarly numbered diseases. At the time of this writing, this research is ongoing.

## Implications for Litigation, Prevention and Health Freedom

In recent years at least three organizations have evolved in the United States in defense of alternative health professionals persecuted by government agencies, especially the Food and Drug Administration (FDA), aided by states attorneys general. Recent prosecutions have involved professionals administering proven oxygenation and bioelectric therapies. Organizations including the World Naturopathic Health Organization (WNHO), and JuriMed—a research and public relations firm that provides "strategies for government-besieged health professionals," have traditionally advanced the defense that oxygenation and bioelectric therapies have been adequately proven safe and effective by early research and mountains of anecdotal reports. State attorney generals have countered and have commonly won cases against practitioners of these therapes with paid "expert witnesses" who charged the defendants with "quackery," and alleged a dearth of sound scientific evidence supporting these "alternative" therapies. With the publication of this book such charades of justice should immediately cease. It is now very clear that electromagnetic and oxygenation therapies fall into the realm of religious observance and spiritual healing. The documentation for this cease and desist warrant comes directly from the authorized King James Bible in the form of the electromagnetic codes in Numbers, Chapter 7.

In essence, so long as governments are obliged to recognize the rapidly diminishing "seperation of church and state," government agents have no right to persecute, under the auspicies of legal prosecution, spiritual/religious observers—health professionals or lay persons who respect the contents of the King James Bible, or the Torah, including the most sacred electromagnetic frequencies published therein.

Freeing health professionals and scientists to practice and investigate such spiritual healing applications should greatly contribute to research and the accumulation of data in several fields of energy medicine. These include acupuncture, homeopathy, herbology, aroma therapy, essential oils, oxygenation, cluster water hydration, biomagnetics, and bioelectric therapies.

Oxygenation, though less obviously a spiritual healing practice, upon closer scrutiny clearly pertains. As discussed in the foreword of this book, oxygen is central to spiritual development and evolution. The Hebrew term for God is "Ya Vah" which means "to breathe is to exist." Many ancient names like Iss*iah*, Ab*rah*am, and Dr. Horowitz's Hebrew name Ar*yah* include God's name. The greetings alo*ha*, in Hawaiian, and *ah*sala*am* in Arabic cultures, similarly declares God's presence. The "prana*[h]*" in Eastern religions, that is, the energy of life, is carried by oxygen and inspired by deep abdominal breathing. The sound made during a belly laugh—"Ha h*ah*," or hearty yawn— "Ha*ah*h," likewise replenishes the lungs, blood, and spirit, and is bioelectrically contagious. God's "covenant" (the word is derived from the Hebrew word "bereat" which means to cut), in fact, implies the shedding of blood and oxygen. Genesis 2:7 says, "God formed a person . . . and breathed into his nostrils the breath of life, so that he became a living being." Thus, like God's grace, forever given, oxygen literally inspires life. The spiritual importance of oxygen is affirmed in all of these ways.

So, besides mounting scientific evidence supporting oxygenation therapies to clean the blood of infectious agents, reduce cell death, and retard aging, it must be first and foremost looked upon as a spiritual healing practice.

## Mixed Reviews From Christians

Though the vast majority of Christians who reviewed the limited edition first printing of this book praised the effort, a few so called "fundamentalist" Christians wrote or called the authors of this work to complain. Two people who purchased the book, for example, demanded refunds stating the authors were obviously "satanic." Kinder Christians took time from their busy schedules to write loving letters that articulated their concerns. One such reader wrote:

> When I read your message regarding musical sounds, waves, vibrations, etc., I became concerned. Not because this might not be true. I believe this could very well be true. I have known, for many years, that certain musical tones can produce certain behaviors in humans and in animals. This is one of the things I teach to teenagers about rock and roll music and its beat and New Age music with its lack of rhythm and/or continuing pattern of sounds and tones. Since Satan was the heavenly choir director before his fall. . . I consider he certainly knows how to use music to keep people, especially teens, in a trance . . . if you know what I mean.

> I also know a little about different groups using music or chanting to call upon the demonic world. Many of them do not realize they are doing this, but they certainly are. Take for example the beating of the drums in Africa, Haiti, or Jamaica. . . . Others who are known for their chanting-type of music are the Krishnas, Hindus, Catholics, New Agers, psychics, witches, etc. I was a psychic/New Ager (into witchcraft) and a Catholic before becoming a Born-again Christian. I remember chanting: sounds, tones and words I used to call up demons. (It sounded much like the "speaking in tongues" that some people do today.) I remember their effect on me and those around me. I also remember a movie I saw years ago—'Close Encounters'—Remember the tones?

> Yes, I would say, there is validity to what you have stated and what your colleagues have written. But here is my point: I can't find this message anywhere in the Word of God! Nothing about sounds, tones, vibrations, secret numbers for healing, chanting, etc. I actually find just the opposite. We aren't even to pray repetitious prayers. Must be annoying to the Lord! They're certainly not what He wants to hear.

> The Masons might know about this, but hey, they worship Lucifer. I know about that also . . . my family is all tied up in the Masonic Lodge and Shriners. . . .

Maybe there is some sort of code in the Word. Mathematically, I know there is a code and possibly there is a correlation between mathematics and sounds or tones. However, is that what the Lord wants from His children? Are we to search for magical tones or numbers to be healed of a disease? Or will that tone heal us anymore than a good dose of echinacea or goldenseal? Aren't we just searching for straws, when it is the Lord who is allowing all this to come to pass anyway? . . . .

I realize that you are doing great work. I understand your zeal. I can understand your frustrations as you watch what these wicked people are doing by spreading disease. But please . . . keep all of this in perspective. Realize that the Lord Jesus Christ knows what they are doing. Our Lord must be feared and placed first in our lives. . . then, we do not need to fear what man can do to us. . . by disease or any other way. We don't need to chant some sort of musical notes to chase the diseases away! God parted the Red Sea. . . Can He not kill a virus or bacteria? . . .

Such concerns were echoed by many "Christians" to whom Dr. Horowitz wrote and suggested they examine their "spiritual ignorance" as explained in 1 Corinthians 2:6-16. These verses, intimately related to the truth offered in this book, and the love of the authors' labors, stated:

Yet there is a wisdom that we are speaking to those who are mature enough for it. But it is not the wisdom of this world, or of this world's leaders, who are in the process of passing away. On the contrary, we are communicating a secret wisdom from God which has been hidden until now which, before history began, God had decreed would bring us glory. Not one of this world's leaders has understood it; because if they had, they would not have executed the Lord from whom this glory flows. But, as the *Tanakh* says,

**"No eye has seen, no ear has heard**
**and no one's heart has imaged**
**all the things that God has prepared**
**for those who love him."**

It is to us, however, that God has revealed these things. How? Through the Spirit. For the Spirit probes all things, even the most profound depths of God. For who knows the inner workings of a person except the person's own spirit inside him? So too no one knows the inner workings of God except God's Spirit. Now we have not received the spirit of the world but the Spirit of God, so that we might understand the things God has so freely given us. These are the things we are talking about when we avoid the manner of speaking that human wisdom would dictate and instead use a manner of speaking taught by the Spirit, by which we explain things of the Spirit to people who have the Spirit. Now the natural man does not receive the things from the Spirit of God — to him they are nonsense! Moreover, he is unable to grasp them . . . But the person who has the Spirit can evaluate everything . . . .

As for me, brothers, I couldn't talk to you as spiritual people but as worldly people, as babies, so far as experience with the Messiah is concerned. I gave you milk, not solid food, because you were not yet ready for it. But you aren't ready for it now either! For you are still worldly! Isn't it obvious from all the jealousy and quarrelling among you that you are worldly and living by merely human standards? . . .

Christ's own teachings, therefore, speak of a level of spiritual deprivation that Joey had described in relation to "matrices of thought" in the early chapters of this book. This work, the authors argue, is of the Spirit of Yeshua. Those without eyes to see or ears to hear the Spirit of this book, and the blessings in its revelations, are much like those counseled in 1 Corinthians. Unfortunately, too many fall into this "human" or "worldly" trap—a trap that includes the "human" *interpretation of scripture* that is vulnerable to human fears, frailties, and spiritually limiting beliefs and attitudes, including those that lead to "jealousy and quarrelling among you that . . . are worldly and living by merely human standards."

The above letter's reference to African, Haitian, and Jamaican music speaks to this divisive human, not Spiritual, mentality. Certain forms of music may be unGodly or spiritually disruptive. This, however, further supports the need for more information and research in this field, not less human inquiry due to professed "Christian" beliefs.

Furthermore, highly relevant to the musical tones, their spiritual meaning and impact, prophetic nature of this work, and the "speaking in tongues" to which this letter referred, 1 Corinthians (13:11;14:1-12) continued:

> When I was a child, I spoke like a child,
> thought like a child, argued like a child;
> now that I have become a man,
> I have finished with childish ways. . . .

> [K]eep on eagerly seeking the things of the Spirit; and especially seek to be able to prophesy. For someone speaking in a tongue is not speaking to people but to God, because no one can understand, since he is uttering mysteries in the power of the Spirit. But someone prophesying is speaking to people, edifying, encouraging, and comforting them. A person speaking in a tongue does edify himself, but a person prophesying edifies the congregation. I wish you would all speak in tongues, but even more I wish you would all prophesy. The person who prophesies is greater than the person who speaks in tongues, unless someone gives an interpretation, so that the congregation can be edified.

> Brothers, suppose I come to you now speaking in tongues. How can I be of benefit to you unless I bring you some revelation or knowledge or prophecy or teaching? Even with lifeless musical instruments, such as a flute or a harp, how will anyone recognize the melody if one note can't be distinguished from another? And if the bugle gives an unclear sound, who will get ready for battle? It's the same with you: how will anyone know what you are saying unless you use your tongue to produce intelligible speech? You will be talking to the air!

> There are undoubtedly all kinds of sounds in the world, and none is altogether meaningless; but if I don't know what a person's sounds mean, I will be a foreigner to the speaker and the speaker will be a foreigner to me. Likewise with you: since you eagerly seek the things of the Spirit, seek especially what will help in edifying [defined as "to instruct or improve in spiritual knowledge"] the congregation."

Let it be known that this is precisely what this book was written to convey—an edification of the congregation. Providing the meaning of God's sounds for the ignorant masses, so that they may once again be heard, intelligible, spiritually uplifting, and globally healing!

Speech, tones, sounds, music, the vibratory essence of Spirit, its mathematics and frequencies, are all most vital areas of growing knowledge during this revolutionary period in human history. Spiritual evolution *is* the Divine focus of this book! Delivering this critical knowledge to the Spiritually mature masses, then empowering those enlightened to act on this wisdom, holds the power to rectify the primary problem that has plagued humanity since the "Tower of Babel." Society fell victim to manipulations by a few evil men who successfully divided the "sheeple" from each other, and from God, by dispensing foreign *dialects*. Thereafter, humanity largely ceased speaking Spiritually uplifting syllables. We were thus immediately cut off from the free flow of Divine love God endlessly bestows. We need to be speaking God's language in harmony once again.

An alternative Christian response to this book came from a leading nutritionist, Valerie Saxion, Ph.D., an avid Bible student. She also proclaimed herself a "fundamentalist." In support of this work, and in reply to the above letter, Dr. Saxion wrote:

> I understand your concern, however I believe it would be wise to read the entire book with an open heart before passing judgment. Perhaps Drs. Horowitz and Puleo are ahead of their time, as most great men are! Truth before its time is often interpreted as heresy!!!

> New truths are often hard to swallow. I'm reminded of my great Aunt Hazel who when I was a child insisted that TV was of the devil and refused to have one in her home. Recently, I visited her. She not only had a very large TV, but sang the praises of Christian programming as her source of hearing the wonderful word of God since she is not getting out to church like she used to.

> Unfortunately, this is the attitude many had concerning television in the early days. I believe this is the reason the airwaves are filled with many undesirable programs. Christians should have been the head and not the tail in the industry. We are to be the ones coming out with new technology and using it to the glory of God.

Consider Daniel 12:4, God told Daniel to seal the book to the end of time. (One thing we all agree, we're at the end of time.) He said knowledge shall be increased.

Knowledge is truly being increased daily in every area. Just look how we're communicating. A hundred years ago this couldn't even be imagined.

Remember, Satan is the creator of nothing. Yes, he was created by God to lead praise and worship in heaven. However, that doesn't make him the creator of it. God clearly states, "He inhabits the praises of His people," no matter what background, color, or quality of voice. God looks at the heart and moves in on the scene when His people praise Him. Whether that be with our voice, an instrument, or giving Him glory for the great things He has done. God's presence brings wisdom, revelation, and healing.

Drs. Horowitz and Puleo's work helped opened my eyes to how Jesus Himself healed in many different ways. He laid hands on the man full of leprosy (Mt. 2:3), and the man was made clean. In Luke 6:8 the man with the withered hand was healed on the Sabbath when Jesus spoke the word. Luke 7:12 says Jesus was moved with compassion and the widows son was raised from the dead. In Luke 8:49 Jesus said to fear not, only believe, and healing came forth. In Matthew 14:36, all those that touched the hem of His garment were made whole. Mark 7:32-33, Jesus put His fingers in the deaf man's ears and spit and touched his tongue (QUITE RADICAL) and immediately he was healed. Mark 8:23 is an awesome creative miracle when Jesus spit on the blind man's eyes and a creative miracle took place.

Jesus healed multitudes in many ways, and the healing didn't stop in Jesus' ministry. In Acts 5:15 the sick were brought out so that Peter's shadow might pass by them, and they were healed. Acts 19:11-12 talks about special miracles when Paul sent handkerchiefs to the diseased, and possessed, and they were delivered.

In the book by the great Christian healer, *John G. Lake: His Life, His Sermons, His Boldness of Faith*, Minister Lake revealed, as Drs. Horowitz and Puleo argue, that "Atonement through the grace of God is scientific in its application. Jesus used many methods of healing the sick. All were scientific. According to Lake, "Science is the discovery of how God does things."

Minister Lake's book further recalled:

Jesus laid His hands upon the sick in obedience to the law of contact and transmission. Contact of His hands with the sick one permitted the Spirit of God in Him to flow into the sick person.

The sick woman who touched His clothes found that the Spirit emanated from His person. "She touched the hem of his garment [Matthew 9:20] and the Spirit flashed into her. She was made whole." This is a scientific process.

Paul, knowing this law, laid his hands upon handkerchiefs and aprons. . . . The Spirit of God emanating from Paul transformed the handkerchiefs into storage batteries of Holy Spirit power. When they were laid upon the sick they surcharged the body, and healing was the result. (Read Acts 19:12.)

This demonstrates, firstly: The Spirit of God is a tangible substance, a heavenly materiality. Secondly: It is capable of being stored in the substance of cloth as demonstrated in the garments of Jesus or the handkerchiefs of Paul. Thirdly: It will transmit power . . . His love and power in them redeems them from sin and sickness . . . and establishes the kingdom of Heaven."

*Healing Codes for the Biological Apocalypse* relays much of the science behind this healing Spirit in those who serve God.

Dr. Saxion continued:

God is the same yesterday, today, and forever. God is still doing special miracles through His people.

However, Mark 6:5-6 says Jesus could do no mighty works because of their unbelief. Obviously, faith in God moves the hand of God on our behalf in whatever way He chooses.

It is the traditions of men that make the word of God of no effect. Let us not limit God with our traditions. God is as big as our hunger is!

Praise God, His mercy always overrides judgment, or where would any of us be!

Other pertinent Bible verses that support this book include Psalms 40:3—"He hath put a new song in my mouth, even praise unto our God, many shall see it and fear and shall trust in the Lord"; and Psalms 96:1—"Oh sing unto the Lord a NEW SONG, sing unto the Lord all the Earth."

Regarding concerns that "chanting" is not of God, or in the Bible, a review of Revelation 4:8-9 shows that four beasts—God's angels— did not rest day or night saying, "Holy, Holy, Holy, Lord God Almighty, which was, and is, and is to come." This is repeated, some might say chanted, like a mantra, throughout eternity.

"So back we go to the Lord's prayer," Dr. Saxion concluded. "If it's in heaven its for the Earth! *Healing Codes for the Biological Apocalypse* reveals and discusses God's heavenly tones that need to be known, further investigated, and used here and now on Earth during this most amazing and critical time in history."

## Returning King Solomon's Greatest Treasure

When Dr. Horowitz, whose Hebrew name is Aryah-ben-Schlomo-ha-Levi, which translated means Lion of God, son of Solomon, the Levi, was a child, his mother, a holocaust survivor, told him,"You should be proud. You are of royal blood." She explained that Len's father, grandfather, great grandfather, and earlier ancestors were all "sons of Solomon" dating back to King Solomon. To be the "son of Solomon," and a Levi, meant that one of Dr. Horowitz's ancient grandfathers, from the tribe of Judah, likely married out of his tribe—a Levi priest's daughter. Not being royally wealthy, he never thought about it again until he began to edit Chapter 3 of this book.

While reviewing the text on King James and the Templars insurgence into the Holy Land to steal the gold, Ark of the Covenant, and ancient arcana from King Solomon's Temple, his mother's early words returned. It occurred to him that his great Levi priest ancestors initially hid these powerful codes in the Bible. Later, the Knights Templar stole the same from beneath the Temple built by his royal ancestor, Solomon, as a tribute to God. Soon thereafter, the knowledge was used by the Illuminati to manipulate the masses along with world financial markets. By so doing, the Templars stole this sacred treasure directly from Dr. Horowitz's family in the Dividian blood line, from God, and from God's people. In essence, it occurred to him that with this book's publication, he was fulfilling a unique calling to return this sacred hidden and later stolen knowledge to God's people on God's behalf.

Realizing all of this, it dawned on him why he had been Divinely guided to meet and work with Dr. Puleo, and complete this unique effort. It also explained the Spiritual guidance the two men received while rapidly completing this book.

Dr. Puleo's transition into this service was detailed in the preface and earliest chapters of this book. For Dr. Horowitz, this unique calling began, most noticeably, in 1990 when he began to investigate the infamous Florida dentist, Dr. David Acer, known to have infected six patients with the AIDS virus. Following the publication of his ninth book, *Deadly Innocence*, that documented this investigation, he was spiritually directed to study the origins of AIDS and Ebola viruses as detailed in his 1997 publication, his first best-seller, *Emerging Viruses: AIDS & Ebola—Nature, Accident or Intentional?*

Since revealing the most horrific facts concerning the manufacture, and vaccine transmission, of numerous immune–system–destroying microorganisms, Dr. Horowitz had frequently prayed to God to reveal the Achilles heal of the Illuminati. He frequently recalled the story of King David and Goliath. He remembered how Solomon's brave father felled the Hebrews' greatest nemesis with one small stone shot directly at Goliath's forebrain. "Dear God, give me the Achilles heal. There has got to be an Achilles heal!" he prayed.

In response to his prayers, Len was directed to move his family to Sandpoint, Idaho to work with Dr. Puleo. As a result, this text strikes a central nerve of the Illuminati.

To the extent that this text helps fulfill Len's destiny, it is destined to serve humanity's Spiritual evolution similarly. This effort returns a major part of the ancient arcana to its rightful owner(s)—God's loving masses. In so doing, this work bears witness to God's direction, the power of His word, and the fulfillment of Bible prophecy. It heralds the dawning of a new and far more Godly age.

Human efforts are currently underway to further investigate the codes discussed herein and their practical applications. Divine efforts are concurrently underway to assemble the force of 144,000 people who will be empowered by this knowledge, and God's calling, to sing in the coming New Age of Atonement for a millennium of world peace. This *is* our destiny.

# Acknowledgments

Drs. Puleo and Horowitz are extremely grateful to the following people who provided so much, and asked for so little, in contributing to this work: Dr. James Dussualt, President of the World Natural Health Organization, for his encouragement and support for this research; Mike and Phyllis Stene, for their donations, kindness, and spiritual support for Dr Puleo's clinical research and patient care requirements; Marvin and Annette Berning for their generous donations and physical help with numerous related projects: Bill Coombs, Vice President of Sunshine Co. Electronics, for donating his experimental equipment to Dr. Puleo's clinic along with his technical expertise; Steve Youngdahl, President of the Sandpoint Mortgage Company for his careful eye in helping to edit and assemble earlier manuscripts upon which this work is based; Don Harkins, Editor of The Idaho Observer, for his steadfast support for this work as well as his numerous contributions to the final edited manuscript; to Steve Moreland for his assistance, encouragement, and research efforts; Mike Fitzpatrick for his faith, contributions, and activity along with Tom Kooyman in helping to assemble "those who have eyes to see and ears to hear," Errol Owen for bringing Drs. Horowitz and Puleo together, and always being there to lend a helping hand; to Dan Anderson for his advice, encouragement, and leadership; to the dozens of people throughout the world—our intelligence network—who sent valuable articles, emails, tapes, and books which contributed greatly to this work, as well to the dozens of other well- wishers who offered suggestions; and to our colleagues of kindred spirits who are likewise laboring to improve healthcare.

# Index

# Index

# Index

# Index

Rudin, Ernst, 98, 228, 229, 230
Russell, Bertrand, 231
Russian Academy of Science's Englehardt
    Institute, 359
Ryan, Clarence, 354
Ryter, Jon Christian, 438


## S

Salk Institute, 241
Salmonella, 327, 328
Sanders, Carl W., 361
Sandpoint, 9, 10, 150, 154, 178, 203, 204,
    205, 336, 513, 515
Sanger, Margaret, 228, 230, 236
Sarcoidosis, 268, 411
Sarnoff, David, 403
Saskatchewan, Canada, mad elk and deer
    outbreak in, 310
Satan, 26; satanic cult, 451
scatter back, 405
Schaw, William, 79
Schmitz, Hermann, 448
Schröder Bank of New York, 90
Schwarzkopf, Norman, 265
Schwend, Friederich, 95
science-based systems engineering (SBSE),
    450
Scientific American, 249
Scientists' Institute for Public Information,
    241
SCMV [simian (monkey) cytomegalovirus],
    247
Scott, P.D., 93
Scottish Rite, 47, 101
scrapie, 207, 225, 226, 246, 249, 259, 284,
    310, 321, 322, 323, 326
secret organizations and societies, 372, 451
Sencer, David, 219
sheep, prion disease in, 226, 328, 331
sickle cell anemia, 285; hemoglobin, 285
Gottlieb, Sidney, 411
Silva Mind Control, 436
Skull & Bones, 70, 83, 116, 117, 402
slavery, 396, 405
Sloan, Alfred P. 448
Sloan Foundation, 122, 211, 241, 444, 446,
    447, 448, 455
slow viruses, 245
Small, Donald, 442
smart chips, 441
SmithKline Beecham, 506
solar plasma, 369
Solfeggio, 57, 58-61, 68, 70, 72, 83, 144,
    153, 154, 165, 166, 168, 169, 172, 176,

177, 181, 184, 334, 397, 458, 459, 460,
    461, 462, 463, 470, 477, 482, 484
Solomon, King, 67
Song of Degrees, 61
Sorenson, William, 358
South Dakota, mad elk disease outbreak in,
    310
Sovereign Military Order of Malta (SMOM),
    86, 90, 91, 92, 93, 94, 101, 210
Soviet scientists, 433
Special Virus Cancer Program, 207, 411
SPECTRE, 78
spiroplasmas, 261
spongiform encephalopathies, 245
Spongiform Encephalopathy Advisory
    Committee (SEAC), 319
Stachybotrys atra, 357, 358
Stephenson, William, 402
Strong, Kenneth, 402
Standard Oil of New Jersey, 90, 97, 98, 116,
    230, 371, 448, 505, 506; see also
    Rockefeller oil
Stead, W. T., 110
"stealth virus," 246, 247, 262, 266, 268, 323,
    324, 325, 326, 353
Steiner, Rudolf, 86
Stevenson, William, 93
Stevens, Vernon, 227
Stockholm International Peace Research
    Institute, 432
supergerm, 248
surveillance, 363, 371, 396, 405, 418, 437
Sweet, Benjamin, 235
swine, prion agents in 312, 313, 315, 320,
    322, 323, 325, 327, 328, 329, 330, 331,
    332, 333, 338; see also pig(s) and
    hog(s)
Szmuness, Wolf, 223


## T

Tanox Biosystems of Houston, 270, 282
Tavistock Institute, 403
Teets, John W., 297
technological slavery, 405
Teledyne Company, 361
Templar Order, 75
Templars, 81, 82, 84, 85, 86, 87, 91, 105,
    121, 149, 150, 153, 156, 512; see also
    Templar Order and Masonic Order and
    Freemasonry
Temple of Set, 451
Ten Commandments, 468
Tenen, Stan, 348
Tesla, Nikola, 24, 73, 74, 156, 169, 183, 184,
    187, 198, 255, 256, 401, 406

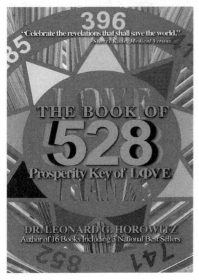

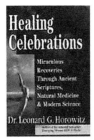
# Order Other Titles in This Genre by Dr. Len Horowitz.

Take control of your health and quick recovery. *Healing Celebrations* reveals the fundamentals of natural and spiritual healing. These truths, applied in your life, can help you turn illnesses into blessings and life threatening diseases into supernatural recoveries. Health in body, mind, emotions and spirit is freely available to everyone. Dr. Horowitz guides this process by delivering 5 basic steps for rejuvenation and hope. Learn to use: 1) detoxification, 2) alkalinization, 3) immunity normalization, 4) oxygenation, and 5) bioenergization in this easy-to-read book.

Only $22.85

Dr. Horowitz advances astonishing revelations about Divine inspiration, startling proof of "intelligent design," with revolutionary new healing implications. *Walk on Water* proves "heaven on earth is right here" with the mathematical-musical manifestation of the material world through spirit. Learn about the mathematics and music of Love connecting your heart to the center of creation!

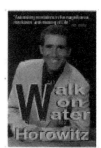

Only $16.55

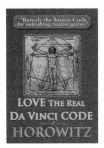

The musical-mathematics of Divine sustenance and karmic justice is explained herein. *LOVE the Real Da Vinci CODE* will change your life by demystifying the technology that makes life happen. It provides practical direction and instruction in how to apply the "Perfect Circle of Sound" for a new paradigm. The Spiritual Renaissance is ongoing. Forthcoming acceleration of this natural process is predicted from these revelations and technological innovations. Herein is the secret set of ancient symbols and numbers needed to free humanity from the earthly impositions of ignorance and resulting illnesses. The real Da Vinci code unlocks the gates to Heaven.

Only $22.85

The greatest gift you can give yourself is an operations manual explaining how to produce the healthy/positive outcomes you desire. *Taking Care of Yourself* gives easy to follow instructions to guide you to succeed in developing powerful immunity against common illnesses from cancers to colds. Each of us is different. You need to diagnose and treat your own unique issues. This self-help package guides your next most important steps to health and higher-level wellness. By making these common sense recommendations part of your daily routine, you will dramatically improve the quality of your life. Let the miracles begin! You deserve them! **5 hours on CD plus workbook**.

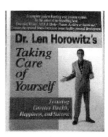

Only $49.40

# Other Books by Dr. Len Horowitz

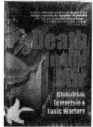
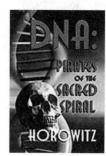
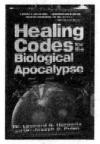
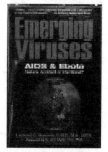